HUMAN ANATOMY AND PHYSIOLOGY

THE BIOLOGY AND MEDICAL DYNAMICS OF HUMAN REPRODUCTION

HUMAN ANATOMY AND PHYSIOLOGY

Additional books in this series can be found on Nova's website
under the Series tab.

Additional e-books in this series can be found on Nova's website
under the e-book tab.

HUMAN ANATOMY AND PHYSIOLOGY

THE BIOLOGY AND MEDICAL DYNAMICS OF HUMAN REPRODUCTION

LAURENCE A. COLE, PH.D.

NOVA BIOMEDICAL

New York

For permission to use material from this book please contact us:
Telephone 631-231-7269; Fax 631-231-8175
Web Site: http://www.novapublishers.com

Additional color graphics may be available in the e-book version of this book.

Library of Congress Cataloging-in-Publication Data

ISBN: 978-1-62948-832-5

Library of Congress Control Number: 2013956179

Published by Nova Science Publishers, Inc. † New York

Contents

Preface

Laurence Cole started his career in England working on an M.D. degree from 1971-1975 at Southampton University Medical School. After three long years he had a major stroke which placed him in a coma for three months. When he left the hospital almost one year later, he was told by Dean Acheson that he had major brain damage and was in no shape to finish medical school or practice medicine. While in England Laurence tried to complete undergraduate degrees in Biochemistry and Genetics. In both cases with his extreme brain damage he could not pass a single examination or complete a first semester. He then left England and took up residency in Israel. In Israel he met his first wife Linda. Linda took Laurence from Israel to Milwaukee WI, USA.

In Milwaukee, Laurence tried working as a clerk in industry. It was not medicine, it was not science, and it just did not work. Laurence enrolled in a Biochemistry Ph.D. program at the Medical College of Wisconsin, part of Marquette University in Milwaukee. Unfortunately, in his first year, with his severe brain damage he flunked everything. Fortunately, the chairman Professor Alan Mehler Ph.D. gave Laurence a second chance, a year to retake everything. In that year Laurence took extensive course notes. He came home and studied them and studied them virtually all night, but regardless of how many hours he spent studying he absorbed nothing. Then one night after midnight Laurence found himself shouting his notes aloud. For some reason something changed and somehow he started absorbing the notes. Laurence somehow made it through the Ph.D. program with flying colors.

He sought opinions from neurosurgeons and psychiatrists on how he was able to somehow study and complete his Ph.D. They said that he was left-handed and that the stroke had destroyed the central areas of the right side of his brain, or his active brain. Somehow, shouting notes aloud was leading to the absorption by the left side, the other side of his brain. By some means Laurence had developed the left side as his active side and had become right-handed. They said that the odds of this happening were remote; about 1 in 1,000 brain damaged individuals.

Laurence obtained a Ph.D. and passed all the needed coursework exams in 1981. the achievement was, regardless of the physiology, some kind of miracle. With his Ph.D. and a dissertation on "hCG Production by Cervical Cancer" he went to the University of Michigan in Ann Arbor to work on a post-doctoral fellowship on hCG and cancer. Somehow, at the University of Michigan he obtained three major million-dollar grants to study hCG and cancer, two R01s from the National Institutes of Health and one from the American Cancer Society. He was then "grabbed" (approached) by Yale University in 1984 as a promising grant recipient. In Obstetrics, Gynecology, and Reproductive Biology at Yale University, Laurence worked his way up from an Associate Professor to an Assistant Professor to a Full Professor.

Laurence's research interest at this time was the hormones hCG and LH, and reproductive biology. He spend 5 years at Yale University investigating hCG as a tumor marker and LH as a reproductive agent. Then he discovered the molecules that we now call hyperglycosylated hCG and hCG free β-subunit, and spent almost 10 years working on hyperglycosylated hCG and hCG free β-subunit function, and hyperglycosylated hCG and hyperglycosylated hCG free β-subunit and cancer.

In 1999 Laurence moved to the University of New Mexico in Albuquerque, New Mexico. Laurence was offered by this university a tenured full professorship, along with the position of Division Chief of the new division of Women's Health Research. At the University of New Mexico Laurence continues the hyperglycosylated hCG and hyperglycosylated hCG free β-subunit studies, studying biological functions in normal and failing pregnancies and in cancer.

In 2006 Linda and Laurence divorced, and in the following year Laurence married Dava, who guides him to this day.

In 2012 the university closed the division of Women's Health Research for unclear financial reasons. Laurence was laid off. He now runs a special clinical laboratory service, the USA hCG Reference Service based in the mountains of Angel Fire, New Mexico, consulting for physicians treating women with gestational trophoblastic diseases and cancers, and positive hCG tests outside of pregnancy.

Laurence writes this book in 2013 with a love and fascination for human reproductive biology. He remembers teaching an undergraduate course at the University of New Mexico from 2003 to 2007 on human reproduction. He loved teaching it, and the hundreds of students enrolled were also seemingly fascinated by the subject!

Glycopeptins

Chapter 1

Structure and Function of Glycopeptins

Four independent hormones, follicle stimulating hormone (FSH), thyroid stimulating hormone (TSH), luteinizing hormone (LH), and human chorionic gonadotropin (hCG), have as a group always been called the glycoprotein hormones. All four hormones share a common 92 amino acid α-subunit, coded for by a single gene on chromosome 6. All four have genetically-related but separate β-subunits, coded for by four separate sets of genes, 112-145 amino acids; hCGβ and LHβ are on chromosome 19, FSHβ on chromosome 11 and TSHβ on chromosome 1 [1]. Three of these hormones, hCG, LH and FSH, primarily stimulate the human ovary and testes or gonads and are together called the gonadotropins or gonad-stimulators.

These names, the glycoproteins hormones and the gonadotropins, all went astray with recent science when it was discovered that hCG does much more than just stimulate the gonads. It primarily promotes hemochorial placentation in the placenta of pregnancy [2], blocks macrophage phagocytosis of the feto-placental unit, blocks uterine myometrial contractions during pregnancy, promotes uterine growth, acts on the brain, and promotes fetal growth and development [3-8]. These names also became meaningless in recent years, when it was discovered that hCG and α- and β-subunit peptides are actually the peptide roots of four completely independent molecules, each varying in overall structure. There is hCG the hormone as produced by syncytiotrophoblast cells, which acts on an LH/hCG hormone receptor. There is hyperglycosylated hCG the autocrine produced by cytotrophoblast cells, that antagonizes a transforming growth factor-β (TGFβ) receptor [9-11]. Thirdly, there is pituitary sulfated hCG, the hormone produced by pituitary gonadotrope cells [12,13]. Finally, there is hyperglycosylated hCGβ, the single subunit autocrine that also acts on a TGFβ receptor. Hyperglycosylated hCGβ is produced by most human cancers [9,10,14-16]. As such, this group of molecules is not all hormone, or not all glycoprotein hormones, and is not all gonad-stimulators or gonadotropins. A new name is suggested for this entire group of inter-related molecules, the glycopeptins (Table 1.1). The new name reflects the fact that these are all glycoproteins and a mixture of both hormones and autocrines or other molecules.

As shown in Table 1.1 the seven glycopeptins vary greatly in size and in extent of glycosylation. The least glycosylated are TSH and LH. N-linked and O-linked oligosaccharide side chains, whether monoantennary, biantennary or triantennary, terminate in one, two or three acidic sugars, sialic acid. As such, the increasing proportion of sugars make the glycopeptins more and more acidic, TSH, isoelectric point, pI, pI=7.0, LH pI= 8.4, FSH pI=5.0, and hCG pI=3.5. The higher the proportion of the sugars, the higher the acidity, the greater the blood circulating half-life. So that TSH ½ life=50 min, LH ½ life=20 min, FSH ½ life=210 min and hCG ½ life=2160 min. So that the hCG group, the most recent evolutionary members of this family of molecules [17,18], is comprised of the most glycosylated molecules, and the longest circulating. This article focuses on human reproductive biology. TSH is produced by pituitary thyrotrope cells and controls thyroid hormone production, so it is not examined further. Here we examine and compare the structure, function, biology and receptors of the 6 other glycopeptins carefully.

Table 1.1. The physical and biological properties of the glycopeptins. The percentage of sugar is the percentage of the molecular weight due to the oligosaccharides [2-5]

Glycopeptin	Cell Source	Molecular weight			Count Amino acids		Oligosaccharides		% sugar
		α-subunit	ß-subunit	Dimer	α-subunit	ß-subunit	N-linked	O-linked	
TSH	Thyrotropes	13,500	15,000	28,500	92	118	3	0	16%
LH	Gonadotropes	13,500	15,400	28,900	92	121	3	0	16%
FSH	Gonadotropes	13,800	17,100	30,900	92	118	4	0	23%
Pituitary Sulfated hCG	Gonadotropes	14,000	20,000	34,000	92	145	4	4	26%
Placental hCG	Syncytiotrophoblast	14,690	22,490	37,180	92	145	4	4	30%
Hyperglycosylated hCG	Cytotrophoblast	16,300	26,500	42,800	92	145	4	4	39%
Hyperglycosylated hCGβ	Malignancy cells	-	26,500	-	-	145	2	4	42%

FSH

FSH is produced by pituitary gonadotrope cells. It is secreted under the control of a releasing signal, gonadotropin releasing hormone (GnRH), as described in Chapter 3. FSH is a glycoprotein with a unique β-subunit and four N-linked sugar side chains (Table 1.1). The molecular weight of FSH is 30,900. The three dimensional crystal structure of FSH has been determined [19]. As demonstrated, FSH α-subunit and β-subunit both show a common cystine-knot structure to TGFβ, suggesting a common evolutionary heritage in both subunits (see Chapter 2). Similar folding is shown in FSH α-β dimer, LH and hCG [19,20].

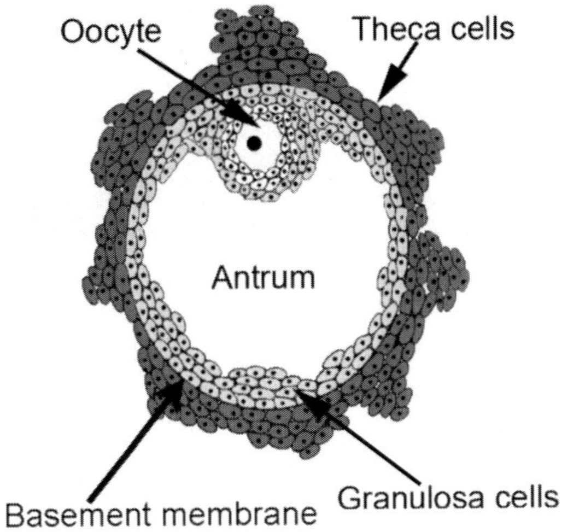

Figure 1.1. Structure of ovarian follicles.

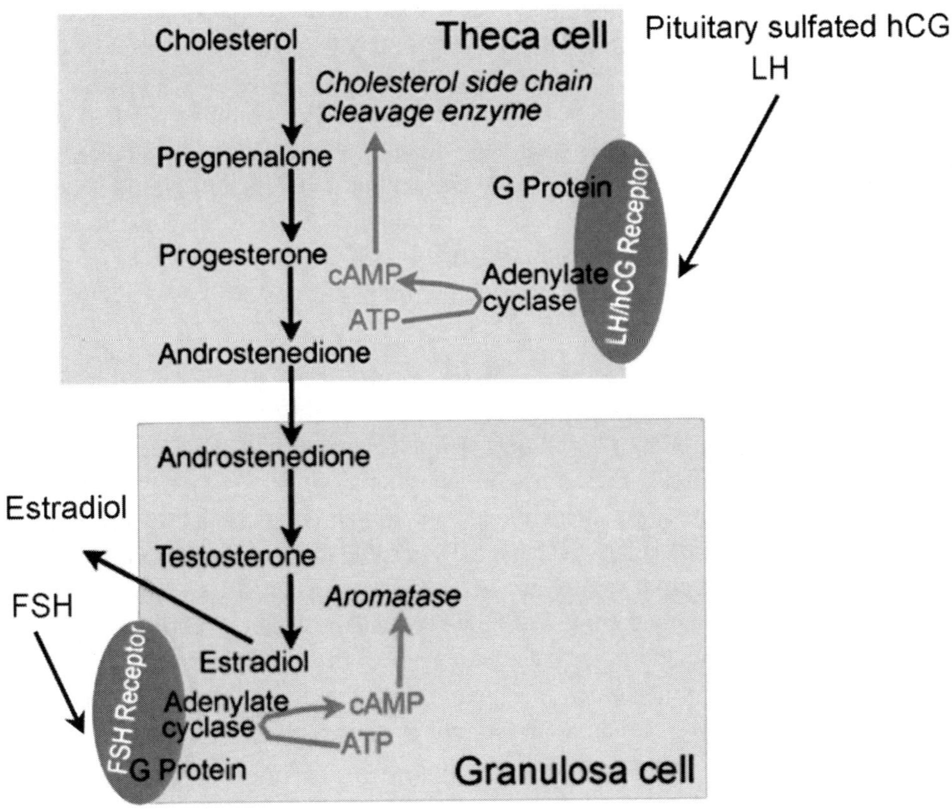

Figure 1.2. Cooperative steroidogenesis in theca cells and granulosa cells.

FSH functions in women during the menstrual cycle to promote estrogen production. The ovarian follicle, or oocyte case, contains granulosa cells which surround the oocyte, and surround the theca cells which wrap the granulosa cells (Figure 1.1). As illustrated in Figure 1.2, the theca cells produce the steroid intermediate androstenedione from root steroid cholesterol is made under the control of LH or pituitary sulfated hCG. These hormones act on cholesterol side-chain cleavage enzyme, the limiting step in the pathway. The granulosa cells, under the hormonal control of FSH, use the androstenedione to make the steroid estradiol. Androstenedione is enzymatically converted to testosterone, which is aromatized (aromatic on steroid ring 1) to produce estradiol. FSH acts on the enzyme aromatase (testosterone > estradiol), the limiting step in the granulosa cell pathway.

FSH has other non-tropic roles during the menstrual cycle. FSH in the early part of the follicular phase is used to promote the construction of multiple primordial follicles within the ovary [21,22]. During the late follicular phase, FSH has functions in promoting competitive growth among antral follicles (those having fluid-filled space), promoting granulosa cell growth, to determine which follicle is to be the dominant follicle and will be ovulated [23,24]. Larger follicles have more FSH receptors. It is thought that for this reason they are promoted further and are more likely to win the dominant follicle race.

Pituitary gonadotrope cell FSH also has functions in men. FSH promotes testicular production of an androgen binding protein, which is critical to testosterone steroidogenesis in men [25,26]. FSH also promotes the growth of testosterone receptors on Sertoli cells and seminiferous tubules in men [27,28]. These are seemingly two side functions in men. The role of FSH in spermatogenesis is less certain. FSH is seemingly mandatory in males for maintaining full fertility following a hypophysectomy. FSH seemingly both regulates the sperm production rate and promotes spermatogenesis in the seminiferous tubules. Optimally the male without pituitary FSH should receive frequent doses of FSH if fertility is desired.

FSH acts on a specific FSH receptor on ovarian granulosa cells. It is a G protein receptor using a cyclic AMP (cAMP) mechanism [29,30].

LH

LH is a glycopeptin produced by pituitary gonadotrope cells. It is also secreted under the control of a releasing signal, gonadotropin releasing hormone (GnRH), as described in Chapter 3. LH is a glycoprotein with a unique β-subunit and three N-linked sugar side chains [31,32] (Table 1.1). The molecular weight of LH is 28,900 (Table 1.1). The three dimensional X-ray crystallography structure of LH has not been determined. It is thought, however, to have a structure similar to gonadotrope cell FSH [19], and placental hCG (Figure 1.7) [2].

LH has numerous functions in men and women beyond its menstrual cycle tropic steroidogenic functions. As illustrated in Figure 1.2, LH and FSH, and theca and granulosa cells work together to make estradiol, LH promoting theca cell androstenedione production, and FSH promoting the conversion of androstenedione to estradiol. Estradiol production occurs in the fallopian phase of the menstrual cycle. In the luteal phase of the menstrual cycle, after ovulation and formation of a corpus luteum, LH promotes luteal phase progesterone production (Figure 1.3). Once more, cholesterol side-chain cleavage enzyme is the limiting enzyme, or that controlled by LH.

LH is also critical for steroidogenesis in men, with LH acting on Leydig cells to produce testosterone production (Figure 1.4) [33, 34]. Once more, cholesterol side-chain cleavage

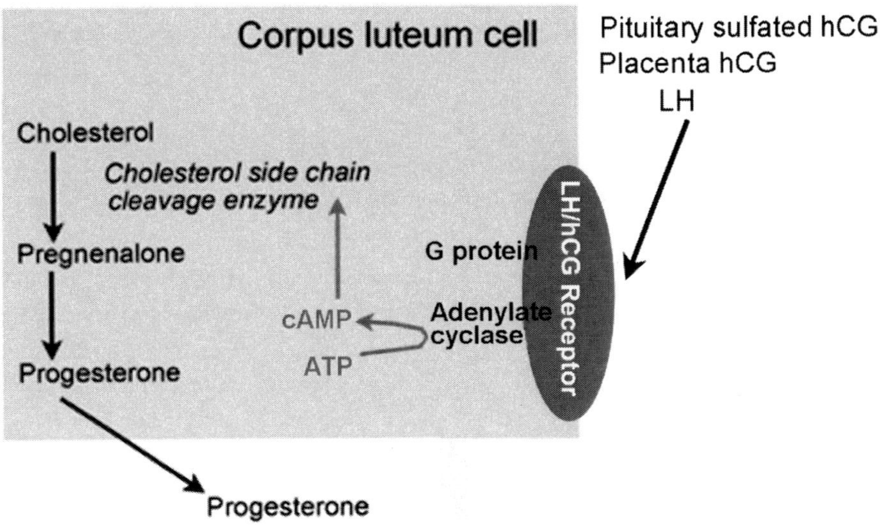

Figure 1.3. Progesterone production in corpus luteal phase of menstrual cycle.

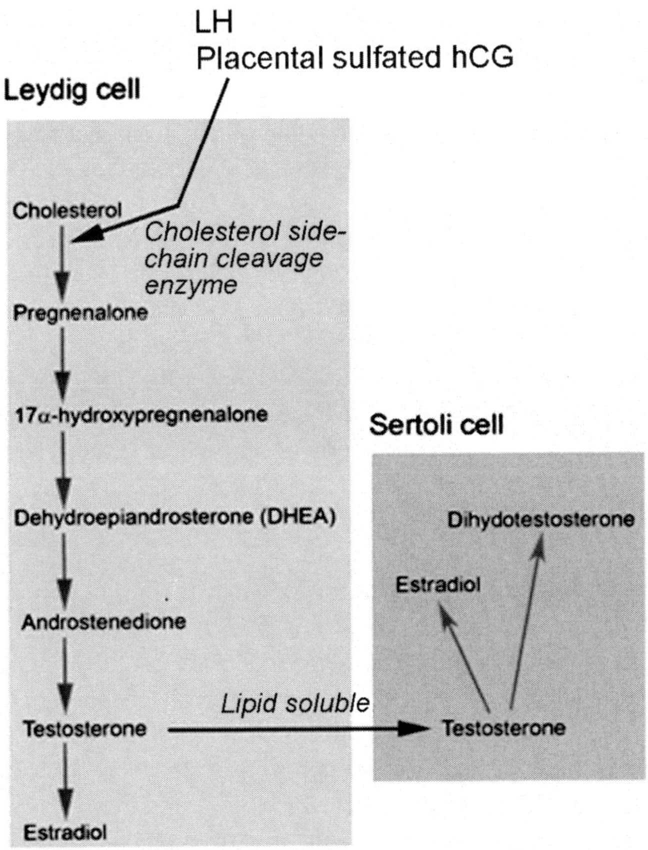

Figure 1.4. Testosterone production by Leydig cells.

enzyme is the limiting enzyme, or that controlled by LH. As illustrated (Figure 1.4), testosterone can pass the cellular barrier and migrate into nearby Sertoli cells, where dihydrotestosterone and estrogen are produced (Figure 1.4) [35]. All LH steroidogenesis function can ber mimicked by pituitary sulfated hCG (see next section).

LH and pituitary sulfated hCG have been shown to be critical to spermatogenesis in men; both LH, and FSH and pituitary sulfated hCG enhance sperm growth and production in men. LH binds Leydig cells, which act on interstitial cells to enhance sperm growth (Figure 1.5) [36,37]. In women LH plays a major role in follicle development and preparation of oocytes for ovulation. Around day 4-5 of the menstrual cycle an LH/hCG receptor appears on granulosa cells of antral follicles (having an antrum, the section of follicle filled with liquid) [38,39]. An LH/hCG receptor is always present on theca cells. LH (or sulfated hCG) promotes a surge in follicular growth promoting both granulosa and theca cell growth [40]. Around day 11-12 of the menstrual cycle LH (or sulfated hCG) levels start to rise to a peak. The rising LH (or hCG) levels cause a surge in growth of the largest follicle or dominant follicle [41]. Around this same time, LH (or sulfated hCG) promotes meiosis, so that the diploid genetic set in the dominant follicle, one half of the diploid chromosome set having come from the mother and one half from the father, generates a haploid set, a half set with a mixture of maternal and paternal genes [42,43]. This is just the first stage of meiosis, and the haploid set resulting is inactive until meiosis is completed upon fertilization of the oocyte (see Chapters 14 and 17). The residual chromosome materials from meiosis are discarded in a small container in the follicle called the first polar body. At this time, around day 12 of the average menstrual cycle, LH promotes growth in the follicle to cause a pronounced stigma or bulge to appear on the oocyte [44]. This comprises a thin layer of theca and granulosa cells to permit bursting of the follicle upon ovulation. Around day 14 of the menstrual cycle ovulation occurs (Figure 1.6). The peak LH (or sulfated hCG) level causes ovulation by promoting production of collagenase, plasminogen activator and other proteases [45,46]. These burn a hole in the stigma, leading the follicle to burst open, and the oocyte within the follicle is released, or spat out. The oocyte or egg is captured by the fimbia of the fallopian tube (Figure 1.6). Blood vessels then invade the empty follicle and, under the influence of LH (or sulfated hCG), the follicle then hemorrhages [47]. The theca and granulosa cell undergo hypertrophy or differentiation and the process of luteinization occurs. Theca cells differentiate into small corpus luteal cells under the influence of LH and granulosa cells differentiate into large corpus luteal cells under the influence of LH [48,49].

LH binds a joint transmembrane receptor with hCG and sulfated pituitary hCG. It is a G protein-coupled receptor using a cyclic AMP (cAMP) mechanism. Its activation is necessary for the hormonal functioning during reproduction [29,30,50]. Upon binding of LH to the external part of the membrane spanning receptor, a transduction of the signal takes place that activates the G protein that is bound to the receptor internally. Upon hormone binding the receptor shifts conformation and thus mechanically activates the G protein, which detaches from the receptor and activates the cAMP system. Cyclic AMP-dependent protein kinases (protein kinase A) are activated by the signal chain coming from the G. These protein kinases are present as tetramers with two regulatory units and two catalytic units. Upon binding of cAMP to the regulatory units, the catalytic units are released and initiate the phosphorylation of proteins leading to the physiologic action. In a feedback mechanism, these activated kinases phosphorylate the receptor. The longer the receptor remains active, the more kinases are activated and the more receptors are phosphorylated.

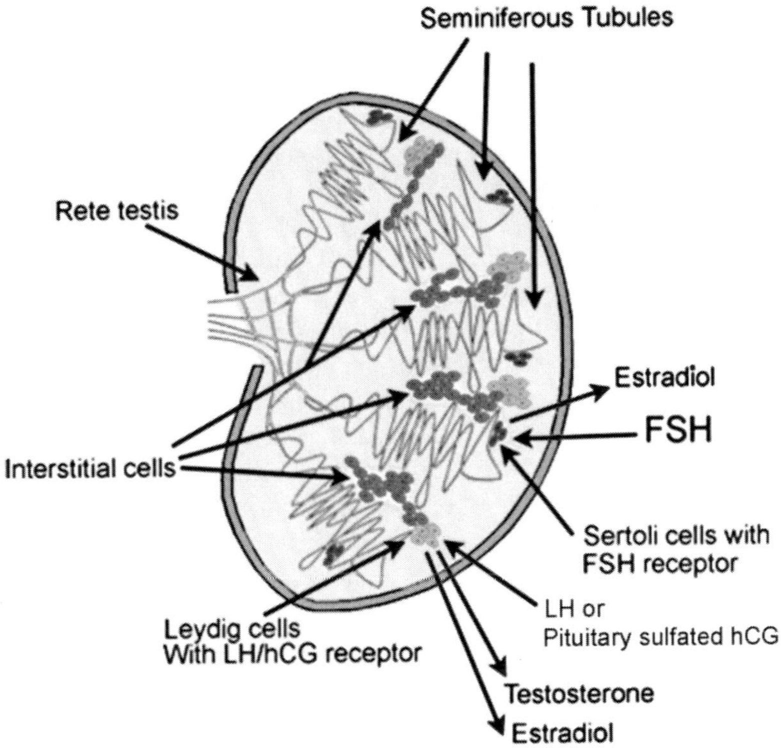

Figure 1.5. Action of LH, sulfated pituitary hCG, and FSH on the testes. LH (or hCG) acts on Leydig cells associated with interstitial cell compilations between seminiferous tubules. LH(or hCG) promotes testosterone and estradiol production. LH or sulfated pituitary hCG also aids in spermatogenesis. FSH acts on Sertoli cells which are part of the seminiferous tubules. FSH promotes estradiol production and promotes the generation of sperm in seminiferous tubules.

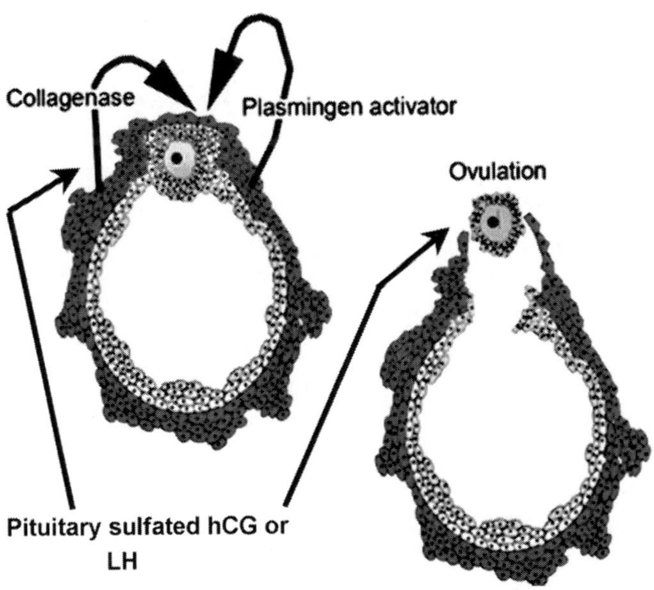

Figure 1.6. Ovulation in the female menstrual cycle.

Pituitary Sulfated hCG

As discussed in Chapter 3 regarding GnRH, gonadotrope cell pituitary sulfated hCG production may be an incidentally produced molecule [12,13]. GnRH may incidentally promote an hCG β-subunit gene in the process of promoting the one small LHβ gene buried among eight copies of hCGβ genes on chromosome 19.

Pituitary sulfated hCG and LH both bind the same LH/hCG receptor and both have identical functions in men and women, promoting androstenedione (follicular phase) and progesterone (luteal phase) production in women, and testosterone production in men, promoting the multiple stages of ovulation in women and enhancing sperm growth in men (Figure 1.5) [12,13]. Pituitary sulfated hCG production, which may be incidental, is tiny compared to LH production. In women, serum concentrations of pituitary sulfated hCG are approximately one-fiftieth of LH concentration, and in men are as little as one two-hundredth of LH concentration. Blood levels in women are 0.05 – 3.0 mIU/ml, and in men are 0.01 – 0.5 mIU/ml [12,13]. Pituitary sulfated hCG is unique in that the complex N- and O-linked-oligosaccharides terminate (non-reducing terminal) with an N-acetylgalactosamine residue and a sulfate group. Placental sulfated hCG, in contrast, terminates with a galactose sugar and acidic sialic acid sugar [12]; thus, the name sulfated hCG. As shown, pituitary sulfated hCG is not as acidic as placental hCG, having approximately one-half the circulating ½-life, 20 hours vs. 36 hours, and biological activity as placental hCG [12].

At the time of the ovulation LH peak in women, around 14 days of the menstrual cycle, pituitary sulfated hCG levels also peaks, averaging (mean and standard deviation of 277 peak menstrual cycle measurements) 1.54 ± 0.90 IU/L mIU/ml [51]. This level is approximately one-fiftieth average LH peak mean measurements (75 mIU/ml). Bearing in mind the 20-hour circulating ½-life of pituitary sulfated hCG, this is about 50x greater than the circulating ½-life of LH (20-25 minutes) [12]. Considering the 50x lower blood concentration of pituitary sulfated hCG, and the 50x higher circulating ½-life of pituitary sulfated hCG, pituitary sulfate hCG may play an equal role to LH in controlling androstenedione and progesterone steroidogenesis in women, and in controlling the process of ovulation. It is inferred that LH and pituitary sulfated hCG may have equal roles in female human reproduction, and that pituitary sulfated hCG also likely plays a major role in male human reproduction.

Pituitary sulfated hCG may become most evident in perimenopausal women, menopausal women, oophorectomized women and castrated men. In these women ovarian estrogen may be minimal (perimenopause) or halted (menopause). Pulsed GnRH promotion of pituitary FSH and LH, normally regulated by estrogen hypothalamic feedback, may be maximal when estrogen js withdrawn. At this perimenopausal, menopausal or agonadal stage high levels of FSH and LH may be promoted, and incidental production of pituitary sulfated hCG (Eight hCGβ genes aside one LHβ gene) may be consequential.

The USA hCG Reference Service has been referred over 100 cases of menopausal, perimenopausal or agonadic (post-oophorectomy) women producing serum hCG. The serum hCG in these women ranged from 1.8 mIU/ml – 39 mIU/ml [52]. As shown, these women were hyper-LH (LH >20 mIU/ml) and hyper-FSH (FSH >30 mIU/ml). As reported, FSH (>30 mIU/ml) is a good marker of menopausal and agonadal women producing pituitary sulfated hCG production [54]. Pituitary sulfated hCG can be demonstrated by placing women on a high estrogen oral contraceptive for three weeks and showing complete suppression of hCG [52].

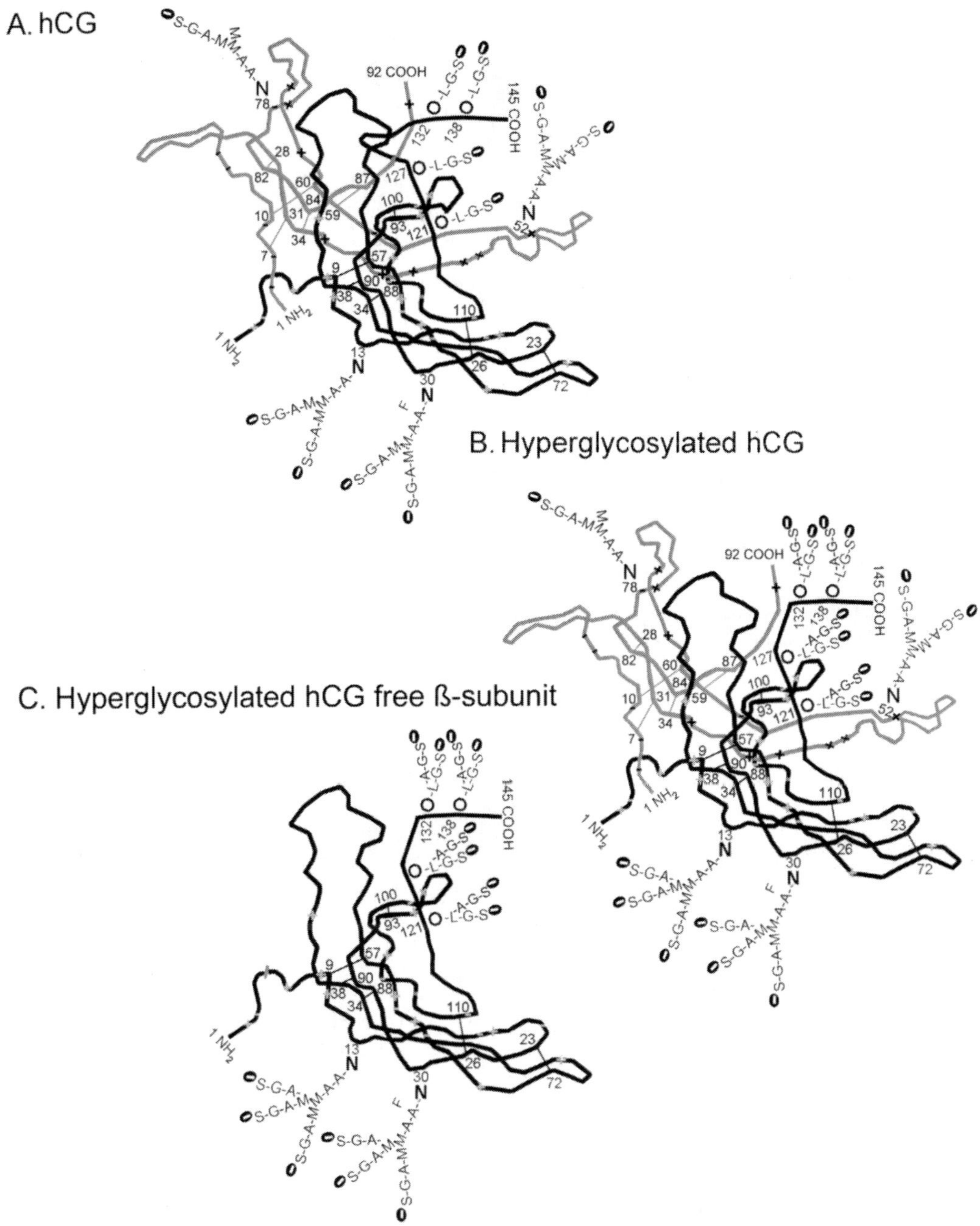

Figure 1.7. Proposed structures for independent hCG variants as determined by Butler et al. (paper uin prepaeration). Panel 1 is regularly glycosylated hCG, with a ß-subunit C-terminal peptide. Panel 2 is hyperglycosylated hCG, with a ß-subunit C-terminal peptide. Panel 3 is hyperglycosylated hCGß with a C-terminal peptide, determined from the intact hyperglycosylated hCG structure.

Placental hCG

Placental hCG is a hormone secreted by placental syncytiotrophoblast cells. Cytotrophoblast cells are the root growing trophoblast cells which produce the autocrine hyperglycosylated hCG and not any of the hormone placental hCG. Cytotrophoblast cells fuse and differentiate to make multi-nuclear, 3-50 nucleus syncytiotrophoblast cells. Only these cells produce placental hCG [3,55]. As described in Chapter 2, hCG ß-subunit evolved from LH ß-subunit in lower simian primates. In syncytiotrophoblast cells with hCG, as in pituitary gonadotrope cells with LH and FSH, the α-subunit of a glycopeptin is produced in excess, and is unregulated. The β-subunit of hCG is limiting on active hCG αβ dimer formation.

Lapthorn et al. [20] and others have examined the three dimensional structure of placental hCG. The problem was that they had to remove all eight carbohydrate structures from placental hCG, and remove the β-subunit C-terminal peptide from placental hCG before they could form crystals [20]. Looking at placental hCG (30% carbohydrate, 11% β-subunit C-terminal) and hyperglycosylated hCG (39% carbohydrate, 11% β-subunit C-terminal), effectively one-half of the molecular weight or structure had to be removed before anything was examined [20]. Is this meaningful? Does this half three dimensional structure mean anything? In determining the FSH three dimensional structure Fox et al. only found that they had to remove one β-subunit oligosaccharide to make crystals [19]. Fortunately, the stripped down hCG structure still resembled that of FSH [19], suggesting some three dimensional correctness. We have examined the half-hCG and the FSH structure carefully, and suggested how the removed oligosaccharides could affect placental hCG structure [53]. Most notably these oligosaccharides structurally distinguish placental hCG and hyperglycosylated hCG, and explain why hyperglycosylated hCG binds a TGFβ receptor. Our proposed structures are shown in Figure 1.7 (Proposed structures from hCG and hyperglycosylated hCG thermodynamic models, Butler et al, paper in preparation).

Placental hCG acts on a common LH/pituitary sulfated hCG/placental hCG hormone receptor. It therefore promotes androstenedione and progesterone production in women and testosterone production in men exactly as done by LH. Placental hCG has no known independent biological functions to LH.

The placental hormone hCG is produced by syncytiotrophoblast cells in line with hyperglycosylated hCG which is produced by cytotrophoblast cells. Hyperglycosylated hCG starts pregnancy by initiating implantation of the placenta tissue of the conceptus into the uterus. Cytotrophoblast cells then fuse to form syncytiotrophoblast cells, and placental hCG is produced. Pregnancy is always started or marked by production of hyperglycosylated hCG, followed by production of placental hCG 1-4 days later [52].

Placental hCG has, like LH, many steroidogenic and non-tropic functions. Placental hCG takes over from LH in promoting ovarian corpus luteal progesterone production at 4 weeks – 8 weeks of gestation. Placental hCG then works side by side with hyperglycosylated hCG in promoting the development of hemochorial placentation or development ad support of the fetal nutrient mechanism [2]. Hyperglycosylated hCG promotes growth of cytotrophoblast cells, and placental hCG promotes their fusion to syncytiotrophoblast cells. Together they form the villous trophoblast structure in hemochorial placentation [2]. Placental hCG then promotes the growth of maternal uterine arteries to meet the hemochorial placentation structure [5,6]. Similarly, umbilical vessel growth is promoted by placental hCG, linking the placenta and fetus. Starting at approximately 10 weeks of pregnancy, hemochorial placentation starts to function linking the oxygen, glucose nutrients of the mother and fetus [2]. Other functions of hCG include suppression of macrophage response to the foreign feto-placental unit [4], and suppression of myometrial contractions and uterine growth during the course of pregnancy [7,8]. Other evidence suggests that placental hCG like hormone is produced in the fetus and promotes fetal organ growth and development [73,74].

Hyperglycosylated hCG

Hyperglycosylated hCG is a super-glycosylated variant of hCG (39% sugar by molecular weight) produced by root cytotrophoblast cells. While placental hCG has 11 and 12 (with fucose) sugar residue biantennary N-linked oligosaccharides, hyperglycosylated hCG has 14 and 15 (with fucose) sugar residue triantennary N-linked oligosaccharides [17,18]. Placental hCG has trisaccharide and tetrasaccharide (NeuAc-Gal (NeuAc) GalNAc-Ser) O-linked oligosaccharides, while hyperglycosylated hCG has pentasaccharide and hexasaccharide (NeuAc-Gal (NeuAc-Gal-GlcNAc) GalNAc-Ser) O-linked oligosaccharide structures [17,18]. Interestingly, placental hCG and hyperglycosylated hCG share a common hCG α-subunit and β-subunit peptide structure, 92 and 145 amino acid sequences.

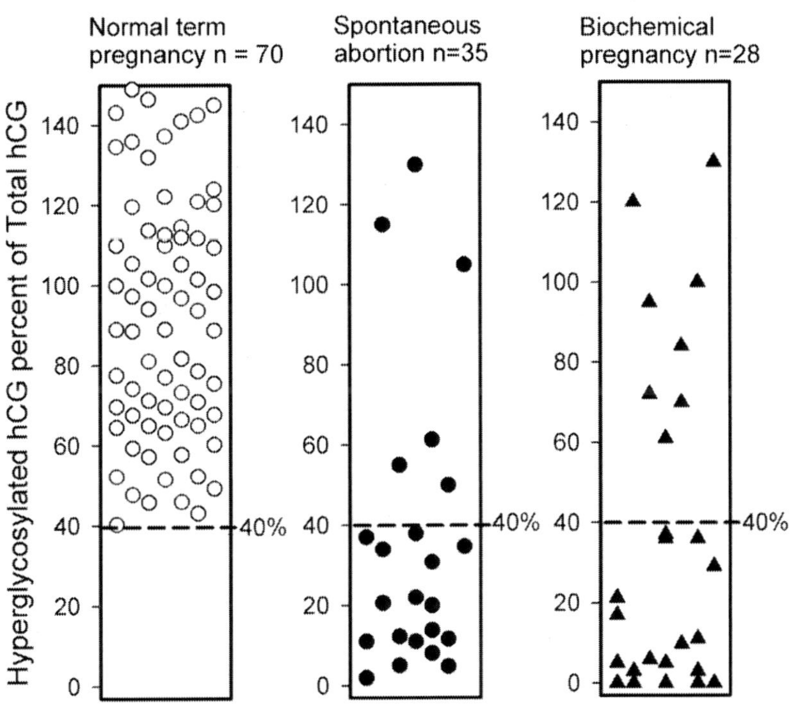

Figure 1.8. Proportion hyperglycosylated hCG (% of total hCG) on the day of implantation in 70 normal term outcome pregnancies, and 35 spontaneous abortion outcome pregnancies (SAB), and 28 biochemical outcome pregnancies [57,58].

While placental hCG is a hormone acting on the LH/pituitary sulfated hCG/placental hCG receptor, hyperglycosylated hCG is very different, being an autocrine, and antagonizing a cytotrophoblast cell TGFβ receptor [9-11]. It was known for years that hCG subunits contained a unique 4 disufide bridge cystine loop peptide region common to TGFβ and inherided from TGFß [20]. With hyperglycosylated hCG receptor the TGFß receptor was found to play a role in hCG biology. The proposed structure of super glycosylated hyperglycosylated hCG is shown in Figure 1.7, panel 2.

Hyperglycosylated hCG, through its TGFβ antagonism action, drives placental implantation. It literally in implantation drives cytotrophoblast growth and cancer-like invasion through cytotrophoblast production and secretion of metalloproteinases and collagenases, intracellular digestion enzymes [55,56].

As shown in Figure 1.8, 70 women with normal term outcome pregnancy, 35 with spontaneous abortion outcome pregnancies and 28 women with biochemical outcome pregnancies were tested on the day of implantation of pregnancy. As shown and confirmed by others, biochemical and spontaneous abortion outcome pregnancies are due to inappropriate implantation [71,72]. As shown (Figure 1.8), 70 of 70 with normal term outcome pregnancies produced sufficient hyperglycosylated hCG (>40% hyperglycosylated hCG of total hCG). In contrast, 29 of 35 spontaneously aborting pregnancies and 21 of 28 biochemical pregnancies produced insufficient hyperglycosylated hCG (<40%), causing failure [57,58]. Clearly, sufficient hyperglycosylated hCG is essential for normal term outcome pregnancy. The 6 spontaneously aborting pregnancies with sufficient hyperglycosylated hCG production, and the 7 biochemical pregnancies producing sufficient hyperglycosylated hCG, are presumed to be trisomies, monosomies and other chromosomally-abnormal pregnancies (see Chapter 26).

Hyperglycosylated hCG has a role in first and second trimester placental tissue growth [59]. In the second trimester of pregnancy, insufficient hyperglycosylated hCG can cause inappropriate placental growth, leading to forced maternal hypertension and preeclampsia [59,60]. Both placental hCG and hyperglycosylated hCG are essential molecules to pregnancy.

Hyperglycosylated hCGβ

Back in the 1970s and early '80s, while working on a PhD, I examined the structures of the forms of hCG free β-subunit produced by two cell lines of cervical epidermoid carcinoma, DoT and CaSki cell line. As published, the free β-subunit was an overly glycosylated or hyperglycosylated variant of hCG free ß-subunit [61,62]. As found, most cancers produced a hyperglycosylated hCG free β-subunit (hyperglycosylated hCGβ) [9]. A possible structure for hyperglycosylated hCG free β-subunit is shown in Figure 1.7, panel 3. This hyperglycosylated hCG free ß-subunit antagonizes the TGFβ-2 receptor on the cancer cells. The antagonism leads to promotion of cancer cell growth, blockage of apoptosis, and promotion of cancer cell invasion [9,10]. Seven independent groups have now shown, confirmed and double-confirmed that this is the mechanism driving most human cancers [9,10,14,15,16,63].

We start by asking why cancers produce hyperglycosylated hCG free β-subunit and not just the αβ dimer or hyperglycosylated hCG. As shown by Ruddon and colleagues and Beebe and colleagues (64,65), a unique placental disulfide isomerase completes the final two disulfide bridges of β-subunit, β26-110 and β93-100. If these disulfide bridges are not completed the β-subunit will not combine with α-subunit to form αβ dimer (64,65). Cancer cells seem to lack this disulfide isomerase, not completing these disulfide bridges, as αβ dimer may not form, and cancer cells secrete only free hCG α- and β-subunits.

Table 1.2. Use of serum total hCGß and urine hCG ß-core fragment as tumor markers for detection of malignancies. Average sensitivities are determined by combining total positive cases from multiple reports [66-69]

	Serum hCGß		Urine hCG ß-core fragment	
Malignancy	Cases	Sensitivity (>3 fmol/ml)	Cases	Sensitivity (>3 fmol/ml)
Choriocarcinoma	20	100%		
Testicular germ cell cancer	17	100%		
Ovarian germ cell cancer	30	100%		
TOTAL	67	100%		
Ovarian adenocarcinoma	150	38%	207	70%
Cervical cancer	60	37%	410	48%
Endometrial cancer	55	33%	53	47%
Vulvar	50	38%	8	50%
Bladder cancer	170	35%	102	48%
Uterine cancer			9	67%
Lung cancer	143	18%	90	28%
Colorectal cancer	136	17%		
Pancreatic cancer			29	55%
TOTAL	764	226 Positive (30%) Detection 17 - 38%	908	495 Positive (55%) Detection 24 - 70% Range

In our own studies in the 1980s and '90s we examined production of hyperglycosylated hCGβ (total hCGβ assay) and their degradation product β-core fragment by large numbers of cancers (Table 1.2). As shown, a total of 1,672 individual cancer cases were investigated; 764 serum samples and 908 urine samples [66-69]. As found, hCGβ-related molecules are produced by 100% of trophoblastic malignancies (cells adopting cytotrophoblast morphology), including choriocarcinoma, testicular germ cell malignancies and ovarian germ cells malignancies, and by a variable percentage of other non-trophoblastic malignancies. Trophoblastic malignancies produce high concentrations of hyperglycosylated hCG while other malignancies produce only low concentrations of the hyperglycosylated hCG free β-subunit which clears the circulation rapidly. As indicated by β-core fragment levels, a terminal degradation product of hCG free ß-subunit, is produced by 70% of ovarian malignancies, 67% of uterine malignancies, 55% pancreatic, 50% vulvar, 48% cervical and bladder, 47% endometrial and 28% lung malignancies. Overall 55% of malignancies produced hCG variants.

Does this 55% indicate that 55% of malignancies function through a hyperglycosylated hCGβ mechanism? Our own studies with 15 non-trophoblastic cell lines show that 15 of 15 or 100% of cancers respond to hyperglycosylated hCGβ [9]. Acevedo et al. [70] used cancer cells and flow cytometry methods to investigate production of hCG β-subunit. As found, all (100%) cancer cells produce an hCG free β-subunit, but some produced miniscule concentrations.

There are seemingly two types of autocrine TGFβ antagonism systems, simple autocrine and complex autocrine. Simple autocrine cells produce miniscule concentrations of signal; these act directly on the autocrine TGFβ receptor. Complex autocrine cells produce high concentrations of signal, which are secreted and circulate through the blood system before feeding back to the same cells' TGFβ receptor. It is inferred that trophoblast malignancies are probably complex autocrine, while most non-trophoblastic malignancies produce tiny concentrations or are likely simple autocrines. It is inferred that all or most human cancers produce hyperglycosylated hCG free β-subunit which functions as a simple or complex autocrine antagonist, promoting the cancer.

Recently, we have investigated the use of a specific antibody to block hyperglycosylated hCGβ, and block cancer growth and progression. Mouse B152 is a specific monoclonal antibody to hyperglycosylated hCG and hyperglycosylated hCGβ [71]. As found, 9 of 9 cancer cell lines regress or seemingly apoptose when treated with varying doses of antibody B152 (when X cells are treated for 24 hours they become 65%-78% cell number) (9, paper submitted). Similarly, when cancer cells are transplanted into nude mice cancers they metastasize rapidly. Treatment of nude mice with B152, vs. non-specific IgG, blocks the cancer completely leading to oncostasis (55, paper submitted). Mouse B152 shows great promise in human cell culture models and human nude mouse models as a potential new treatment for human cancers. B152 will need to be humanized by recombinant DNA technology before humans can receive this therapy and clinical trials can be started with this possible new human cancer therapy.

References

[1] Dos Santos S, Mazan S, Venkatesh B, Cohen-Tannoudji J, Quérat B. Emergence and evolution of the glycoprotein hormone and neurotrophin gene families in vertebrates. *BioMed Cent Evol Biolo* 2011;11:332-340.

[2] Cole LA. hCG and Hyperglycosylated hCG, Promoters of Villous Placenta and Hemochorial Placentation. *Placenta: Functions, Development and Disease,* Nicholson R. (ed), Nova Publishers, 2013, Ch 8.

[3] Shi QJ, Lei ZM, Rao CV, Lin J, Novel role of human chorionic gonadotropin in differentiation of human cytotrophoblasts. *Endocrinol* 1993; 132: 387-395.

[4] Wan H, Marjan A, Cheung VW, Leenen PJM, Khan NA, Benner R, Kiekens RCM, Chorionic gonadotropin can enhance innate immunity by stimulating macrophage function. *J Leukocyte Biol* 2007; 82: 926-933.

[5] Zygmunt M, Herr F, Keller-Schoenwetter S, Kunzi-Rapp K, Munstedt K, Rao CV, Lang U, Preissner KT, 2002. Characterization of human chorionic gonadotropin as a novel angiogenic factor, *J Clin Endocrinol Metab* 87: 290-5296.

[6] Rao CV, Li, X, Toth P, Lei ZM, Cok VD, Novel expression of functional human chorionic gonadotropin/luteinizing hormone receptor in human umbilical cords. *J Clin Endocrinol Metab* 1993; 77:1706-1714.

[7] Reshef E, Lei ZM, Rao CV, Pridham DD, Chegini N, Luborsky JL, The presence of gonadotropin receptors in nonpregnant human uterus human placenta fetal membranes and decidua. *J Clin Endocrinol Metab* 1990; 70: 421-430.

[8] Eta E, Ambrus G, Rao V, Direct regulation of human myometrial contractions by human chorionic gonadotropin. *J Clin Endocrinol Metab* 1994; 79: 1582-1586.

[9] Cole LA, Butler SA, Hyperglycosylated hCG, hCGß and hyperglycosylated hCGß: interchangeable cancer promoters. *Molec Cellul Endocrinol* 2012; 349: 232-238.

[10] Butler SA, Ikram MS, Mathieu S, Iles RK, The increase in bladder carcinoma cell population induced by the free beta subunit of hCG is a result of an anti-apoptosis effect and not cell proliferation. *Brit J Cancer* 2000; 82: 1553-1556.

[11] Berndt S, Blacher S, Munuat C, Detilleux J, Evain-Brion D, Noel A, Fournier T, Foidart JM. Hyperglycosylated human chorionic gonadotropin stimulates angiogenesis through TGF-ß receptor activation. *FASEB J* 2013;27:1309-1321.

[12] Birken S, Maydelman Y, Gawinowicz MA, Pound A, Liu Y, Hartree AS, Isolation and characterization of human pituitary chorionic gonadotropin. *Endocrinol* 1996; 137: 1402-11.

[13] Odell WD, Griffin J, Pulsatile secretion of human chorionic gonadotropin in normal adults. *New Engl J Med* 1987; 317: 1688-1691.

[14] Carter WB, Sekharem M, Coppola D, Purified hCG induces apoptosis in breast cancer. *Breast Cancer Res Treatm* 2006; 100: S243-S244.

[15] Jankowska A, Gunderson SI, Andrusiewicz N, Burczynska B, Szczerba A, Jarmolowski A, Nowak-Markwitz E, Warchol JB. Reduction of human chorionic gonadotropin beta subunit expression by modified U1 snRNA caused apoptosis in cervical cancer cells. *Molec Cancer* 2008;7:26-29.

[16] Li D, Wen X, Ghali L, Al-Shalabi FM, Docherty SM, Purkis P, Iles RK, hCG beta expression by cervical squamous carcinoma-in vivo histological association with tumour invasion and apoptosis. *Histopathol* 2008; 53: 147-55.

[17] Elliott MM, Kardana A, Lustbader JW, Cole LA, Carbohydrate and Peptide structure of the α- and β-subunits of human chorionic gonadotropin from normal and aberrant pregnancy and choriocarcinoma. *Endocrine* 7: 1997; 15-32.

[18] Valmu L, Alfthan H, Hotakainen K, Birken S, Stenman UH, Site-specific glycan analysis of human chorionic gonadotropin beta-subunit from malignancies and pregnancy by liquid chromatography - electrospray mass spectrometry. *Glycobiol* 2006; 16: 1207-1218.

[19] Fox KM, Dias JA, Van Roey P, Three dimensional structure of human follicle-stimulating hormone. *Molec Endocrinol;* 2001; 15:378-389.

[20] Lapthorn AJ, Harris DC, Littlejohn A, Lustbader JW, Canfield RE, Machin KJ, Crystal structure of hCG. *Nature* 1994; 369: 455-461.

[21] de Jong D, Macklon NS, Eijkemans MJ, Mannaerts BM, Coelingh Bennink HJ, Fauser BC, Dynamics of the development of multiple follicles during ovarian stimulation for in vitro fertilization using recombinant follicle-stimulating hormone (Puregon) and various doses of the gonadotropin-releasing hormone antagonist ganirelix (Orgalutran/Antagon). *Fertil Steril* 2001;75:688-693.

[22] Devroey P, Fauser BC, Platteau P, Beckers NG, Dhont M, Mannaerts BM. Induction of multiple follicular development by a single dose of long-acting recombinant follicle-Stimulating hormone (FSH-CTP, corifollitropin alfa) for controlled ovarian stimulation before in vitro fertilization. *J Clin Endocrinol Metab* 2004;89:2062-2070.

[23] Kumar TR, Wang Y, Naifang L, Matzuk MM. Follicle stimulating hormone is required for ovarian follicle maturation but not male fertility. *Nature Genetics* 1997;15:201-204.

[24] Wolfsdorf KE, Diaz T, Schmitt EJ, Thatcher MJ, Drost M, Thatcher WW, The dominant follicle exerts an interovarian inhibition on FSH-induced follicular development. *Theriogenology* 1997;48:435-447.

[25] Hall SH, Conti M, French FS, Joseph DR, Follicle-stimulating hormone regulation of androgen-binding protein messenger RNA in sertoli cell cultures. *Mol Endocrinol* 1990; 4:349-355.

[26] Hansson V, Weddington SC, Petrusz P, Ritzen EM, Nayfeh SN, French FS. FSH stimulation of testicular androgen binding protein (ABP): comparison of ABP response and ovarian augmentation. *Endocrinol* 1975;97:469-473.

[27] Walker WH, Cheng J, FSH and testosterone signaling in Sertoli cells. *Reprod* 2005;130:15-28.

[28] Verhoeven G, Cailleau J, Follicle-stimulating hormone and androgens increase the concentration of the androgen receptor in Sertoli cells. *Endocrinol* 1988;122:1541-1550.

[29] Heitman LH, Ijzerman AP, G protein-coupled receptors of the hypothalamic-pituitary-gonadal axis: a case for Gnrh, LH, FSH, and GPR54 receptor ligands. *Med Res Rev* 2008 28:975-1011.

[30] Arey BJ, Stevis PE, Deecher DC, Shen ES, Frail DE, Negro-Vilar A, Lopez FJ, Induction of promiscuous G protein coupling of the follicle-stimulating hormone (FSH) receptor: a novel mechanism for transducing pleiotropic actions of FSH isoforms. *Mol Endocrinol* 1997 11:517-526.

[31] Baenziger JU, Green ED, Pituitary glycoprotein hormone oligosaccharides: structure, synthesis and function of the asparagine-linked oligosaccharides on lutropin, follitropin and thyrotropin. *Biochim Biophys Acta* 1988;947:287-306.

[32] Green ED, Baenziger JU, Asparagine-linked oligosaccharides on lutropin, follitropin, and thyrotropin. II. Distributions of sulfated and sialylated oligosaccharides on bovine, ovine, and human pituitary glycoprotein hormones *J Biol Chem* 1988;263:36-44.

[33] Keeney DS, Sprando RL, Robaire B, Zirkin BR, Ewing LL, Reversal of long-term LH deprivation on testosterone secretion and Leydig cell volume, number and proliferation in adult rats. *J Endocrinol* 1990;127:47-58.

[34] Ewing LL, Wing TY, Cochran RC, Kromann N, Zirkin BR, Effect of luteinizing hormone on Leydig cell structure and testosterone secretion. *Endocrinol* 1983;112:1763-1769.

[35] Krishnamurthy H, Kats R, Danilovich N, Javeshghani D, Sairam MS, Between Sertoli cells and Leydig cells in the absence of follicle-stimulating hormone-receptor signaling. *Biol Reprod* 2001;65:1201–1207.

[36] Sriraman V, Sairam MR, Jagannadha Rao A. Evaluation of relative role of LH and FSH in restoration of spermatogenesis using ethanedimethylsulphonate-treated adult rats. *Reprod Biomed Online* 2004;8:167-174.

[37] Johnson L, Blanchard TL, Varner DD, Scrutchfield WL, Factors affecting spermatogenesis in the stallion. *Theriogenology* 1997;48:1199–1216.

[38] Gagné RC, Lussier JG, Bousquet D, Barnes FL, Sirard MA. Presence of LH receptor mRNA in granulosa cells as a potential marker of oocyte developmental competence and characterization of the bovine splicing isoforms. *Reprod* 2003;125:437-446.

[39] Flynn MP, Maizels ET, Karlsson AB, McAvoy T, Ahn J-H, Nairn AC, Hunzicker-Dunn M. Luteinizing Hormone Receptor Activation in Ovarian Granulosa Cells Promotes Protein Kinase A-Dependent Dephosphorylation of Microtubule-Associated Protein 2D. *Mol Endocrinol* 2008; 22:1695–1710.

[40] Ayabe T, Tsutsumi O, Momoeda M, Yano T, Mitsuhashi N, Taketani Y. Impaired follicular growth and abnormal luteinizing hormone surge in luteal phase defect. *Fertil Steril.* 1994;61:652-656.

[41] Christenson LK, Gunewardena S, Hong X, Spitschak M, Baufeld A, Vanselow J. Research Resource: Preovulatory LH Surge Effects on Follicular Theca and Granulosa Transcriptomes. *Molec Endocrinol* 2013;7:1153-1171.

[42] Norris RP, Freudzon M, Mehlmann LM, Cowan AE, Simon AM, Paul DL, Lampe PD, Jaffe LA. Luteinizing hormone causes MAP kinase-dependent phosphorylation and closure of connexin 43 gap junctions in mouse ovarian follicles: one of two paths to meiotic resumption. *Developm* 2008;135:3229-3238.

[43] Hegele-Hartung C, Grützner M, Lessl M, Grøndahl C, Ottesen JL, Brännström B.Activation of Meiotic Maturation in Rat Oocytes After Treatment with Follicular Fluid Meiosis-Activating Sterol In Vitro and Ex Vivo. *Biol Reprod* 2001;64:418-424.

[44] Dhont M, Serreyn R, Duvivier P, Vanluchene E, De Boever J, Vandekerckhove D. Ovulation stigma and concentration of progesterone and estradiol in peritoneal fluid: relation with fertility and endometriosis. *Fertil Steril* 1984;41:872-877.

[45] Zhang T, Guo CX, Hu ZY, Liu YX. Localization of plasminogen activator and inhibitor, LH and androgen receptors and inhibin subunits in monkey epididymis. *Mol Hum Reprod.* 1997;3:945-952.

[46] Reich R, Miskin R, Tsafriri A. Follicular plasminogen activator: involvement in ovulation. *Endocrinol* 1985;116:516-521.

[47] Wuttke W, Pitzel L, Seidlová-Wuttke D, Hinney B. LH pulses and the corpus luteum: the luteal phase deficiency LPD). *Vit Horm* 2001;63:131-158.

[48] Chen SU, Chen RJ, Shieh JY, Chou CH, Lin CW, Lu HF, Yang YS. Human chorionic gonadotropin up-regulates expression of myeloid cell leukemia-1 protein in human granulosa-lutein cells: implication of corpus luteum rescue and ovarian hyperstimulation syndrome. *J Clin Endocrinol Metab.* 2010;95:3982-3992.

[49] Gibson N. Corpus Luteum. Gynecology and Obstetrics, Sciara JJ, Dooley S, Depp R, Lurain JL, Kaunitz A, Eschenbach DA (eds), *Lipincott Williams and Wilkins,* 2004, Ch 14.

[50] Dufau ML. The luteinizing hormone receptor. *Ann Rev Physiol.* 1998;60:461-496.

[51] Cole LA, Ladner DG, Cole LA, Gutierrez JM, Production of hCG during the menstrual cycle *J Reprod Med* 2009; 54: 245-250.

[52] Cole LA, Laidler L, Muller C, USA hCG Reference Service 10 year report, *Clin Biochem* 2010; 43: 1013-1022.

[53] Cole LA, Butler SA, The biological function of hyperglycosylated hCG. *Asian Pacific J Reprod* 2012;1:7-12.

[54] Gronowski AM, Fantz CR, Parvin CA, Sokoll LJ, Wiley CL, Wener MH, Grenache DG, Use of serum FSH to identify perimenopausal women with pituitary hCG. *Clin Chem* 2008; 54: 652-656.

[55] Cole LA, Dai D, Leslie KK, Butler SA, Kohorn EI, Gestational trophoblastic diseases: 1. Pathophysiology of hyperglycosylated hCG-regulated neoplasia. *Gynecol Oncol* 2006; 102:144-149.

[56] Murphy G, Reynolds JJ, Whitham SE, Docherty AJ, Angel P, Heath JK, Transforming growth factor beta modulates the expression of collagenase and metalloproteinase inhibitor. *Euro Molec Biol Org J* 1987; 6: 1899-1904.

[57] Sasaki Y, Ladner DG, Cole LA, Hyperglycosylated hCG the source of pregnancy failures. *Fertil Steril* 2008; 89: 1871-1786.

[58] Cole LA, Hyperglycosylated hCG and pregnancy failures. *J Reprod Immunol* 2012; 93: 119-122.

[59] Brennan MC, Wolfe MD, Murray-Krezan CM, Cole LA, Rayburn WF. First Trimester Hyperglycosylated Human Chorionic Gonadotropin and Development of Hypertension. *Prenat Diagn* 2013; in press.

[60] Bahado-Singh RO, Oz, AU, Kingston JM, Shahabi S, Hsu CD, Cole LA. The role of hyperglycosylated hCG in trophoblast invasion and the prediction of subsequent pre-eclampsia. *Prenat Diagn* 2002;22:478-481.

[61] Cole LA, Birken S, Sutphen S, Hussa RO, and Pattillo RA, Absence of the COOH-terminal peptide on ectopic human chorionic gonadotropin ß-subunit (HCG-ß). *Endocrinol* 1982; 110: 2198-2200.

[62] Cole LA, Hussa RO, Use of glycosidase digested human chorionic gonadotropin ß-subunit to explain the partial binding of glycoprotein hormones to Con A. *Endocrinol* 1981; 109: 2276-2279.

[63] Iles RK, Ectopic hCGß expression by epithelial cancer: Malignant behavior metastasis and inhibition of tumor cell apoptosis. *Molec Cellul Endocrinol* 2007; 264-270

[64] Beebe JS, Huth JR, Ruddon RW, Combination of the chorionic gonadotropin free beta-subunit with alpha. *Endocrinol* 1990;126:384-391.

[65] Ruddon RW, Hanson CA, Bryan AH, Putterman GJ, White E.L. Synthesis and secretion of human chorionic gonadotropin subunits by cultured human malignant cells. *J Biol Chem* 1980;255:1000-1007.

[66] Nam JH, Cole LA, Chambers JT, and Schwartz PE Urinary gonadotropin fragment a new tumor marker: I. Assay development and cancer-specificity. *Gynecol Oncol* 1990; 36: 383-390.

[67] Schwartz PE, Chambers JT, Taylor KJ, Cole LA, and Makuch R, Urinary gonadotropin fragments. *Anticancer Res* 1993; 13:1722-1725.

[68] Cole LA, β-core fragment (β-core UGP or UGF). *Tumor Marker Upd* 1994; 6: 69-75.

[69] Cole LA, Nam J-H, Park S-Y, Koh MW, Tanaka A, Urinary Beta Core Fragment: 7 years later. *J Tumor Marker Onc* 1994; 9:53-60.

[70] Acevedo HF, Krichevsky A, Campbell-Acevedo EA, Galyon JC, Buffo MJ, Hartsock RJ, Flow cytometry method for the analysis of membrane-associated human chorionic gonadotropin, its subunits, and fragments on human cancer cells. *Cancer* 1992;69:1818-1828.

[71] Norwitz ER, Schust DJ, Fisher SJ, (2001). Implantation and the survival of early pregnancy, *New Engl J Med* 2001;345, 1400-1408.

[72] Semprini AE, Simon G. Not so efficient reproduction. *Lancet* 2000;356, 257-258.
[73] Goldsmith PC, McGregor WG, Raymoure WJ, Kuhn RW, Jaffe RB. Cellular localization of chorionic gonadotropin in human fetal kidney and liver. *J Clin Endocrinol Metab* 1983;57:54-61.
[74] Abdallah MA, Lei ZM, Li X, Greenwold N, Nakajima ST, Jauniaux E, Rao CV. Human Fetal nongonadal tissues contain human chorionic gonadotropin/ luteinizing hormone receptors. *J Clin Endocrinol Metab* 2004;89:952-956.

Key Points

1. The glycopeptins are the glycoprotein hormones, TSH, FSH, LH and placental hCG, plus the pituitary hormone sulfated hCG, and the TGFβ antagonists, hyperglycosylated hCG and hyperglycosylated hCG free β-subunit.
2. All the glycopeptides are glycoproteins comprising 16% - 42% sugar. The sugar side chains add an acidic element to the molecule making it more acidic. This repels the glomerular basement membrane charge barrier, extending circulating half-life from 20 minutes (LH) to 36 hours (placental hCG).
3. Glycopeptins range from hormones (TSH, LH, FSH, placental hCG, pituitary sulfated hCG) to TGFβ antagonizing autocrines (hyperglycosylated hCG and hyperglycosylated hCG free β-subunit). Glycopeptins act on receptors on throid gland cells, gonads, placenta, uterus, and cancer cells.

Chapter 2

Evolution of Glycopeptins

The glycopeptins group of molecules is a clear group of molecules that all evolved together from transforming growth factor-β (TGFβ), an evolutionary source including the glycopeptin αβ ancestral α-subunit root, and a stem of gonadotropin ancestral hormone in fish (GAH) (Figure 2.1).

TGFβ Ancestral Glycopeptin Root

TGFβ is an ancient protein found in all animals, bacteria, fungi and mycoplasma [1-9]. Somehow TGFβ evolved to platelet-derived growth factor (PDGF), to nerve derived growth factor (NGF) and vascular endothelial growth factor (VEGF) key cell promotion signals. The root of the glycopeptide family of protein also evolved from TGFβ (Figure 2.1). The glycopeptin subunits all contain the same unique TGFβ cystine knot structure.

Around 500 million years ago TGFβ evolved into the ancestral α-subunit, the forefather to both glycoprotein hormone α-subunit and β-subunit (Figure 2.1). As demonstrated, α-subunits and β-subunits both show a common cystine-knot structure to TGFβ, suggesting a common evolutionary heritage in both subunits. A single root ancestry involving both glycopeptin subunits is proposed. First a gonadotropin ancestral hormone (GAH) evolved in early fish from a duplication of the ancestral α-subunit to form a new β-subunit and αβ dimer. Then approximately 500 million years ago a TSH evolved (Figure 2.1). Approximately 200 million years ago an LH β-subunit evolved along with an FSH β-subunit from GAH (Figure 2.1) with the α-subunit and the β-subunit mutating or diverging into different peptides. The most recent member of the cystine knot proteins to evolve is Chorionic Gonadotropin (CG), approximately 37 million years ago, with the appearance of early simian primates. Amazingly, CG has a cystine knot ring virtually identical to that which was part of TGFβ [10,11] (Figure 2.1). The α- and β-subunits of TSH, LH and FSH changed slowly with evolution, becoming the sequences we know today.

Evolution of Lower Simian CG and hyperglycosylated CG

Prosimians produced a form of LH with its two subunits. The α-subunit contained 2 N-linked oligosaccharides, and the β-subunit had just one N-linked oligosaccharide and no O-linked oligosaccharide sugar structures. Lower Simian LH was quite a basic hormone, pI 8.4,, with a 20-25 minute circulating ½-time. While LH was a pituitary gonadotrope hormone controlling steroidogenesis and ovulation it had no placenta function. A deletion mutation occurred with the evolution of lower simian primates in the LH β-subunit gene (Figure 2.2) [12,13]. As illustrated, the triplet codon corresponding to amino acid 114, DNA -C-A-A-, coding for Gln lost a nucleotide, making the codon C-A-BLANK. This put the subsequent DNA sequence out of order. The resulting frame shift took a C from the adjacent codon making -C-A- into -C-A-C- coding for Arg. Examining the LHβ codon sequence, -C-A-A- (Residue 114) CTC TCA GGC CTC CTC TTC CTC TAA coding for the peptide Gln, Leu Ser, Gln, Leu, Leu, Phe, Leu STOP (Figure 2.2). The peptide frame shifted to CAC TCT CAT GAG GCC TCC TCT TCC TCT AAG or to a different amino acid sequence, Arg, Phe, Gln, Asp, Ser, Ser, Ser, Ser, Lys. With the absence of a -T-A-A- STOP or termination codon the sequence read on and on for 24 additional codons up to amino acid 145, after which a new -T-A-A- termination codon was found (Figure 2.2) [12,13].

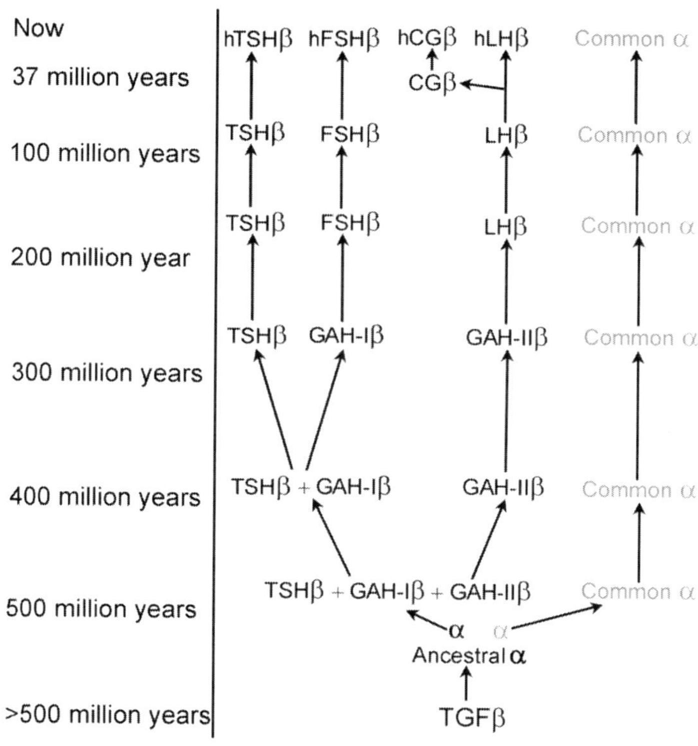

Figure 2.1. The evolution of in glycoprotein hormones. TSH is thyroid stimulating hormone, FSH is follicle stimulating hormone, LH is leuteinizing hormone and CG is chorionic gonadotropin. The abbreviation GAH is gonadotropin ancestral hormone. The figure follows the evolutionary guidelines proposed for glycoprotein hormones [10,11].

Thus, there came about the new glycopeptin that today we call lower simian chorionic gonadotropin (CG). CG adopted placental trophoblast cells rather than pituitary gonadotrope cells as a home. In root cytotrophoblast cells hyperglycosylated CG was made and in the fused syncytiotrophoblast cells the same β-subunit genes made placenta CG.

Up to this point, mammals and early primates, such as prosimian primates (e.g. Lemurs), had mothered babies through epitheliochorial placentation, a grossly inefficient placentation method (Figure 2.3). Epitheliochorial placentation involved a placenta loosely hooked onto the inner lining of the uterus which permitted the transfer of nutrients by passage through multiple layers of tissue, through the maternal vasculature, connective tissue and the epithelium of the uterus, then across and through the epithelium of the placenta, more connective tissue, and finally across the fetal umbilical vasculature into the fetus (Figure 2.3). This was a grossly inefficient way of transferring oxygen and glucose to the fetus. It was because of this inefficiency that the fetal body had the limited nutrient supplies to build a limited brain. The brain was roughly 0.1% of the mass of the body, a thousandth of the weight of the animal. This was the case in most mammals and in prosimian primates, which had a brain just 0.07% of body weight, or one thousand three-hundredth of body weight.

Early simian LH ß-subunit, 121 amino acids

CCC **CA**A **C**TC TCA GGC CTC CTC TTC CTC **TAA**
Pro Gln Leu Ser Gln Leu Leu Phe Leu
113 114 115 116 117 118 119 120 121 stop

The deletion mutation

deletion

CCC **CA/ C** TCT CAT CAG GCC TCC TCT TCC TC**T AA**G

The result, Early Simian CG ß-subunit. 145 amino acids

CCC **CAC** TCT CAG GCC TCC TCT TCC TC**T AA**G GCC CCT
Pro **Arg** Phe Gln Asp Ser Ser Ser Ser Lys Ala Pro
113 **114** 115 116 117 118 119 120 121 122 123 124

CCC CCC AGC CTT CCA AGT CCA TCC CGA CTC CCG GGG
Pro Pro Ser Leu Pro Ser Pro Ser Arg Leu Pro Gly
125 126 127 128 129 130 131 132 133 134 135 136

CCC TCG GAC ACC CCG ATC CTC CCA CAA **TAA**
Pro Ser Asp Thr Pro Ile Leu Pro Gln stop
137 138 139 140 141 142 143 144 145

Figure 2.2. Point mutation in LHβ gene leading to the evolution of CG [12,13]. TAA is the termination codon.

Then came the evolution of lower simian primates. It is with this evolution that placental CG and hyperglycosylated CG emerged. CG and hyperglycosylated CG would change the way that placentation occurred. Lower simian primate placenta CG was going to use its CG/LH and TGFβ receptor skills to build on everything, permitting greater nutritional efficiency and very much needed brain growth.

In lower simian primates a new placentation system developed, hemochorial placentation (Figure 2.4). With hyperglycosylated CG the placenta started invading the uterus for the first time, and implanted to a depth of 1% of uterine thickness. With hyperglycosylated CG cytotrophoblast cells grew, making villous sticks of hyperglycosylated CG. With placental CG the cytotrophoblast cells on the villous sticks fused to become syncytiotrophoblast cells. Placental hCG also extended the maternal uterine spiral arteries to reach the hemochorial placentation, and developed the umbilical circulation linking the hemochorial placentation and the fetus. Maternal blood flowed into the hemochorial placentation tank of placenta, then passed through the syncytiotrophoblast cells and into the umbilical circulation to reach the fetus (Figure 2.4). A new, more efficient placentation fetal nutrition system was started (Table 2.1) as a result of the expression of CG. With the more efficient nutrition system the brain grew from the size of the prosimian primate brain's 0.07% of the animal's total weight to the lower simian primate's brain, 0.17% of the animal's total weight.

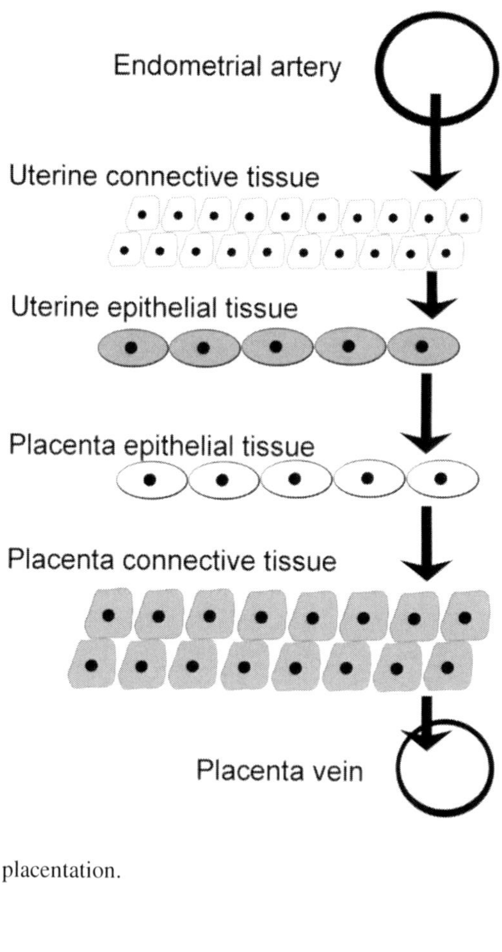

Figure 2.3. Epitheliochorial placentation.

Table 2.1. Fetal nutrition in mammals, primates and humans [12,13]

Species	Implantation characteristics	Depth of implantation	Sugar structures and pI of CG (blood 1/2-life)	Brain mass % body weight
Humans	Hemochorial	40%	8 oligosaccharides, pI 3.5 (36 h)	2.4%
Advanced Simian Primate	Hemochorial	10%	6 oligosaccharides, pI 4.9 (6.0 h)	0.74%
Lower Simian Primate	Hemochorial	1%	5 oligosaccharides, pI 6.3 (2.4h)	0.17%
Prosimian Primate	Epitheliochorial	No implant	No CG produced	0.07%
Horse, Mammal	Epitheliochorial	No implant	No CG produced	0.12%
Pig, Mammal	Epitheliochorial	No implant	No CG produced	0.09%

Evolution of CG and Hyperglycosylated CG, Lower Simian Primates – Humans

With the evolution of advanced simian primates (i.e. chimpanzee) mutations took place in the CG β-subunit molecule, such that it now had a third O-linked oligosaccharides, or 6 oligosaccharides in total vs. 5 oligosaccharides in lower simian primates. The pI or acidity of CG was increased from pI 6.3 to pI 4.9. This also increased the circulating ½-life from 2.5 hours to approximately 6.0 hours, effectively more than doubling the potency of placental CG and hyperglycosylated CG or making super-placental CG and super-hyperglycosylated CG molecules. The end result was that under the influence of super-hyperglycosylated CG the placenta invaded deeper, to 10% of uterine thickness, and that super-hyperglycosylated CG promotes larger, more efficient villous structures. Super-placenta CG more efficiently promoted villous structure differentiation, more efficiently promoted maternal spiral arteries connecting with the hemochorial placentation structure, and more efficiently promoted connection to the fetus through an umbilical circulation.

As illustarted in Figures 2.4 and 2.5, a completely more efficient form of hemochorial placentation was developed in advanced simian primates (Table 2.1). In advanced simian primates with the much more efficient hemochorial placentation system a larger-brained primate developed, with a brain weight of 0.74% of its total weight (Table 2.1). Advanced simian primates produced super-CG molecules leading to super hemochorial placentation.

With the evolution of humans multiple additional mutations occurred in the CG β-subunit molecule leading to the addition of one further N-linked oligosaccharide and one further O-linked oligosaccharide. The human CG molecule then contained a total of 8 oligosaccharides compared to 6 oligosaccharides in the advanced simian species (Table 2.1). With the additional acidic sugars the pI was increased from pI 4.9 to pI 3.5. This improved the circulating ½-life from approximately 6 hours to 36 hours, or 6-fold boosted placental and hyperglycosylated CG bioactivity, making an ultra-super-placenta and hyperglycosylated CG. The end result was that under the influence of ultra-super-hyperglycosylated CG the placenta invaded very much deeper to 40% of uterine thickness, and that ultra-super-hyperglycosylated

CG promoted the formation of very much more efficient villous structures. Ultra-super-placenta CG more efficiently promoted the villous differentiation and of the hemochorial placentation structure, and very much more efficiently promoted connection to the fetus through an umbilical circulation; this was ultra-super hemochorial placentation.

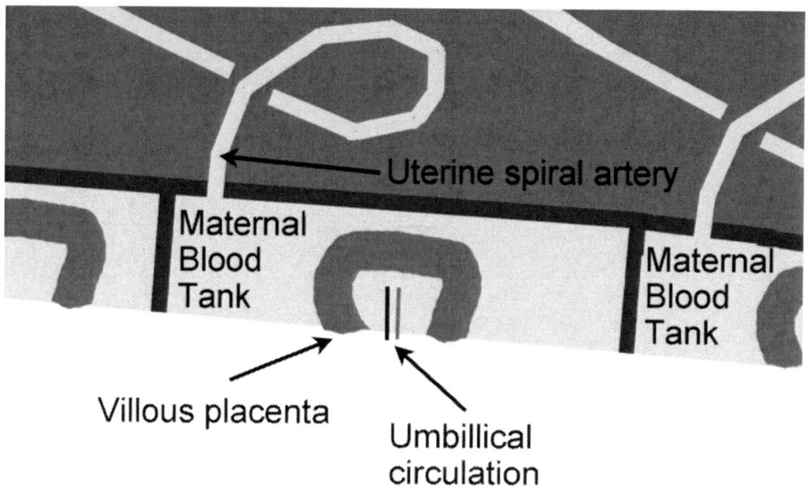

Figure 2.4. Hemochorial placentation in lower simian primate.

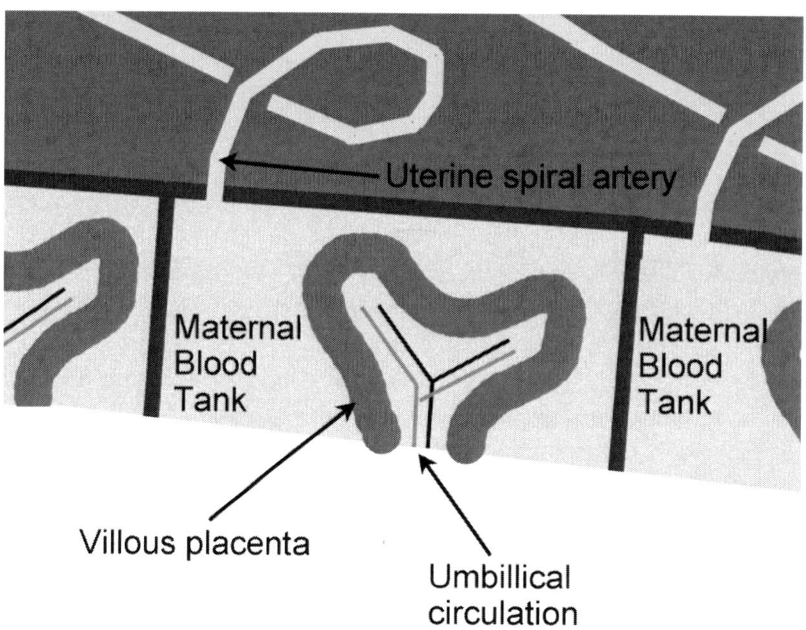

Figure 2.5. Hemochorial placentation in advanced simian primate.

As shown in Figure 2.6, an extremely more efficient form of hemochorial placentation was developed in humans (Table 2.1). In humans this placentation system led to the development of a very much larger brain, with a brain weight of 2.4% of the total weight (Table 2.1). This is how the human brain developed through the evolution of placental CG and hyperglycosylated CG, and the extreme evolutionary development of these powerful promoters. The evolution of CG (placental CG and hyperglycosylated CG) led to the development of hemochorial placentation, the extreme evolutionary development of super-CG and ultra-super-CG led to the placentation mechanism needed to support a human-size brain. As described below, deficiencies of these ultra-super-promoters can cause major problems during pregnancy. Furthermore, ultra-super-hyperglycosylated CG and its invasion and growth pathways are stolen or misused by human cancers. The detailed story of CG and evolution is published [14,15].

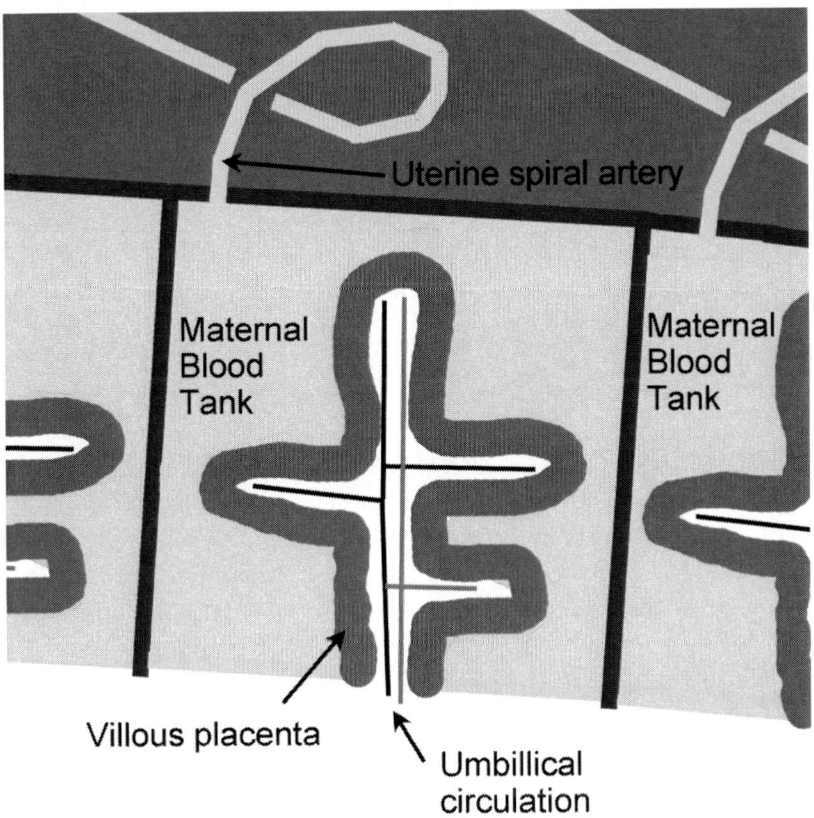

Figure 2.6. Hemochorial placentation in humans.

Consequence of Hyperglycosylated hCG Evolution

The consequence of ultra-super-hyperglycosylated hCG and the need to produce adequate concentrations is major in human pregnancies. If a person does not produce sufficient ultra-super hyperglycosylated hCG, a pregnancy is destined to failure. As described in Chapter 1, adequate production of hyperglycosylated hCG is mandatory for a pregnancy to implant appropriately and go to term without aborting. As shown in Figure 1.8, 70 of 70 pregnancies producing adequate hyperglycosylated hCG will go to term. Twenty-nine of 35 pregnancies spontaneously aborting are producing deficient hyperglycosylated hCG. Twenty-one of 28 biochemical pregnancies will be producing deficient hyperglycosylated hCG. The balance of spontaneous abortion and balance of biochemical pregnancies seemingly failed due to major genetic abnormalities [14-17]. As described in Chapter 1, pregnancy hypertension and preeclampsia are other complications of deficient hyperglycosylated hCG production during the course of pregnancy.

Possibly the biggest complication of CG and its evolution is that human cancers use the ultra-super-promotion model of hyperglycosylated hCG and its free β-subunit to drive human cancers. As described in Chapter 1, hyperglycosylated hCG and its free β-subunit function through a TGFβ receptor to drive most human cancers. Through a TGFβ antagonism model they drive cancer growth, block cancer apoptosis and drive cancer invasion [18-23]. This has now been confirmed and double-confirmed by seven independent laboratories [18-23]. In this respect hCG-related molecules do good, as in the evolution of humans, and are also used for evil, as in driving human cancers.

References

[1] Pang K, Ryan JF, Baxevanis D, Martindale MQ. Evolution of the TGF-β signaling pathway and its potential role in the Ctenophore, Mnemiopsis leidyi. *Plos One* 2011:6:1-15.

[2] Derynck R, Zhang YE. Smad-dependent and Smad-independent pathways in TGF-β family signaling. *Nature* 2003;425:577-584.

[3] Newfeld S, Wisotzkey RG, Kumar S. Molecular evolution of a developmental pathway: Phlogenetic analyses of transforming growth factor-β family ligands, receptors and Smad signal trasducers. *Genetics* 1999;152:783-795.

[4] Kohll G, Hu S, Clelland E, Di Mucclu T, Rothenstein J, Peng C. Cloning of transforming growth factor-β1 (T and its type II receptor from zebrafish ovary and role of TGFβ1 in oocyte maturation. *Endocrinol* 2003;144:1931-1941.

[5] Runyan CE, Schnaper HW, Pocelet AC; The role of internalization in transforming growth factor beta1-induced Smad2 association with Smad anchor for receptor activation (SARA) and Smad2-dependent signaling in human mesangial cells. *J Biol Chem* 2005;280:8300-8308.

[6] Massangue J, Chen YG. Controlling TGF-beta signaling. *Genes Dev* 2000;14;627-644.

[7] Murphy G, Reynolds JJ, Whitham SE, Docherty AJ, Angel P, Heath JK. Transforming growth factor beta modulates the expression of collagenase and metalloproteinase inhibitor. *Euro Molec Biol Org J* 1987;6:1899-1904.

[8] Herpin A, Lelong C, Favrel P. Transforming growth factor-beta-related proteins: an ancestral and widespread superfamily of cytokines in metazoans. *Dev Comp Immunol* 2004;28:461-485.

[9] Lyons SM, Prasad A. Cross-Talk and Information Transfer in Mammalian and Bacterial Signaling. *Plos One* 2012;7: e34488.

[10] Cole LA, Khanlian SA, Kohorn EI. Evolution of the Human Brain, Chorionic Gonadotropin and Hemochorial Implantation of the Placenta: Insights into Origins of Pregnancy Failures, Preeclampsia and Choriocarcinoma. *J Reprod Med* 2008;53:449-557

[11] Sun PD, Davies DR. The cystine-knot growth-factor superfamily. *Ann Rev Biophys Biomol Struct* 1995;24:269-291.

[12] Fiddes JC, Goodman HM.The cDNA for the ß-subunit of human chorionic gonadotropin suggests evolution of a gene by readthrough into the 3'-untranslated region. *Nature* 1980;286:684-687.

[13] Maston GA, Ruvolo M. Chorionic gonadotropin has a recent origin within primates in an evolutionary history of selection. *Mol Bio Evol* 2002;19:320-335.

[14] Cole LA, Khanlian SA, Kohorn EI, Evolution of the Human Brain Chorionic Gonadotropin and Hemochorial Implantation of the Placenta: insights into origins of pregnancy failures preeclampsia and choriocarcinoma. *J Reprod Med* 2008; 53: 449-557.

[15] Cole LA, hCG and hyperglycosylated hCG in the establishment and evolution of hemochorial placentation. *J Reprod Immunol* 2009; 82: 111-117.

[16] Sasaki Y, Ladner DG, Cole LA, Hyperglycosylated hCG the source of pregnancy failures. *Fertil Steril* 2008; 89: 1871-1786.

[17] Cole LA, Hyperglycosylated hCG and pregnancy failures. *J Reprod Immunol* 2012; 93: 119-122.

[18] Carter WB, Sekharem M, Coppola D, Purified hCG induces apoptosis in breast cancer. *Breast Cancer Res Treatm* 2006; 100: S243-S244.

[19] Jankowska A, Gunderson SI, Andrusiewicz N, Burczynska B, Szczerba A, Jarmolowski A, Nowak-Markwitz E, Warchol JB. Reduction of human chorionic gonadotropin beta subunit expression by modified U1 snRNA caused apoptosis in cervical cancer cells. *Molec Cancer* 2008;7:26-29.

[20] Li D, Wen X, Ghali L, Al-Shalabi FM, Docherty SM, Purkis P, Iles RK, hCG beta expression by cervical squamous carcinoma-in vivo histological association with tumour invasion and apoptosis. *Histopathol* 2008; 53: 147-55.

[21] Cole LA, Butler SA, Hyperglycosylated hCG hCGß and hyperglycosylated hCGß: interchangeable cancer promoters. *Molec Cellul Endocrinol* 2012; 349: 232-238.

[22] Butler SA, Ikram MS, Mathieu S, Iles RK, The increase in bladder carcinoma cell population induced by the free beta subunit of hCG is a result of an anti-apoptosis effect and not cell proliferation. *Brit J Cancer* 2000; 82: 1553-1556.

[23] Iles RK, Ectopic hCGß expression by epithelial cancer: Malignant behavior metastasis and inhibition of tumor cell apoptosis. *Molec Cellul Endocrinol* 2007; 264-270

Key Points

1. CG and hyperglycosylated CG first evolved in lower simian primates. With this evolution came the first hemochorial placentation. It was with further mutations and the evolution of hCG and hyperglycosylated hCG that the human brain developed.
2. All mammalian species prior to the lower simian primate used epitheliochorial placentation and other less efficient fetal nutritional mechanisms.

Chapter 3

Gonadotropin Releasing Hormone (GnRH) and Inhibins, Regulators of Glycopeptins

Here we examine gonadotropin releasing hormone (GnRH) and the intricate mechanisms by which gonadotropin production - more specifically, pituitary luteinizing hormone (LH), pituitary follicle stimulating hormone (FSH) and pituitary sulfated human chorionic gonadotropin (sulfated hCG) - are controlled [1-3].

Since gonadotropins are control hormones themselves, controlling estrogen, progesterone and testosterone production, GnRH and the hypothalamic-pituitary axis is the overlord system that regulates the entire human reproductive system [1-3]. It initiates and then controls the menstrual cycle in women and spermatogenesis and steroidogenesis in men. Here we also examine one other group of critical hormone, inhibins, which control FSH production by the pituitary.

GnRH

GnRH is a strange molecule, synthesized in the brain hypothalamus and acting on pituitary gonadotrope cells [1-3]. A gene on chromosome 8 codes for the GnRH precursor molecule, GnRH-associate peptide (GAP), a 56 amino acids long peptide (Figure 3.1) [4-6]. Hypothalamic neuron proteases cleave GAP to make GnRH, which is a decapeptide amide, just 10 amino acids long (Figure 3.1).

The GnRH sequence starts with a remote amino acid, pyro-glutamic acid, a Glu amino acid containing a pentagonal ring structure. The sequence ends with the amino acid Gly and an amide structure, making it a rare decapeptide amide. The molecular weight of GnRH is just 1167 [4-6].

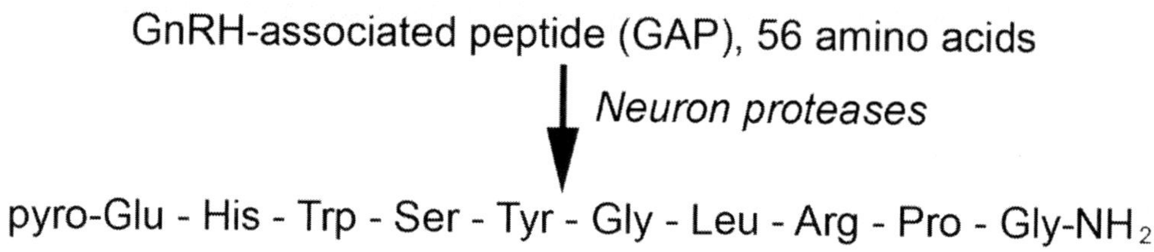

Figure 3.1. GnRH and its precursor molecule GAP.

The hypothalamus is an area of the brain with a number of small nuclei having a variety of functions. The lateral and penfornical nuclei, for instance, control hunger and thirst. The ventromedial nucleus modulates food intake and satiety. The posterior preoptic nucleus modulates body temperature, the preoptic and paraventricular nuclei control libido and penis erection, the posterior nucleus controls shivering, the medial preoptic nucleus controls bladder contraction, the anterio-hypothalamic nucleus controls sweating and the paraventricular nucleus seemingly controls sleep. It could be said that the hypothalamus of the brain controls thirst, hunger, libido, body temperature, urination and sleep. The preoptic nucleus, in addition to controlling libido and erection, seemingly controls GnRH production or release of the hormone that regulates human reproduction.

GnRH is a neurohormone since it is released by neurons and not endocrine tissue. It is released into the hypophyseal-hypothalamic tract (see Figure 2.3), a portal vascular plexus tract linking the hypothalamus and the pituitary [1-6]. GnRH is released in a pulsatile fashion by neurons, roughly one pulse every 0.5 to 3 hours. Both the pulse frequency and the amplitude of the pulse are important in GnRH action. They act on receptors on pituitary gonadotrope cells to promote the release of all three gonadotropins, LH, FSH and sulfated hCG [1-6].

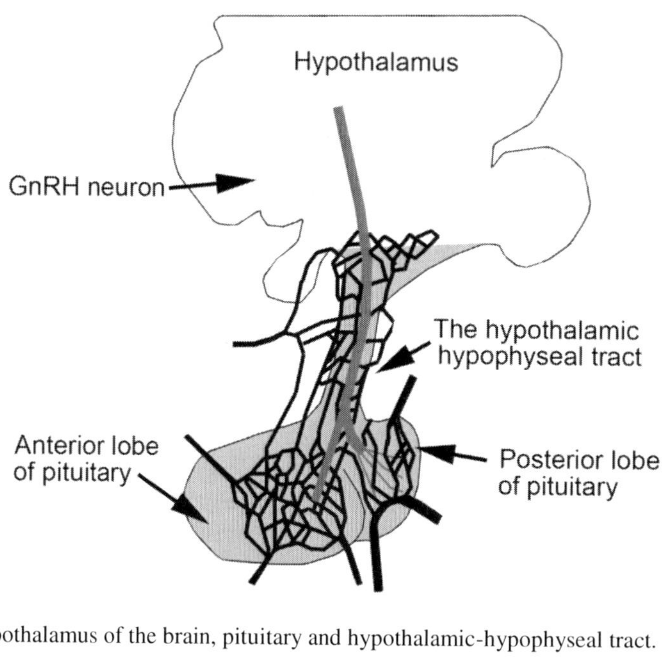

Figure 3.2. The hypothalamus of the brain, pituitary and hypothalamic-hypophyseal tract.

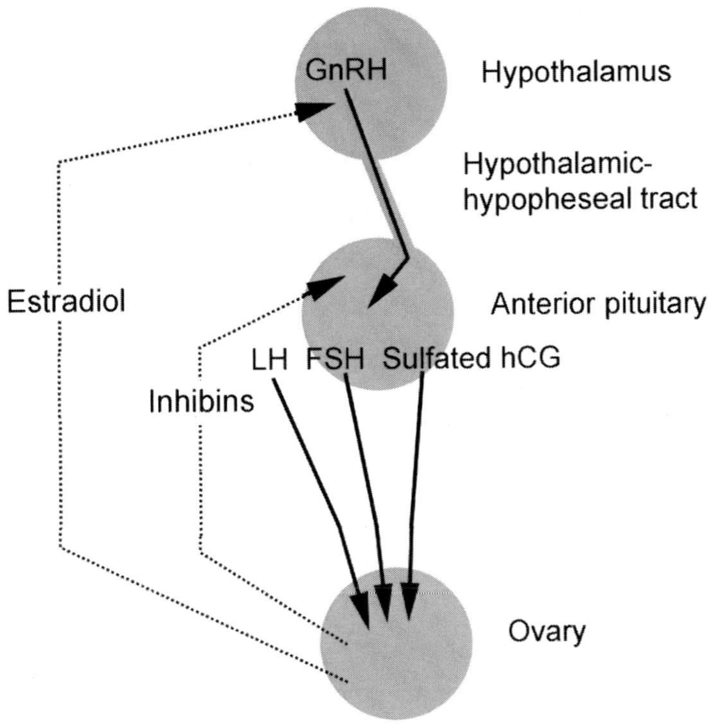

Figure 3.3. The hypothalamic-pituitary-gonad axis in women. The hypothalamus produces GnRH pulses, these promote pulses of pituitary LH, FSH and sulfated hCG, which promote synthesis of progesterone and estradiol in the ovary. The progesterone and estradiol feed back to the hypothalamus to modulate GnRH synthesis.

As indicated in Figure 3.2, the pituitary gland has 2 lobes. The anterior pituitary contains gonadotrope cells which produce FSH, LH and sulfated hCG, thyrotrope cells which produce thyroid stimulating hormone, lactotrope cells which make prolactin and corticotrope cells which make adrenalcorticotropic hormone. Pulses of GnRH act only on the gonadotrope cells, to cause parallel pulsatile release of pituitary FSH, LH and sulfated hCG. The pituitary also has a posterior lobe. The posterior lobe is a collection of axonal projections from the hypothalamus. These produce oxytocin and vasopressin [7-10].

GnRH promotes both FSH and LH in gonadotrope cells. Promotion of extremely low concentrations of sulfated hCG, about $1/50^{th}$ LH and FSH production, may be incidental [11,12]. Gonadotrope cells produce the common α-subunit in excess, which combines with the limiting concentration of LH, FSH and sulfated hCG. On chromosome 19, the gene for LH β-subunit sits directly aside 8 duplicated copies of genes coding for hCG β-subunit. GnRH stimulates the solitary gene for LH β-subunit. It may not be able to do this without promoting some of the 8 adjacent hCG β-subunit genes, incidentally promoting sulfated hCG. That it is incidental is suggested by the duplication of LH and sulfated hCG; they both perform the same job. They also both bind the same receptor, and the extremely low concentrations of sulfated hCG [11,12].

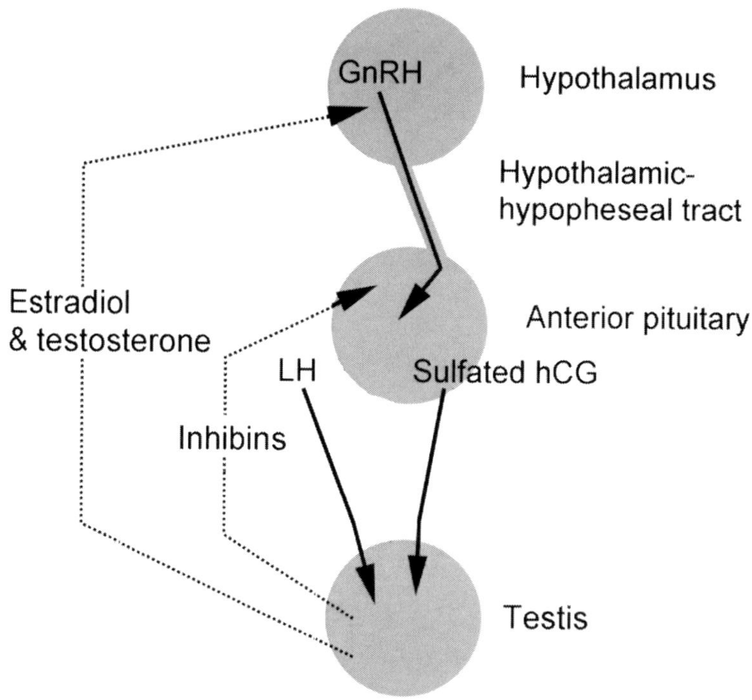

Figure 3.4. The hypothalamic-pituitary-gonad axis in men. The hypothalamus produced GnRH pulses, these promote pulses of pituitary LH and sulfated hCG, which promote synthesis of testosterone and estradiol in the testis. The testosterone and estradiol feed back to the hypothalamus to modulate GnRH synthesis.

GnRH controls LH, FSH and sulfated hCG production, so effectively also controls their sex steroid production during the menstrual cycle in women and syeroidogenesis in men (Figures 3.3 and 3.4). The production of LH and FSH during the follicular phase of the menstrual cycle leads to estradiol production [1-10]. The estradiol peak in the ovulatory phase is promoted in the most advanced follicles by inhibins in addition to LH and FSH (see next section). While estradiol feedback generally controls and inhibits GnRH production (Figure 3.3), in the ovulatory phase of the menstrual cycle it does not inhibit GnRH; it causes a surge in GnRH production. This surge causes the LH peak (FSH secretion is blocked by Inhibin). LH is also produced in the luteal phase of the menstrual cycle when it promotes progesterone production by the corpus luteum [1-10].

The pulse of GnRH during the menstrual cycle mimics resulting pulses of LH and sulfated hCG. Pulses are elevated during the follicular phase and luteal phases of the menstrual cycle, decline to zero just prior to menstrual bleeding, and reach a peak around day 14 or the midpoint of the menstrual cycle [13].

Inhibins

Inhibins are proteins that exist in two forms. Inhibin A is a glycoprotein of molecular weight 32,000, and inhibin B is a larger glycoprotein of molecular weight 54,000 [14,15]. Both molecules are produced by female ovarian granulosa cells in the follicular phase of the menstrual cycle, and by ovarian corpus luteal cells in the luteal phase of the menstrual cycle. They are also produced in men by Sertoli cells. Inhibins have numerous key functions in male and female reproduction. GnRH promotes all 3 gonadotropins not differentiating between LH, sulfated hCG and FSH. Inhibins resolve this issue by specifically blocking pituitary FSH production (Figures 3.3 and 3.4). The inhibin receptor is on the pituitary gonadotrope cells. As such, through this means, inhibins permit the separate modulation of LH and FSH [14,15]. In men, completion of spermatogenesis requires low concentrations of FSH and high relative concentrations of LH and sulfated hCG. GnRH seemingly equally promotes all 3 glycopeptins. This low FSH high LH and sulfated hCG mixture is accomplished by Sertoli cell inhibins, which suppress FSH release from the pituitary (Figure 3.4).

In women, FSH and LH are both produced during the follicular phase of the menstrual cycle to promote estradiol production. Then, FSH is suppressed by rising granulosa cell inhibins around the time of the estrogen peak in the ovulatory phase [16,17]. These inhibins permit an LH peak to dominate during the ovulatory phase. In the luteal phase of the menstrual cycle the corpus luteal cells produce inhibins to continuously suppress FSH (Figure 3.3)[16,17].

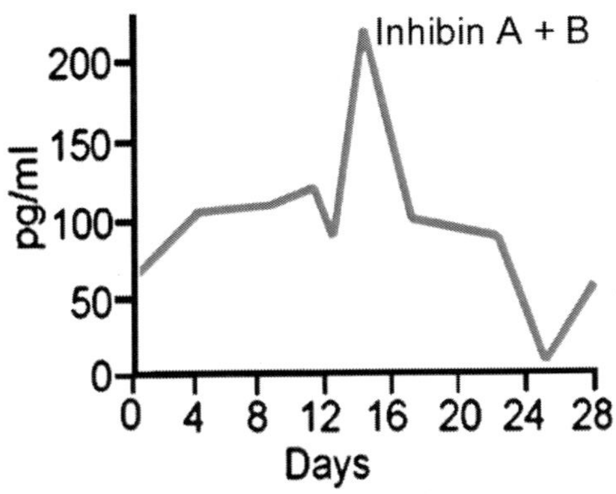

Figure 3.5. Concentration of inhibins (inhibin A + B) during the menstrual cycle.

Inhibins have multiple other biological functions in human reproduction. Just as human reproduction cannot exist with LH and FSH, it also cannot exist with inhibins. In the female ovary follicles compete in growth to become the dominant follicle [18](Chapter 5). LH promotes follicular growth. FSH promotes follicle growth further, starting the race for the dominant follicle. The racing follicles, depending on their size, produce greater and greater amounts of inhibins. In turn, those producing greater amount of inhibins promote their own growth to a greater extent (Chapter 5). The most advanced follicles, under stimulation by FSH, LH and inhibins, raise estradiol levels to a peak around day 11-13 of the menstrual cycle [19]. Inhibins like LH and FSH promote cholesterol side chain cleavage enzyme and aromatase, the two key enzymes in estradiol synthesis (Chapter 4 and Chapter 6) [19].

Figure 3.5 shows mean concentrations of inhibins (inhibin A plus inhibin B) during the menstrual cycle. As shown, concentrations of inhibins are highest at the time of the LH and sulfated hCG peak, when inhibins block FSH production [14,15].

The Hypothalamic-Inhibin, Pituitary-Gonad Axis

The glycopeptins with the assistance of GnRH and inhibins in the hypothalamic-pituitary-gonad axis completely control LH, FSH and sulfated hCG and steroid production in the male and female [1-19]. In males, LH (or sulfated hCG) and FSH promote estrogen and testosterone production. Both LH and FSH promote spermatogenesis (Chapter 9). Inhibins keep LH and FSH in balance by modulating pituitary FSH production (Figure 3.4).

In females, FSH and LH are both stimulated by GnRH during the follicular phase of the menstrual cycle to promote estradiol production. Then, FSH is suppressed by rising granulosa cell inhibins around the time of the estradiol peak in the ovulatory phase. These inhibins permit an LH peak to dominate during the ovulatory phase [2,13]. During most of the menstrual cycle, estradiol modulates or reduces GnRH pulses. At the time of the estradiol peak, the estrogen causes a surge in GnRH production. This surge causes the LH peak. In the luteal phase of the menstrual cycle GnRH pulses the gonadotrope cells. The corpus luteal cells produce inhibin which continuously suppresses FSH during this phase of the menstrual cycle (Figure 3.3)[2,13].

Hypothalamic-Pituitary Disorders

Failure of the hypothalamus to produce GnRH or failure of the pituitary to produce FSH or LH causes secondary amenorrhea. Secondary amenorrhea is the absence of menstrual periods for 6 months or longer in a woman with a history of normal menstrual periods. The hypothalamus and pituitary are common causes of this complaint. Psychiatric medications such as phenothiazide, extreme weight loss or anorexia nervosa, and stress are all causes for hypothalamic malfunction, failure to produce GnRH and secondary amenorrhea. Pituitary adenomas and micro-adenomas cause failure of the pituitary to produce gonadotropins and secondary amenorrhea. In such cases, an MRI or CT scan of the head are indicated, most notably in the region of the sella tursica, or the hypothalamus and pituitary to investigate the possibility of hypothalamic or pituitary tumors. Hypothalamic or pituitary secondary amenorrhea can be treated with exogenously administered gonadotropins. Contraceptive estrogen-progestogen pills suppress hypothalamic GnRH. Occasionally, when a patient stops taking contraceptive pills a menstrual period may not occur for multiple months. This is due to a delay in the brain or hypothalamus restarting production of GnRH pulses.

References

[1] Millar RP, Lu ZL, Pawson AJ, Flanagan CA, Morgan K, Maudsley SR. Gonadotropin-releasing hormone receptors. *Endocr Rev* 2004;25: 235–275.

[2] Charlton H. Hypothalamic control of anterior pituitary function: a history. *J. Neuroendocrinol* 2008;20: 641–646.

[3] Sower SA, Freamat M, Kavanaugh SI. The origins of the vertebrate hypothalamic-pituitary-gonadal (HPG) and hypothalamic-pituitary-thyroid (HPT) endocrine systems: new insights from lampreys. *Gen Comp Endocrinol* 2009;161: 20–29.

[4] Flanagan CA, Millar RP, Illing N. Advances in understanding gonadotrophin-releasing hormone receptor structure and ligand interactions. *Rev Reprod* 1998; 2:113–20.

[5] Janáky T, Juhász A, Bajusz S. Analogues of luteinizing hormone-releasing hormone containing cytotoxic groups. *Proc Natl Acad Sci USA* 1992;89:972–976.

[6] Seeburg PH, Adelman JP. Characterization of cDNA for precursor of human luteinizing hormone releasing hormone. *Nature* 1984;311: 666–668.

[7] Horn AM, Robinson ICAF, Fink G. Oxytocin and vasopressin in rat hypophysial portal blood: experimental studies in normal and Brattleboro rats". *Journal Endocrinol* 1985;104:211-230.

[8] Fliers E, Unmehopa A. *Molec Cellul Endocrinol* 2006; 251;1:1–8.

[9] Knepel W, Homolka L, Vlaskovska M, Nutto D. Stimulation of adrenocorticotropin/beta-endorphin release by synthetic ovine corticotropin-releasing factor in vitro. Enhancement by various vasopressin analogs. *Neuroendocrinol* 1984;38:344-350.

[10] Melmed S. *The pituitary*. Academic Press, 2010.

[11] Birken S, Maydelman Y, Gawinowicz MA, Pound A, Liu Y, Hartree AS, Isolation and characterization of human pituitary chorionic gonadotropin. *Endocrinol* 1996; 137: 1402-11.

[12] Odell WD, Griffin J, Pulsatile secretion of human chorionic gonadotropin in normal adults. *New Engl J Med* 1987; 317: 1688-1691.

[13] Marshall JC, Dalkin AC, Haisenleder DJ, Griffin ML, Kelch RP. GnRH pulses--the regulators of human reproduction. *Trans Am Clin Climatol Assoc* 1993;104:31–46.

[14] Bardin CW, Morris PL, Shaha C, Feng ZM, Rossi V, Vaughan J, Vale WW, Voglmayr J, Chem C-L. Inhibin Structure and Function in the Testis. *Ann NY Acad Sci* 1989;564:10-23.

[15] Deffieux X, Antoine JM. Inhibins, activins and anti-Müllerian hormone: structure, signalling pathways, roles and predictive value in reproductive medicine. *Gynecol Obstet Fertil* 2003;31:900-911.

[16] Lu C, Yang W, Chen M, Liu T, Yang J, Tan P, Li L, Hu X, Fan C, Hu Z, Liu Y. Inhibin A inhibits follicle-stimulating hormone (FSH) action by suppressing its receptor expression in cultured rat granulosa cells. *Mol Cell Endocrinol* 2009;27:48-56.

[17] Chada M, Průsa R, Bronský J, Pechová M, Kotaska K, Lisá L. Inhibin B, follicle stimulating hormone, luteinizing hormone, and estradiol and their relationship to the regulation of follicle development in girls during childhood and puberty. *Physiol Res* 2003;52:341-346.

[18] Guilbault LA, Rouillier P, Matton P, Glencross RG, Beard AJ, Knight PG. Relationships between the level of atresia and inhibin contents (alpha subunit and alpha-beta dimer) in morphologically dominant follicles during their growing and regressing phases of development in cattle. *Biol Reprod* 1993;48:268-276.

[19] Campbell BK, Mann GE, McNeilly AS, Baird DT. The Pattern of Ovarian Inhibin, Estradiol, and Androstenedione Secretion during the Estrous Cycle of the Ewe. *Endocrinol* 1990:127;227-235.

Key Points

1. There are two forms of inhibin.
2. GnRH is decapeptide amide and is made by neurons.
3. GnRH is transmitted to the gonadotrope cells through the hypothalamic-hypophyseal tract. GnRH promotes both LH and FSH.
4. The steroid hormones progesterone and estradiol in women, and testosterone and estradiol in men, can feedback to the hypothalamus and control GnRH pulses.
5. Inhibin is made by Sertoli cells in men, and granulosa cells (in follicular phase) and corpus luteal cells (in luteal phase).
6. Inhibin selective suppresses FSH production by the gonadotrope cells of the pituitary.
7. The combination of GnRH and inhibin controls the menstrual hormone gonadotropin and sex steroid levels during the menstrual cycle.

The Ovary and Female Reproduction

Chapter 4

Estrogens, Progestogens and Androgens

Estrogens, progestogens and androgens are all fatty acid steroids (Figure 4.1). Steroids by definition comprise 4 carbon rings, A, B, C and D, a hexagon, a hexagon, a hexagon and a pentagon. The root steroid in cholesterol (Figure 4.1), with the 4 rings, an 8 carbon tail, carbons 20-27, and 3 methyl group side chains, carbons 18, 19 and 20. All steroids are made starting with cholesterol (Figure 4.1).

Sex Steroids

Sex steroids are androgens, estrogens and progestogens. They are all made from the root steroid cholesterol (Figure 4.1). Cholesterol is always thought about in a negative sense; cholesterol, vascular blockage, cranial vascular accident and myocardial infarction. On the positive side cholesterol is the root or mother steroid; without cholesterol there would be no sex steroids, and there would be no such thing as sex. As illustrated in Figure 4.1, cholesterol is made from cytoplasmic Acetyl CoA. The ingredients come from oxidation of sugars or oxidative degradation of fatty acids such as mitochondrial Acetyl CoA which is transferred to the cytoplasm. Cholesterol carbons are numbered to a convention. This same convention is used in numbering all sex steroids.

There is not just one form of progesterone; there are multiple progestogens. These can all be identified as *21 carbon steroids*. Progestogens include progesterone and 17α-progesterone, the two biologically active natural progestogens (Figure 4.2). Synthetic progestogen agonists used by steroid manufacturers include norpregnene and norethisterone, amongst others (Figure 4.2). Similarly, there is not just one androgen. Natural androgens include testosterone, androstenedione, dehyroepiandrosterone (DHEA) and dihydrotestosterone. Androstanalone is an example of a commercial androgen agonist. All androgens are characteristically *19 carbon steroids* [3-11].

There are three natural forms of estrogen; these are estrone or E1, estradiol or E2 and estriol or E3 (Figure 4.2). To help remember their names, structures and numbers consider the following. As illustrated in Figure 4.3, estrONE or E1 contains one hydroxyl group, estraDIOL or E2 contains two hydroxyl groups and esTRIol or E3 contains three hydroxyl groups. Estrogens have two characteristics; firstly, they are always 18 carbon steroids, and secondly, they always have an aromatized left side ring or ring A. All 3 estrogens are aromatized or produced by the same aromatase enzyme, in the dominant follicle. The racing follicles, depending on their size, are made from different androgen substrates. Estrone (E1) is made by aromatase action on androstenedione, estradiol (E2) by aromatase action on testosterone, and estriol (E3) by aromatase action on 16α-dehydroxyandostenedione. Ethinyl estradiol is an example of a commercial estrogen agonist [1-11].

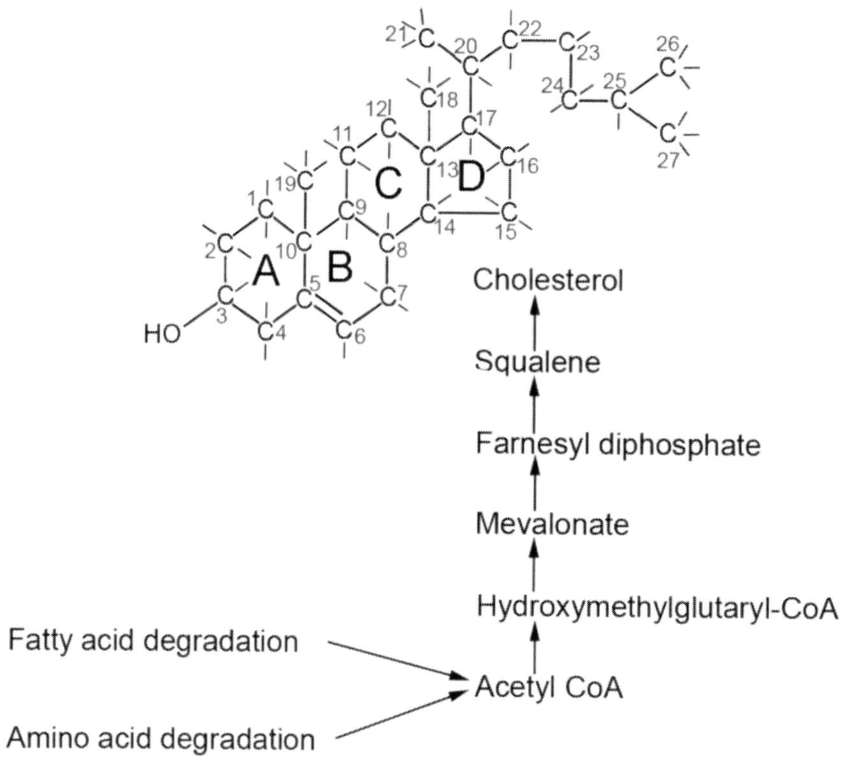

Figure 4.1. The structure, synthesis and carbon numbering of cholesterol. Carbons are numbered according to accepted guidelines. Short lines are hydrogen bonds.

Sex Steroids Synthesized by the Ovary

All female steroids pertinent to normal reproduction are produced in the ovary. In the follicular phase of the menstrual cycle, granulosa and theca cells work side by side in producing the principal estrogen, estradiol (E2). As shown in Figure 4.4, two pathways generate the androgen androstenedione in theca cells. One pathway involves pregnenolone and progesterone and generation of the second form of progestogen, 17α-hydroxyprogesterone. The second pathway bypasses progesterone synthesis, involving 17α-hydroxypregnenolone and the androgen dehydroepiandrosterone (DHEA) (Figure 4.4). The key or rate limiting step in all pathways is generation of pregnenolone from cholesterol by cholesterol side-chain cleavage enzyme. All other enzymes are present, not controlled and fully active. Cholesterol side-chain cleavage enzyme is activated by LH or sulfated hCG binding to a LH/hCG receptor on theca cells [4-9].

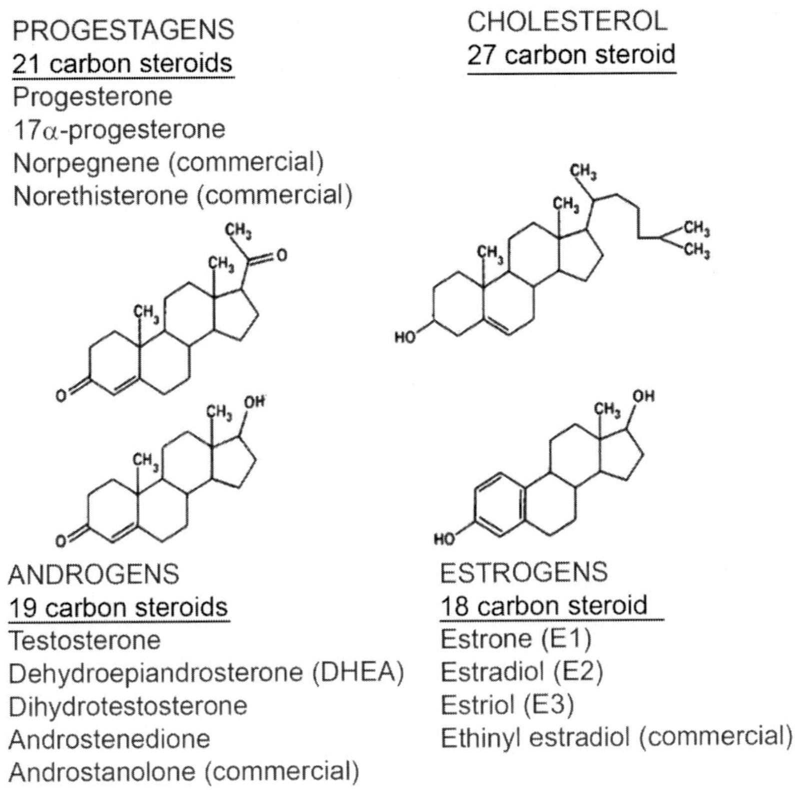

Figure 4.2. Classes of sex steroid as identified by number of carbon atoms.

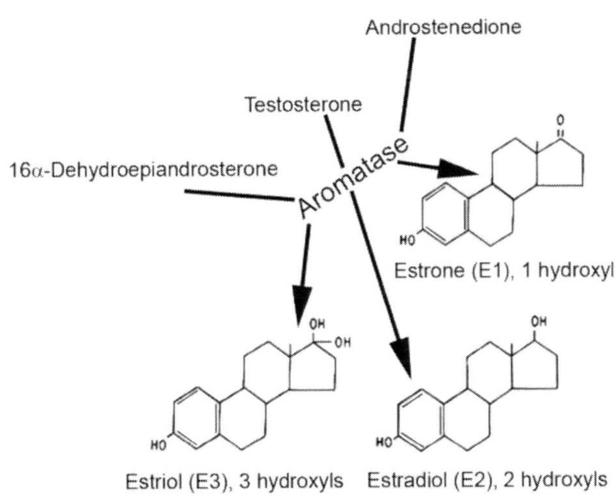

Figure 4.3. Aromatase can make estrone (E1), estradiol (E2) and estriol (E3).

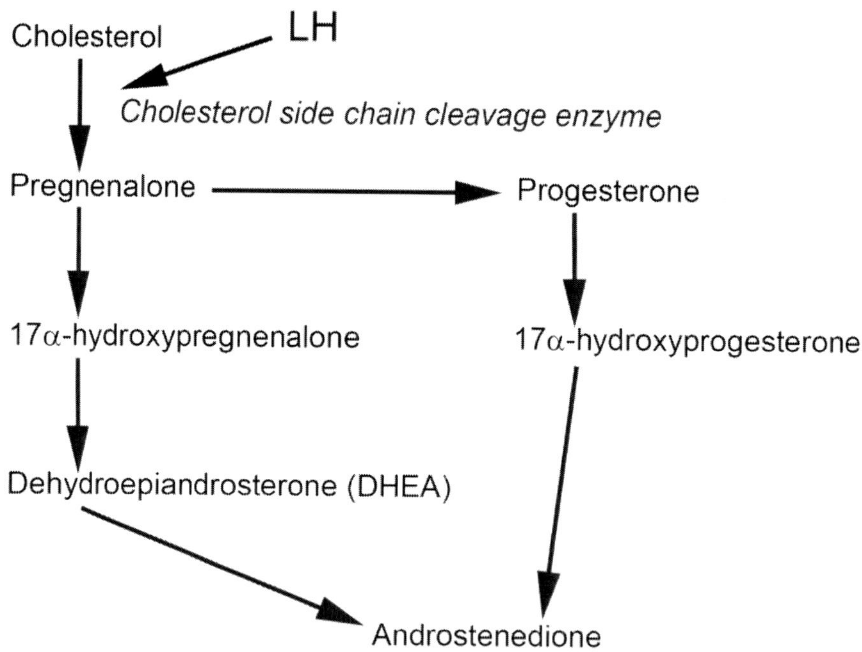

Figure 4.4. Sex steroid production in theca cells during the follicular phase of the menstrual cycle.

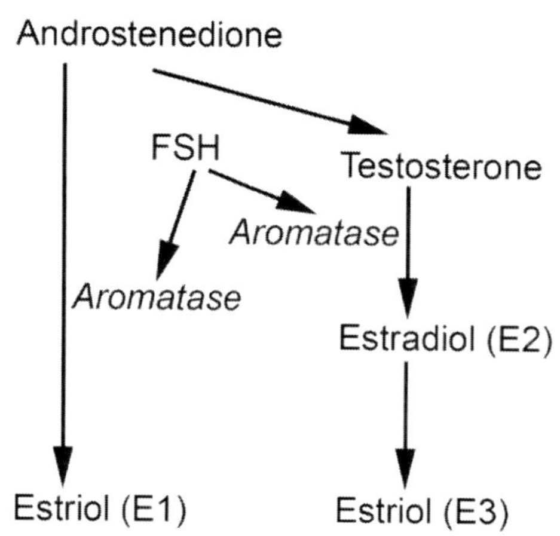

Figure 4.5. Sex steroid production in granulosa cells during the follicular phase of the menstrual cycle.

Theca cells are wrapped around granulosa cells in ovarian follicles. Granulosa cells take up the androgen androstenedione; first, they convert it to testosterone and then aromatize it to the principal estrogen, estradiol (E2) (Figure 4.5). Alternatively, androstenedione can be aromatized directly to estrone (E1). The limiting step in these pathways is aromatase which is promoted by FSH binding its receptor on granulosa cells. Other steps are not regulated. Estradiol and estrone are the principal estrogens made in the menstrual cycle [4-9].

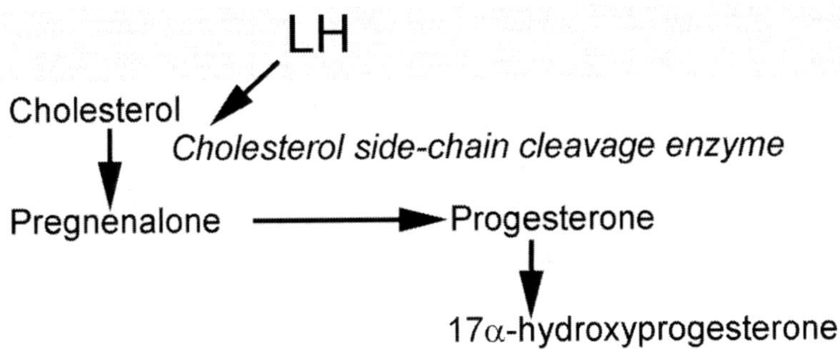

Figure 4.6. Sex steroid production by corpus luteal cells during the luteal phase of the menstrual cycle.

In the luteal phase of the menstrual cycle only progestogens are made. Corpus luteal cells lack the enzyme activities needed to make androgens like androstenedione and just make progesterone and 17α-hydroxyprogesterone (Figure 4.6). Once again, the limiting factor is cholesterol side chain cleavage enzyme which is promoted by LH (Figure 4.6).

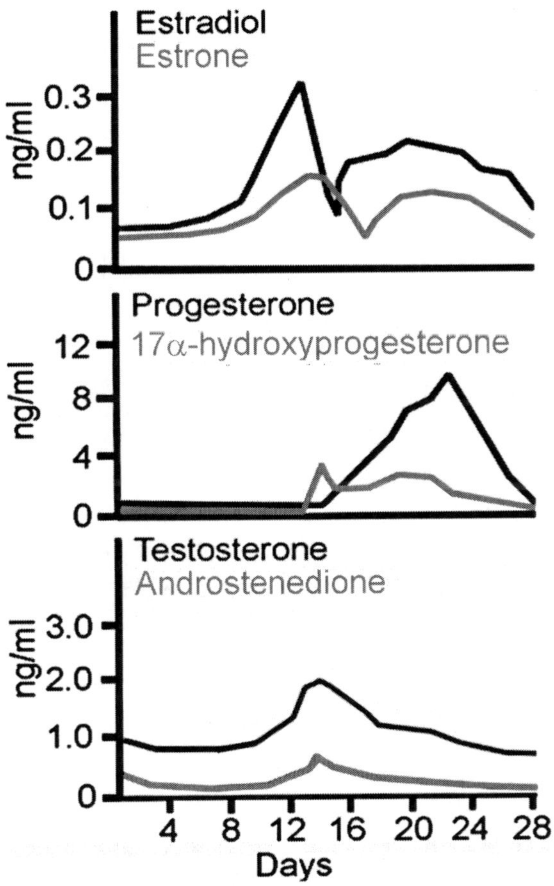

Figure 4.7. Mean sex steroid serum concentrations in women in the menstrual cycle.

With the assistance of LH and FSH the ovary makes primarily estrone (E1) and estradiol (E2) and progesterone and 17α-hydroxyprogesterone during the menstrual cycle. Other intermediates have biological functions [4-7]. A small amount of testosterone enters the blood and is used by the female reproductive biology; for instance, for muscular anabolism and for promoting female libido (see Chapter 13).

Figure 4.7 shows mean sex steroid concentrations during the menstrual cycle. As shown, estradiol (E2) is the principal estrogen detected in serum. Estradiol levels in the follicular phase rise to a peak at around day 11-12. Estrone (E1) concentrations peak at around the time of ovulation at day 14. Both estradiol (E2) and estrone (E1) levels remain elevated in the luteal phase, rising to a climax around day 20 – day 24 and then dropping down. On the progestogen side, progesterone predominates. Progesterone levels are virtually zero during the follicular phase. Starting with the LH peak levels rise continuously and peak around day 23. Levels then drop down after the peak. Levels of 17α- hydroxyprogesterone are very small, peaking with the LH peak and remaining elevated during the luteal phase [1,2,9,10,11]. In women's blood the androgen androstenedione is most evident. This is a weak androgen with 10% of the biological potency of testosterone. Androstenedione concentrations in serum are mostly elevated at around 1 ng/ml during the follicular phase and luteal phase, with a peak around the time of ovulation. A tiny concentration of testosterone is present in serum in women, about 0.2 ng/ml in the follicular and luteal phase and peaking around the time of ovulation.

Sex Steroids Synthesized in Pregnancy

In pregnancy, completely different pathways are activated for sex steroid synthesis (Figure 4.8). A little bit of each steroid synthesis pathway involves the mother, the placenta and different fetal organs (Figure 4.8). Progesterone production is maintained by the placenta from 7 weeks of pregnancy to term, or after corpus luteal progesterone production has finished. The mother provides the placenta with cholesterol, and the placenta makes progesterone using the same pathway as used during the menstrual cycle by the corpus luteum (Figure 4.8). The cholesterol side chain cleavage enzyme is strongly promoted by the high levels of placental hCG made by the placenta during this time [1,2,8,9].

In the synthesis of estrone (E1) and estradiol (E2), the fetal adrenal gland and the maternal adrenal gland produce a dehydroepiandrosterone-sulfate (DHEA-sulfate). This is the substrate. The placenta converts this molecule to androstenedione and then into testosterone. Then an aromatase converts androstenedione and testosterone to estrone (E1) and estradiol (E2) (Figure 4.8). High concentrations of estrogens are produced during pregnancy. The principal form of estrogen made in pregnancy is estriol (E3). Estriol (E3) is an estrogen with little use in the menstrual cycle [2,4,5,6,7]. The fetal adrenal makes dehydroepiandrosterone-sulfate (DHEA-sulfate). This becomes hydroxylated in the fetal liver as 16α-hydroxydehydroepiandrosterone-sulfate. The fetal liver then produces 16α-hydroxyandrostenedione. This passes into the placenta where it is aromatized to estriol (E3) (Figure 4.8).

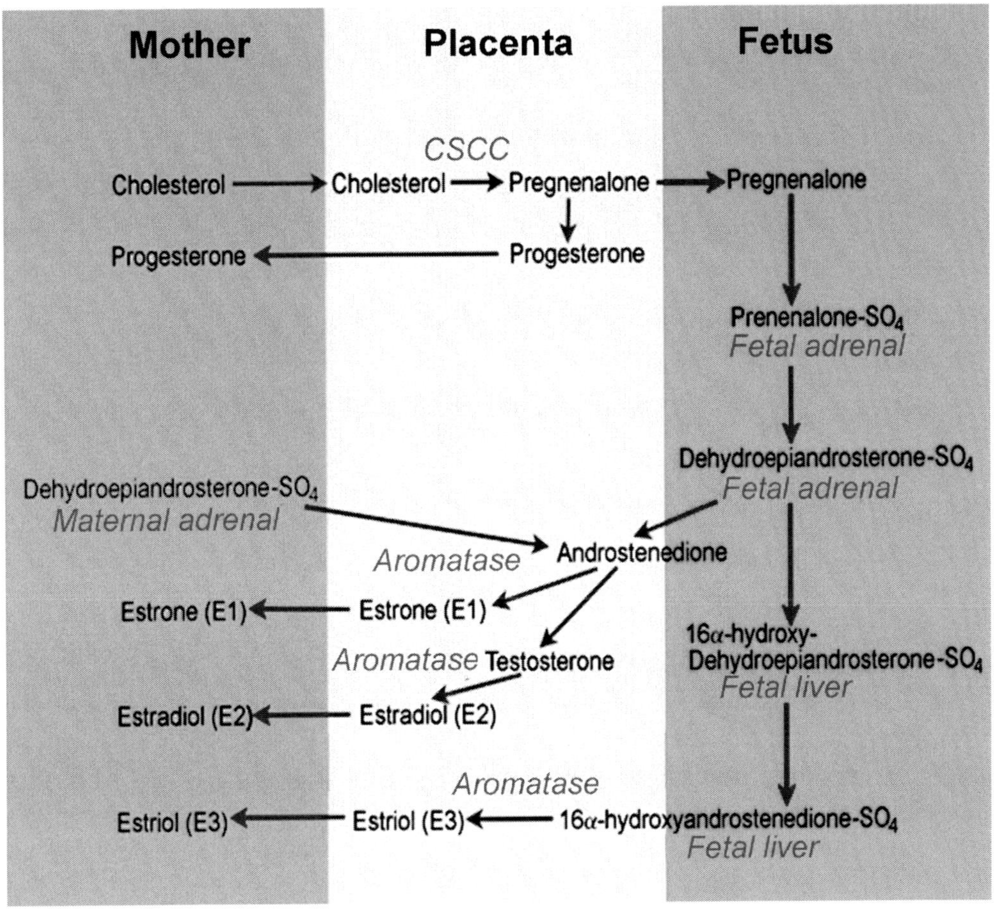

Figure 4.8. Sex steroid synthesis during pregnancy. Figure illustrates the many elements needed to make sex steroids in pregnancy. Cholesterol side chain cleavage enzyme is CSCC.

Levels of progesterone and estriol made in pregnancy rise continuously during the length of the pregnancy. Progesterone levels in serum are approximately 20 ng/ml at 4 weeks' gestation (weeks since last menstrual bleeding) and 180 ng/ml at 40 weeks of gestation. Estriol levels range from approximately 50 ng/ml at 28 weeks to 200 ng/ml at 40 weeks of pregnancy. Estriol assessment is used as a measure of fetal well-being since the production of estriol requires appropriate fetal adrenal and fetal liver function.

Functions of Sex Steroids

The sex steroids have multiple functions in women. Sex steroids are lipids, and so can pass through the lipid bilayer on plasma membranes of cells. All sex steroids act on bivalent receptors within cells (Figure 4.9). Upon binding to the receptor, the hormone-receptor complex is transported to the nucleus and promotes DNA transcription leading to protein production (Figure 4.9) [1,2,9,11].

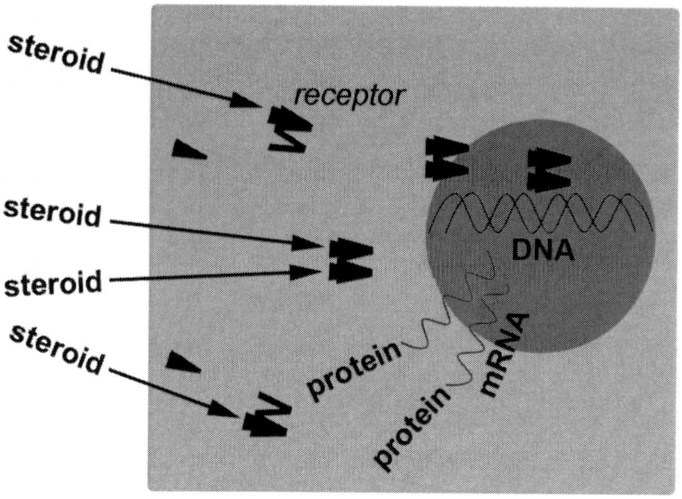

Figure 4.9. Sex steroid interaction with cytoplasmic bivalent receptor.

Sex Steroids in the Menstrual Cycle

Estrogens modulate secondary sexual characteristics. These include enlargement of breasts and erection of nipples as well as growth of body hair, most prominently underarm and pubic hair and a greater development of thigh muscles and widening of the hips. Distribution of weight and body fat deposits around buttocks, thighs and hips is dependent on estrogens. In the follicular phase of the menstrual cycle, estrogens start the growth of the glandular endometrial lining (Figure 4.10). This is a function taken over by progesterone in the luteal phase of the menstrual cycle. At the end of the menstrual cycle all gained lining is lost with the shedding of the endometrial lining of the uterus, or menses [2,4,5].

Estrogens feed back to the hypothalamus in different ways. Low levels of estrogens, like those observed in the follicular phase, feed back to the hypothalamus and inhibit GnRH production. This reduces GnRH stimulation of gonadotropins. In contrast, high levels of estradiol, as seen at the estradiol peak, strongly promote GnRH pulses and pulse amplitude, leading to the LH peak (Chapter 5 and Chapter 6).

Estrogens also have a function in the propulsion of the ovum through the fallopian tubes. Ampullary muscles of the fallopian tube are contracted in unison in response to estrogens, leading to ovum movement. Estradiol, the most potent natural estrogen, is mildly anabolic. It promotes calcium uptake by bones. It is in the absence of this calcium uptake, as occurs in menopause due to the absence of estrogens and estrogen-promoted uptake, that osteoporosis can occur (Chapter 29) (Figure 4.10].

Progestogens are primarily produced in the luteal phase of the menstrual cycle, where they promote the growth of the glandular endometrial lining of the uterus, supported by spiral arteries of the uterus (Figure 4.10). This prepares the uterus for a possible implanting pregnancy [1,2,9-11].

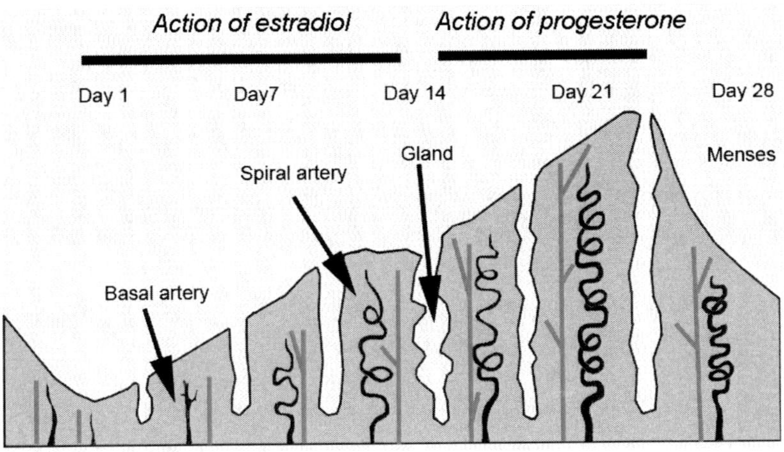

Figure 4.10. Endometrial lining of the uterus.

Androgens also have functions in women. Testosterone is an unconjugated steroid. It is able to cross the blood:brain barrier, where it affects libido, sexual aggressiveness and behavior (see Chapter 13). Androgens can also be anabolic in women, affecting calcium uptake by bone, hair growth and muscle growth.

Sex Steroids in Pregnancy

Estrogens promote growth during pregnancy, mammary growth and fetal nutrition. This is all discussed in Chapters 21 and 25.

References

[1] Ellmann S, Sticht H, Thiel F, Beckmann MW, Strick R, Strissel PL. Estrogen and progesterone receptors: from molecular structures to clinical targets. *Cell Mol Life Sci* 2009 66:2405-2426.

[2] Stormshak F, Bishop CV. Estrogen and progesterone signaling: Genomic and nongenomic actions in domestic ruminants. *J Anim Sci* 2007;86:299-315.

[3] Neumann F. The physiological action of progesterone and the pharmacological effects of progestrogens--a short review. *Postgrad Med J* 1978;54:11–24.

[4] Crews D, Cantú AR, Rhen T, Vohra R. The relative effectiveness of estrone, estradiol-17 beta, and estriol in sex reversal in the red-eared slider (Trachemys scripta), a turtle with temperature-dependent sex determination. *Gen Comp Endocrinol* 1996;102:317-326.

[5] Ryan KJ. Biochemistry of aromatase: significance to female reproductive physiology. *Cancer Res* 1982;42:3342–3344.

[6] Nelson LR, Bulun SE. Estrogen production and action. *J Am Acad Dermatol* 2001;45: S116–S124.

[7] Cui J, Shen Y, Li R. Estrogen synthesis and signaling pathways during aging: from periphery to brain. *Trends Mol Med* 2013;19:197-209.

[8] Siiteri PK, Macdonald PC. Placental Estrogen Biosynthesis During Human Pregnancy. *J Clin Endocrinol Metab* 1966;26:751-761.

[9] Imai Y, Youn MY, Kondoh S, Nakamura T, Kouzmenko A, Matsumoto T, Takada I, Takaoka K, Kato S. Estrogens maintain bone mass by regulating expression of genes controlling function and life span in mature osteoclasts. *Ann N Y Acad Sci* 2009;1173-1178.

[10] Rodd C, Jourdain N, Alini M. Action of estradiol on epiphyseal growth plate chondrocytes. *Calcif Tissue Int* 2004;75:214-224.

[11] Gargett CE, Zaitseva M, Bucak K, Chu S, Fuller PJ, Rogers PA. 17-beta-estradiol up-regulates vascular endothelial growth factor receptor-2 expression in human myometrial microvascular endothelial cells: role of estrogen receptor-alpha and -beta. *J Clin Endocrinol Metab* 2002;87:4341-4349.

Key Points

1. Cholesterol is the root steroid.
2. Two enzymes are key limiting points, cholesterol side chain cleavage enzyme is modulated by LH and hCG, and aromatase which is modulated by FSH.
3. The theca and granulosa cells work together to make estradiol, theca cells convert cholesterol to androstenedione, promoted by LH, and granulosa cells convert androstenedione to estradiol, promoted by FSH.
4. There are 2 molecules that are natural progestogens, progesterone and 17α-hydroxyprogesterone; there are 4 molecules that are natural androgens, testosterone, Dehydroepiandrosterone(DHEA), androstenedione, and dihydrotestosterone; there are 3 molecules that are natural estrogens, estrone (E1), estradiol (E2) and estriol (E3).
5. Corpus luteal cells make progesterone and 17α-hydroxyprogesterone under the stimulus of LH.
6. In pregnancy, progesterone is made by the placenta. Estriol is produced from a combined fetal-placental cooperation. The fetal adrenal makes dehydroepiandrosterone-sulfate (DHEA-sulfate); the fetal liver converts it to 16α-hydroxydehydroepiandrosterone-sulfate. This is then converted to 16α hydroxyandrostenedione-sulfate which is aromatase converted to estriol in the placenta.
7. The estrogen peak occurs at about day 11 of the menstrual cycle.
8. Measurement of estriol in pregnancy serum and urine is used as a test of fetal well-being.
9. Estradiol in the follicular phase promotes growth of the endometrial glandular lining.
10. Progesterone in the luteal phase primarily promotes growth of the endometrial lining.

Chapter 5

Follicular Growth and Selection, Ovulation and Luteinization

Approximately 15-20 follicles in a woman's ovaries compete each month to become the dominant follicle. This is the follicle which is ovulated. In humans usually only one follicle reaches ovulation stage each month. Here under *Follicle Selection* the promoters that drive this follicle competition are described. The ovulation process involves multiple steps; first, the *Estrogen Peak*, then the *LH Peak*, then *Meiosis* of the oocyte. Then a stigma or bulge is formed on the follicle, and the thinning of the follicle occurs in *Preparation of the Follicle for Ovulation*. After *Ovulation* the empty follicle is considered and *Luteinization*, or becoming a corpus luteum, is considered.

Follicular Selection

Here we follow the diagram in Figure 5.1. Initially there are multiple new primordial follicles developed by the action of FSH, and surviving atretic follicles from previous menstrual cycles. In the first stage of development FSH promotes the growth of primordial follicles and recovery of atretic follicles from previous menstrual cycles through a pathway involving insulin-like growth factor (IGF) 1 and 2 [1-3].

Follicles start competing to become the largest follicle or Dominant Follicle (Figure 5.1). Every follicle is promoted by FSH, depending upon how large it is or how many FSH receptors it has. Every follicle, regardless of its size, produces the same set amount of IGF binding protein (IGFBP). IGF1 and 2 are bound by this binding protein. Bound IGF is destroyed by a proteolytic enzyme, deactivating the IGF molecule. Thus, a large follicle producing IGF over and above that set amount bound by IGFBP fairs the best and is promoted to grow the most (Figure 5.1)[1-3].

For example, a small follicle may have just a few FSH receptors and so produces little IGF 1 and IGF2 in response to FSH. This follicle may have all its IGF 1 and IGF2 bound by the follicle's set supply of IGFBP. The bound IGF is destroyed by proteases. The end result

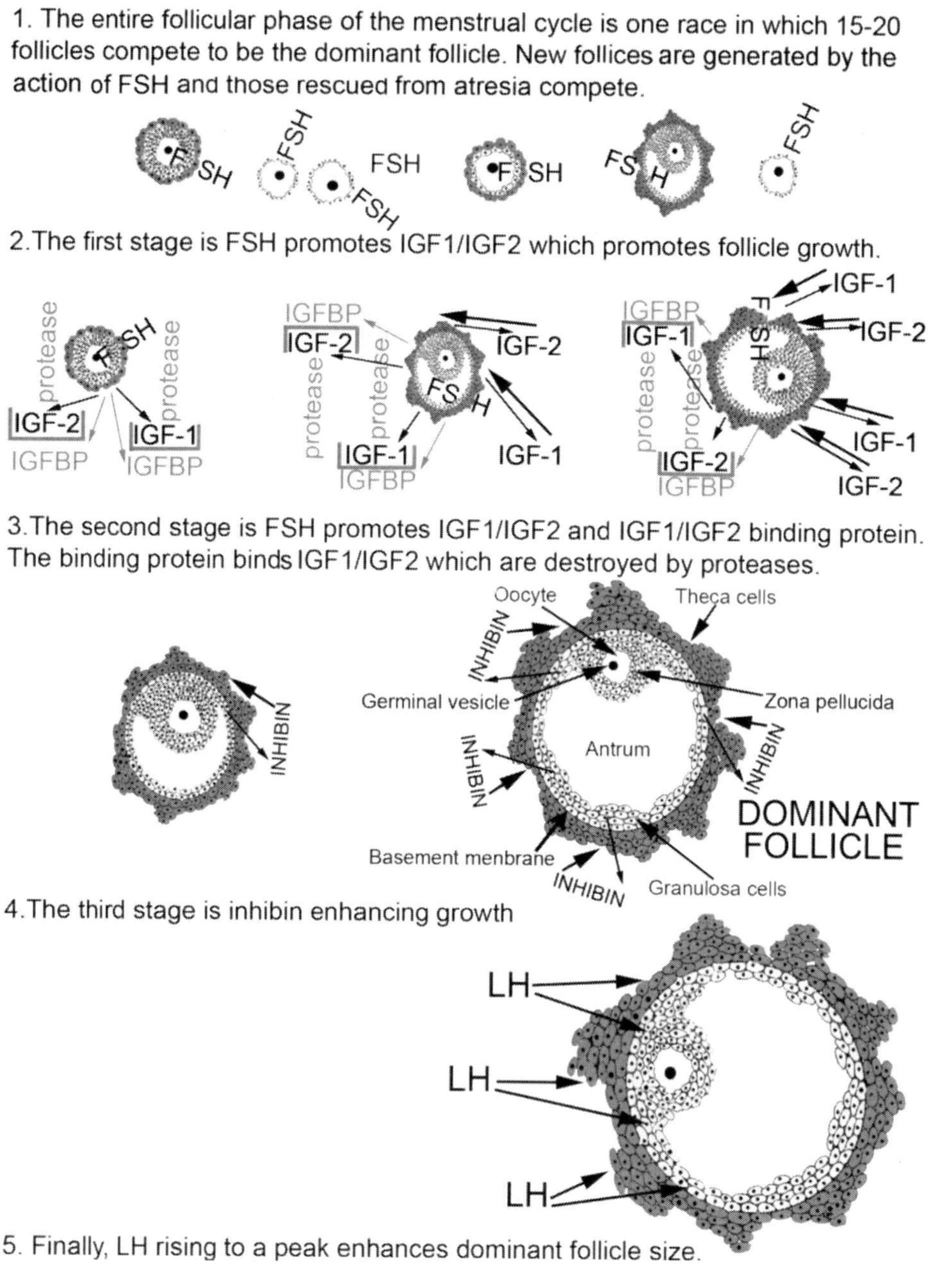

Figure 5.1. Competitive follicle growth during the follicular phase of the menstrual cycle.

is that this small follicle has no remaining active IGF1 and IGF2 to actively stimulate follicle growth. A large follicle, in contrast, may have numerous FSH receptors, and FSH promotes large amounts of IGF1 and IGF2. Only a small proportion of the IGF1 and IGF2 are bound by the set follicle supply of IGFBP, and are destroyed by proteolytic enzyme. The end result is that the large follicle has much non-destroyed IGF, so that its growth can be very much stimulated by IGF-1 and IGF-2 [1-3]. In this stage of competitive follicular growth some follicle will get very much promoted in size (Figure 5.1).

Looking at the example in Figure 5.1, the small follicle (shown on the left side of section 2) is produced the same amount of IGF1 and IGF2 and IGFBP. All the IGF is bound by IFBP and destroyed by proteases. There is no effective IGF to stimulate the growth of this follicle. The medium-sized follicle (in the middle of section 2) produces twice as much IGF1 and IGF2 as IGFBP. Half of the IGF is destroyed after binding and protease action; however, the remaining half of IGF1 and IGF2 promotes follicular growth. The large follicle (on the right side) produces three-fold more IGF1 and IGF2 than IGFBP. Just a third is bound and destroyed; the remaining two-thirds act to promote the extensive growth of this follicle (Figure 5.1).

After this stage, most competing follicles are now antral follicles. This means that they have a liquid filled antrum or interior. In the next stage of follicle growth (shown in section 3 of Figure 5.1), each follicle produces inhibins. The amount of inhibins produced by a follicle is dependent on the follicle size. Inhibins produced by the granulosa cells promote follicle growth. The larger follicles produces more inhibin, and so promote growth to a greater extent than the smaller follicles. This leads to affirmation of a Dominant Follicle between the two ovaries (Figure 5.1)[1-3].

Around day 12-14 of the menstrual cycle, LH levels start to head up towards the midcycle LH peak. The rising LH levels bind the LH/placental hCG receptors on theca and granulosa cells of the dominant follicle and promote a growth surge (Figure 5.1). This is the final step in growth promotion; it makes the Dominant Follicle much larger and ready for ovulation.

Estrogen Peak

A series of events initiates ovulation during the menstrual cycle. Firstly, around day 11-13 of the menstrual cycle estradiol levels rise to a peak. This initiates the hypothalamus to produce rapid potent pulses of GnRH. Around the same time, granulosa cells produce higher levels of inhibin. The inhibins block pituitary production of FSH so FSH cannot promote the estrogen peak. Inhibin ends up directly promoting the estrogen peak itself (Figure 5.2). The end result, with rapid GnRH pulses and higher levels of inhibin, is a tall LH peak following the estrogen peak [4-6]. The LH peak promotes the rupture of the follicle or ovulation. The empty follicle undergoes luteinization.

Around day 11 of the menstrual cycle, the most advanced follicles or the dominant follicles produce estradiol for the estradiol peak. Estradiol is normally made from LH promotion of cholesterol side chain cleavage enzyme (CSCC enzyme) in theca cells and FSH promotion of aromatase in granulosa cells, the two key enzymes in estradiol synthesis. LH and FSH can promote limited concentrations of estradiol. Estradiol promotion through cholesterol side chain cleavage enzyme and aromatase is controlled at this time by inhibins in the granulosa and theca cells of the follicle (Figure 5.2). Estradiol reaches a peak around day 12 of the menstrual cycle [4-6].

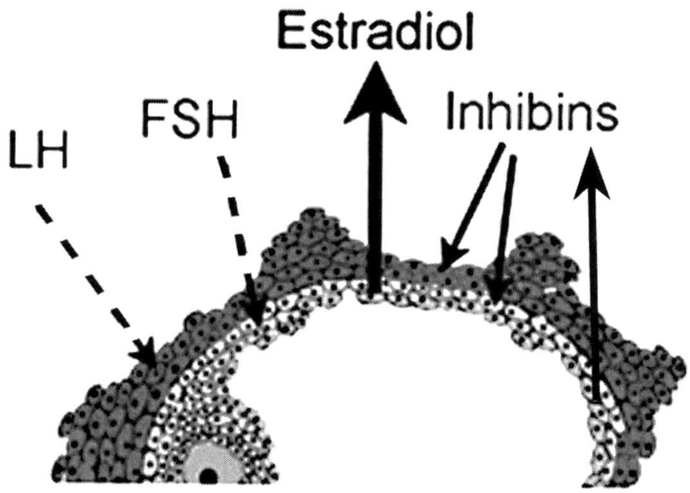

Figure 5.2. Generation of estradiol for estradiol peak.

LH Peak

The estradiol peak promotes hypothalamic production of GnRH, increasing both the pulse frequency and pulse amplitude. The GnRH pulses are received by the pituitary gonadotrope cells. Normally, the pituitary gonadotrope cells would start producing high concentrations of FSH and LH in response to the more frequent and higher amplitude pulses. At this time, however, after about 13-14 days of an average menstrual cycle, the granulosa cells of the dominant follicle are producing higher concentrations of inhibin. This is inhibiting gonadotrope production of FSH. As such, the gonadotrope cells produce primarily LH with a relatively minor FSH peak.

Meiosis

The rising LH at approximately 12 days of the menstrual cycle stimulates dominant follicle growth. LH then promotes meiosis in the oocyte of the follicle. Initially, the oocyte is diploid, with one half set of 23 chromosomes from the woman's mother and one half set of 23 chromosomes from the woman's father. LH then promotes meiosis [7,8]. In meiosis the chromosomes from the mother and father are first duplicated (prophase 1-leptotene, Figure 5.3) and then randomly shuffled up, known as chiasmata (prophase 1-diakineses, Figure 5.3), and finally pulled apart to generate 2 cells (late telophase 1, Figure 5.3) [7,8]. This generates 2 cells in which meiosis is not completed. Meiosis does not go any further in the follicle. It is completed upon penetration of the ovum by sperm (as described in Chapter 17). Figure 5.3 shows this first stage of first meiotic division. Overall, both stages of meiosis allow the resulting ovum to provide a haploid set to be combined with the haploid set provided by a sperm [7,8], making a new diploid set for the new being.

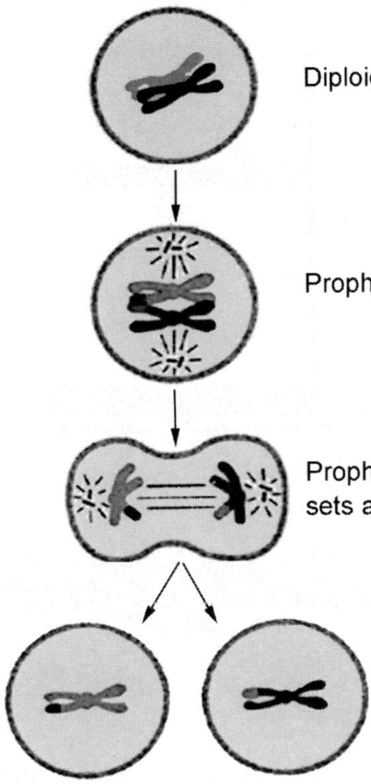

Figure 5.3. First stage of meiosis in oocyte.

Excess chromosome material generated in the first stage of meiosis (generates 2 cells in late telophase, only 1 cell needed) beyond that needed to make the haploid set is thrown out of thc oocyte and discarded in a small cavity called the first polar body in the dominant follicle.

Preparation of the Follicle for Ovulation

As the follicle expands under the influence of LH the follicular fluid increases the size of the antrum. With this the follicular walls (granulosa cells and theca cells) become thinner or more stretched by the antrum. With growth, a bulge appears in the follicle; this is called the stigma (Figure 5.4). The top wall of the stigma region becomes particularly thin in granulosa and theca cells, preparing the follicle for popping or ovulation.

Ovulation

In the last day prior to ovulation, the theca cells under the LH influence produce 3 proteases (proteolytic enzymes), collagenase which breaks down collagen, plasminogen activator, which cleaves and activates procollagenase, the collagenase precursor, and gelatinase, a pepsin-like degradative enzyme (Figure 5.5) [9-11]. These proteases digest their way through the thin theca and granulosa cell wall of the stigma. Once they pierce the wall the follicle literally pops or throws itself open. As the follicular fluid squirts out of the follicle the oocyte is dislodged (Figure 5.5) [9-11]. The oocyte is dislodged towards the fimbria of the fallopian tube. The ovum then starts its journey down the fallopian tube.

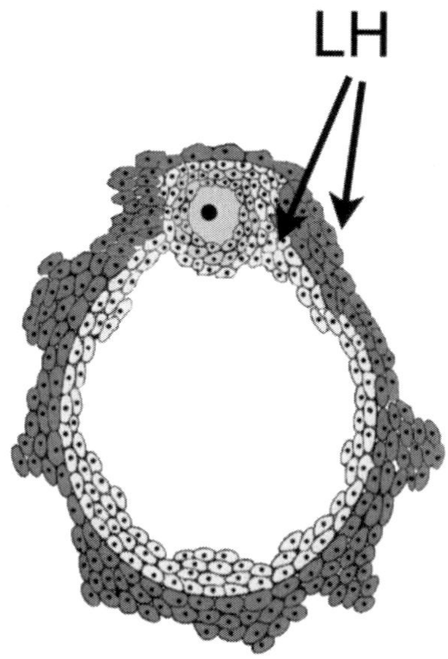

Figure 5.4. Appearance of stigma and thinning on follicle.

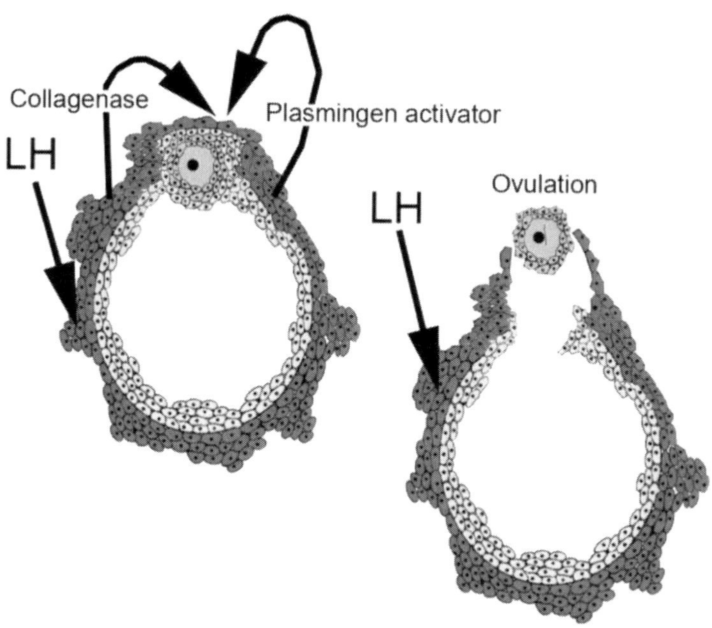

Figure 5.5. Ovulation of follicle.

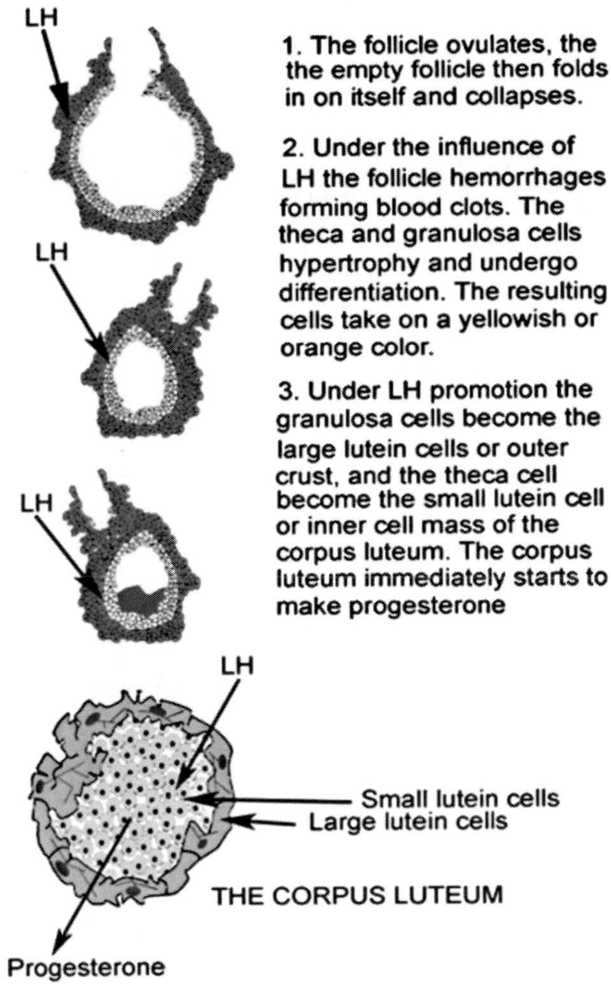

Figure 5.6. Luteinization of the follicle after ovulation.

Luteinization

After ovulation the follicle is empty. A vacuum is created by the expulsion of the follicular fluids. The empty follicle then collapses into the vacuum space left by the fluids (Figure 5.6). Promoted by LH, the membrane propria breaks down and blood vessels invade. The follicle hemorrhages and clots form within the follicle (Figure 5.6) [12,13]. Promoted by LH, luteinization is completed. The granulosa and theca cell hypertrophy and differentiate. The corpus luteum is formed. The corpus luteum takes on a yellow or orangy color. The granulosa cells form the large lutein cells or the outer crust of the corpus luteum (Figure 5.6). The theca cells form the small lutein cells or inner mass of cells within the corpus luteum (Figure 5.6) [12,13]. The corpus luteum immediately starts producing progesterone.

References

[1] Fortune JE. Ovarian follicular growth and development in mammals. *Biol Reprod* 1994; 50:225-232.

[2] Monniaux D, Huet C, Besnard N, Clément F, Bosc M, Pisselet C, Monget P, Mariana JC. Follicular growth and ovarian dynamics in mammals. *J Reprod Fertil* 1997;51:3-23.

[3] Giudice LC. Insulin-like growth factor family in Graafian follicle development and function. *J Soc Gynecol Investig* 2001;8:S26-S29.

[4] Hughes EG, Robertson DM, Handelsman DJ, Hayward S, Healy DL, de Kretser DM. Inhibin and estradiol responses to ovarian hyperstimulation: effects of age and predictive value for in vitro fertilization outcome. *J Clin Endocrinol Metab.* 1990;70:358-364.

[5] Fraser HM, Groome NP, McNeilly AS. Follicle-stimulating hormone-inhibin B interactions during the follicular phase of the primate menstrual cycle revealed by gonadotropin-releasing hormone antagonist and antiestrogen treatment. *J Clin Endocrinol Metab* 1999;84:1365-1369.

[6] Arai K, Watanabe G, Taya K, Sasamoto S. Roles of Inhibin and Estradiol in the Regulation of Follicle-Stimulating Hormone and Luteinizing Hormone Secretion during the Estrous Cycle of the Rat. *Biol Reprod* 1996;55:127-133.

[7] Mehlmann LM, Kalinowski RR, Ross LF, Parlow Af, Hewlett EL, Jaffe LA. Meiotic resumption in response to luteinizing hormone is independent of a $G_i$family G protein or calcium in the mouse oocyte. *Dev Biol* 2006;299:345–355.

[8] Activation of Meiotic Maturation in Rat Oocytes After Treatment with Follicular Fluid Meiosis-Activating Sterol In Vitro and Ex Vivo, Christa Hegele-Hartung C, Grützner M, Lessl M, Grøndahl C, Ottesen JL, Brännström M. Evidence for follicle wall involvement in ovulation and progesterone production by frog (Rana pipiens) follicles in vitro. *Biol Reprod* 2001;418-424.

[9] Schuetz AW, Lessman C._Evidence for follicle wall involvement in ovulation and progesterone production by frog (Rana pipiens) follicles in vitro. *Differentiation.* 1982;22:79-84.

[10] Liu YX, Liu XM, Nin LF, Shi L, Chen SR. Serine protease and ovarian paracrine factors in regulation of ovulation. *Front Biosci* 2013;18:650-664.

[11] Espey LL. Ovarian Proteolytic Enzymes and Ovulation. *Biol Reproduction* 1974;10: 216-235.

[12] Tapanainen JS, Lapolt PS, Perlas E, Hsueh AJ. Induction of ovarian follicle luteinization by recombinant follicle-stimulating hormone. *Endocrinol* 1993;133:2875-2880.

[13] Murphy BD. Models of luteinization. *Biol Reprod.* 2000;63:2-11.

Key Points

1. Approximately 15-20 follicles compete each menstrual cycle to become the dominant follicle. The competing follicles are a mixture of new primordial follicles made under the influences of FSH and recovered atretic follicles from previous menstrual cycles.
2. In phase 1, FSH promotes follicle growth through promotion of IGF-1 and IGF-2. In the principal part of follicle competition to become the dominant follicle a set amount of IGF binding protein (IGFBP) is made by every follicle regardless of size. This binds the IGF. Once bound it is destroyed by protease. A small follicle may produce its set IGFBP and it may bind all IGF, leaving none to promote growth. A large follicle may produce much IGF, and a set amount of IGFBP is produced. This leads to the destruction of just one-quarter of the IGF. The rest stimulates growth of the follicle.
3. Inhibin (the amount produced being related to the size of the follicle) leads to follicular growth. A dominant follicle is then recognized.
4. LH, while rising to a peak, promotes follicular grow. LH, while rising to a peak, promotes meiosis in the oocyte. LH, while rising to a peak, promotes the formation of a bulge in the follicle called the stigma and thinning of the follicle cells. The proteases collagenase, plasminogen activator and gelatinase digest the follicle on the stigma, causing ovulation.
5. The follicular fluid is squirted out of the follicle along with the oocyte. The first stage of ovulation is an estradiol peak. The estradiol peak causes the hypothalamus to produce increased pulses of GnRH at increased altitude. This causes the gonadotrope cell to produce LH needed for an LH peak. FSH production by the pituitary cells is suppressed by inhibins.
6. After ovulation, the follicle folds in on itself. The membrana propia between the theca and granulosa cells breaks down and hemorrhaging occurs. The granulosa and theca cells hypertrophy and differentiate to become the large lutein cells (outer cells of corpus luteum) and small lutein cells (inner cells) of the corpus luteum. The corpus luteum immediately produces progesterone.

Chapter 6

Putting Everything Together: The Menstrual Cycle

The first 5 chapters of this book provide an introduction to the menstrual cycle. They look at the glycopeptins (Chapters 1 and 2), gonadotropin releasing hormone (GnRH) and the menstrual cycle (Chapter 3), sex steroids and steroidogenesis and the menstrual cycle (Chapter 4), growth of the follicle during the menstrual cycle (Chapter 5), and the steps of ovulation and the menstrual cycle (Chapter 5). This chapter is somewhat repetitive of Chapters 1-5; it ties together all this learned information into one intricate model, the menstrual cycle.

Three full-page figures are shown to model the menstrual cycle. Figure 6.1 shows changing blood levels of GnRH, inhibins, LH and FSH and the sex steroids during the course of the menstrual cycle. Figure 6.2 is a diagram illustrating endometrial lining of the uterus during the different stages of the menstrual cycle, and Figure 6.3 is a diagram illustrating the anatomy of the uterus during the menstrual cycle. These three figures guide the description of the menstrual cycle.

Order of the Menstrual Cycle

The start of the menstrual cycle occurs with the start of menstrual bleeding. *During the first week or first 7 days of the menstrual cycle* minimal GnRH pulses (both pulse frequency and amplitude are equally important) are produced in the hypothalamus. These promote minimal luteinizing hormone (LH) and follicle stimulating hormone (FSH) production by gonadotrope cells of the pituitary (Figure 6.1) [1-24]. This combination of signaling leads to low level estradiol and estrone production (Figure 6.1). FSH also starts the promotion of primordial follicle synthesis and growth (Figure 6.1) and the FSH-promoted recovery of certain atretic follicles from the preceding menstrual cycle. Normally about 15-20 follicles start each menstrual cycle together between the two ovaries. The formed estradiol starts the growth of the endometrial lining of the uterus (Figure 6.2) [1-24].

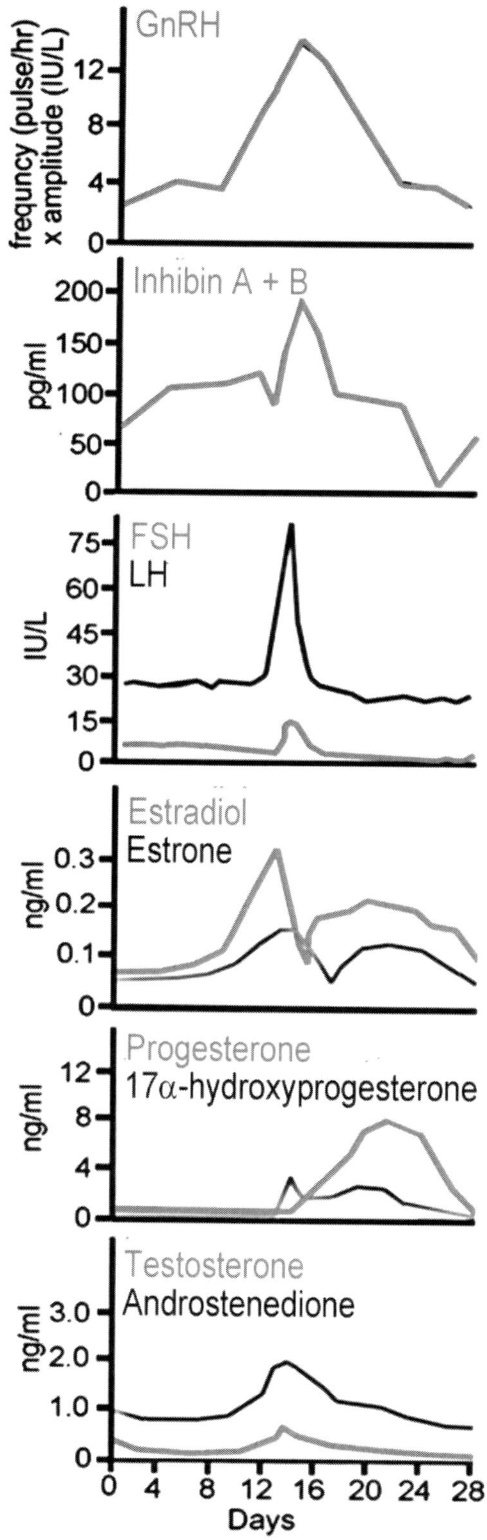

Figure 6.1. Concentration of sex hormones during the menstrual cycle.

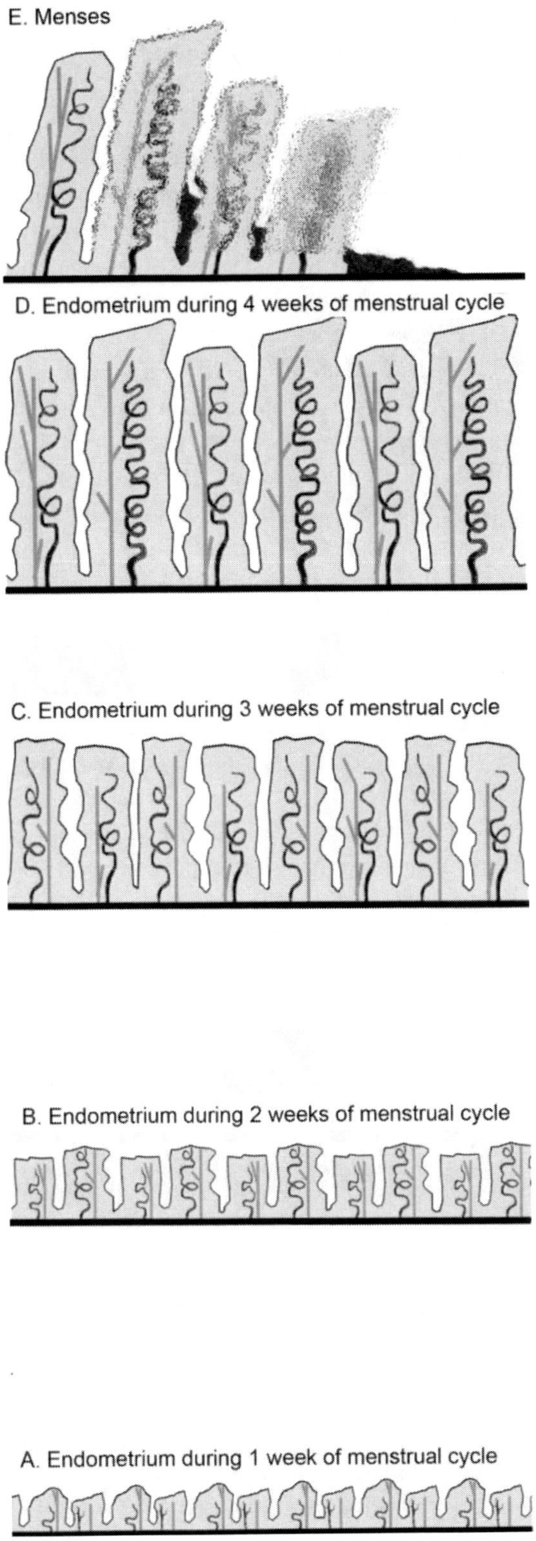

Figure 6.2. Endometrial lining during the menstrual cycle.

In the second week of the menstrual cycle GnRH pulses (pulses + amplitude) start to increase. Under the promotion of the FSH produced by the pituitary, the growth competition starts between follicles, competing to generate the largest follicle or the one dominant follicle generated in humans between the two ovaries each month. FSH promotes follicle growth though promotion of insulin-like growth factor (IGF) 1 and 2 [1-24]. The follicles produce a set amount, regardless of follicle size and regarless of IGF binding protein (IGFBP) production. IGF is bound by the IGFBP and then destroyed and deactivated by protease. The end result is that a small follicle with minimal FSH receptors may produce a small amount of IGF1 and 2 under FSH stimulation, and the small set amount of IGFBP. All IGF may be bound by IGFBP, and deactivated. As a result, there is no IGF1 or IGF2 remaining to promote growth in this small follicle. In contrast, a very big follicle may have numerous FSH receptor sites and may promote large amounts of IGF1 and 2 under FSH stimulation. The set amount of IGFBP may bind a small portion of the total IGF, leading to its deactivation. Most IGF remains functional and strongly promotes growth of the follicle. These are the two extremes. This way the follicles selectively grow to differing extents (Figure 6.3) [1-24].

As the second week passes, levels of inhibins grow and FSH levels are suppressed. Inhibins promote further growth in the developing follicles. Inhibins are produced by the granulosa cells of the follicles; the larger the follicle, the greater the production of inhibins and the greater the growth promotion. Usually at this time a single Dominant Follicle becomes apparent [1-24].

Around day 11 of the menstrual cycle, the most advanced of the follicles or the Dominant Follicle produces estradiol for the estradiol peak. Estradiol is normally made from LH promotion of cholesterol side chain cleavage enzyme (CSCC enzyme) in theca cells and FSH promotion of aromatase in granulosa cells, the two key enzymes in estradiol synthesis. LH and FSH can promote at this time only limited concentrations of estradiol. Estradiol promotion through CSCC enzyme and aromatase is enhanced by inhibins in the granulosa and theca cells of the most advanced follicles or the dominant follicle. Estradiol levels reach a peak around day 12 of the menstrual cycle (Figure 6.1). Around day 12-13 GnRH is slowly elevating (Figure 6.1). The estradiol promotes GnRH further, leading to a GnRH peak. The GnRH peak promotes pituitary LH and FSH with the strongest signal leading to the Day 13 LH peak. Inhibin levels produced in granulosa cells reach a peak also (Figure 6.1), and suppress any FSH peak. The end result is just a major LH peak (Figure 6.1) [1-24].

The LH peak promotes ovulation of the dominant follicle. Rising LH promotes follicle growth, then promotes meiosis in the oocyte of the dominant follicle. Rising LH also causes the follicle to form a bulge or stigma comprising thin layers of granulosa and theca cells. The LH peak promotes protease production, with promotes degrading a hole in the stigma leading to the follicle busting open, releasing follicular fluid and the oocyte (Figure 6.3).

The estradiol also in the second week of the menstrual period promotes growth of the endometrial lining (Figure 6.2) [1-24].

In the beginning of the third week of the menstrual cycle the empty follicle after ovulation collapses and hemorrhages. The granulosa and theca cells hypertrophy and differentiate to make the corpus luteal cells (Figure 6.3). The corpus luteum generates progestogens, under the stimulation of LH. Levels of progesterone and 17α-hydroxyprogesterone rise and strongly promote growth of the endometrial lining, its spiral artery support and formation of glands in the endometrial lining (Figure 6.2). While GnRH promotes the pituitary during the third week of pregnancy, higher levels of inhibins suppress FSH, so that primarily LH is produced to promote progesterone. Any remaining follicles, other than the dominant follicle which ovulated and formed the corpus luteum, undergo atresia or partial destruction (Figure 6.3). Follicles then remain in atresia through the remainder of the menstrual cycle. Atretic follicles may be rescued from atresia by FSH-promoted growth in the next menstrual cycle [1-24].

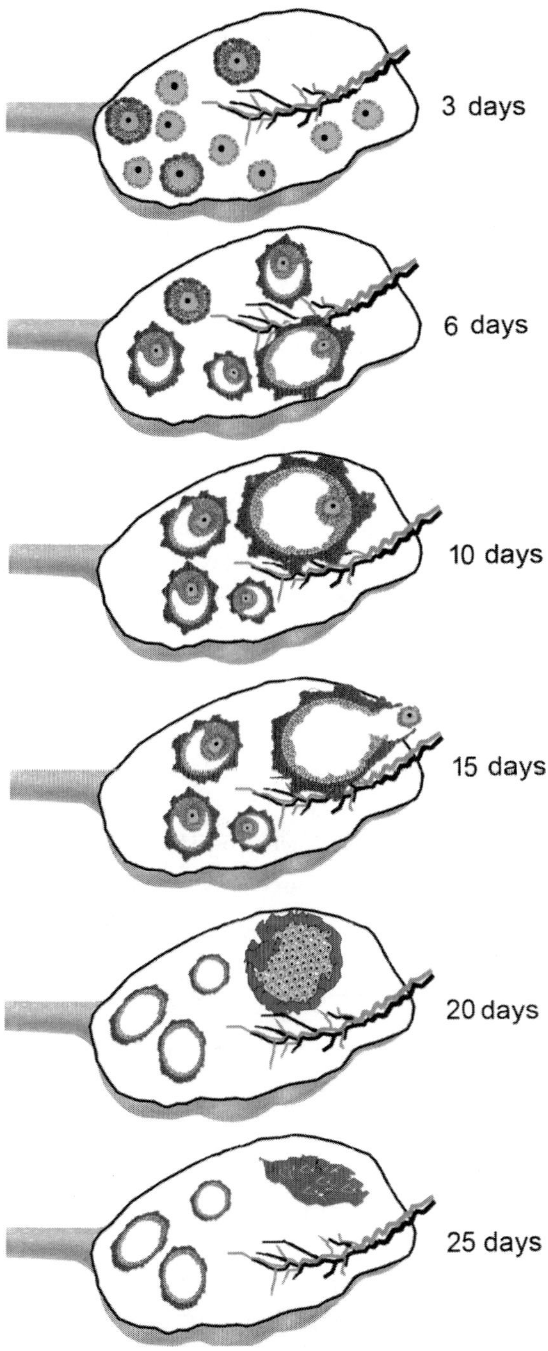

Figure 6.3. The anatomy of the ovary during the menstrual cycle.

In the fourth week of the menstrual cycle, progesterone production peaks around day 24 of the menstrual cycle (Figure 6.1). After day 24, two things occur; GnRH pulses reach a minimum, and the corpus luteum breaks up and atrophies to become a corpus albicans. With the failure of the corpus luteum, progesterone production dies. Slowly, the progesterone support of the growing endometrial lining and its spiral arteries fails. On the last day of the menstrual cycle, with diminution of spiral artery support, the lining fails and is shed, or menses occurs (Figure 6.2) bringing the endometrial lining back to its day 0 start. This is the menstrual cycle [1-24].

Regularity of the Menstrual Cycle

In our charts and tables we describe the menstrual cycle according to old standards, with the LH peak occurring on day 13, ovulation occurring on day 14 and the menstrual cycle length being 28 days. Is this real? Do women really have consistent 28-day menstrual cycles? The answer is "occasionally, but not normally." We quote Laurence Cole's 2009 paper on the normal variabilities of the menstrual cycle, listed under further reading. Four hundred and fifty-eight menstrual cycles were investigated in 210 women. The investigation involved daily urine samples and daily measurement of LH and hCG in urine samples, and determination (in note books) by volunteers of the first day of menstrual bleeding. The average timing of the LH peak was on day 14.7 ± 2.4 (standard deviation) days. The range of LH peaks was on day 9 to day 20. The average length of menstrual periods was 27.7 ± 2.4 days. The range of menstrual cycles was 20 days to 34 days. The timing of implantation in menstrual cycle leading to pregnancy was also investigated. Implantation occurred at 24.6 ± 3.1 days, with a range of 16 to 30 days [1-24].

Most women had variable length menstrual periods; for instance, 29 days, then 27 days, then 30 days, then 26 days, then 28 days. Yes, these numbers may average 28 days, but there is clear individual variation, with some women hitting the extremes of 20 and 24 days on occasions. In conclusion, our use of 13 days for LH peak, 14 days for ovulation and 28 days for menstrual cycle length are simply approximations as a guide.

References

[1] Ellmann S, Sticht H, Thiel F, Beckmann MW, Strick R, Strissel PL. Estrogen and progesterone receptors: from molecular structures to clinical targets. *Cell Mol Life Sci* 2009 66:2405-2426.

[2] Stormshak F, Bishop CV. Estrogen and progesterone signaling: Genomic and nongenomic actions in domestic ruminants. *J Anim Sci* 2007;86:299-315.

[3] Neumann F. The physiological action of progesterone and the pharmacological effects of progestrogens - a short review. *Postgrad Med* J 1978;54:11–24.

[4] Crews D, Cantú AR, Rhen T, Vohra R. The relative effectiveness of estrone, estradiol-17 beta, and estriol in sex reversal in the red-eared slider (Trachemys scripta), a turtle with temperature-dependent sex determination. *Gen Comp Endocrinol* 1996;102:317-326.

[5] Ryan KJ. Biochemistry of aromatase: significance to female reproductive physiology. *Cancer Res* 1982;42:3342–3344.

[6] Nelson LR, Bulun SE. Estrogen production and action. J Am Acad Dermatol 2001;45: S116–S124.

[7] Cui J, Shen Y, Li R. Estrogen synthesis and signaling pathways during aging: from periphery to brain. *Trends Mol Med* 2013;19:197-209.

[8] Siiteri PK, Macdonald PC. Placental Estrogen Biosynthesis During Human Pregnancy. *J Clin Endocrinol Metab* 1966;26:751-761.

[9] Imai Y, Youn MY, Kondoh S, Nakamura T, Kouzmenko A, Matsumoto T, Takada I, Takaoka K, Kato S. Estrogens maintain bone mass by regulating expression of genes controlling function and life span in mature osteoclasts. *Ann N Y Acad Sci* 2009;1173-1178.

[10] Rodd C, Jourdain N, Alini M. Action of estradiol on epiphyseal growth plate chondrocytes. *Calcif Tissue Int* 2004;75:214-224.

[11] Gargett CE, Zaitseva M, Bucak K, Chu S, Fuller PJ, Rogers PA. 17-beta-estradiol up-regulates vascular endothelial growth factor receptor-2 expression in human myometrial microvascular endothelial cells: role of estrogen receptor-alpha and -beta. *J Clin Endocrinol Metab* 2002;87:4341-4349.

[12] Fortune JE. Ovarian follicular growth and development in mammals. *Biol Reprod* 1994; 50:225-232.

[13] Monniaux D, Huet C, Besnard N, Clément F, Bosc M, Pisselet C, Monget P, Mariana JC. Follicular growth and ovarian dynamics in mammals. *J Reprod Fertil* 1997;51:3-23.

[14] Giudice LC. Insulin-like growth factor family in Graafian follicle development and function. *J Soc Gynecol Investig* 2001;8:S26-S29.

[15] Hughes EG, Robertson DM, Handelsman DJ, Hayward S, Healy DL, de Kretser DM. Inhibin and estradiol responses to ovarian hyperstimulation: effects of age and predictive value for in vitro fertilization outcome. *J Clin Endocrinol Metab.* 1990;70:358-364.

[16] Fraser HM, Groome NP, McNeilly AS. Follicle-stimulating hormone-inhibin B interactions during the follicular phase of the primate menstrual cycle revealed by gonadotropin-releasing hormone antagonist and antiestrogen treatment. J *Clin Endocrinol Metab* 1999;84:1365-1369.

[17] Arai K, Watanabe G, Taya K, Sasamoto S. Roles of Inhibin and Estradiol in the Regulation of Follicle-Stimulating Hormone and Luteinizing Hormone Secretion during the Estrous Cycle of the Rat. *Biol Reprod* 1996;55:127-133.

[18] Mehlmann LM, Kalinowski RR, Ross LF, Parlow Af, Hewlett EL, Jaffe LA. Meiotic resumption in response to luteinizing hormone is independent of a $G_i$family G protein or calcium in the mouse oocyte. *Dev Biol* 2006;299:345–355.

[19] Activation of Meiotic Maturation in Rat Oocytes After Treatment with Follicular Fluid Meiosis-Activating Sterol In Vitro and Ex Vivo, Christa Hegele-Hartung C, Grützner M, Lessl M, Grøndahl C, Ottesen JL, Brännström M. Evidence for follicle wall involvement in ovulation and progesterone production by frog (Rana pipiens) follicles in vitro. *Biol Reprod* 2001;418-424.

[20] Schuetz AW, Lessman C. Evidence for follicle wall involvement in ovulation and progesterone production by frog (Rana pipiens) follicles in vitro. *Differentiation.* 1982;22:79-84.

[21] Liu YX, Liu XM, Nin LF, Shi L, Chen SR. Serine protease and ovarian paracrine factors in regulation of ovulation. *Front Biosci* 2013;18:650-664.

[22] Espey LL. Ovarian Proteolytic Enzymes and Ovulation. *Biol Reproduction* 1974;10: 216-235.

[23] Tapanainen JS, Lapolt PS, Perlas E, Hsueh AJ. Induction of ovarian follicle luteinization by recombinant follicle-stimulating hormone. *Endocrinol* 1993;133:2875-2880.

[24] Murphy BD. Models of luteinization. *Biol Reprod.* 2000;63:2-11.

Key Points

1. It is important to understand all aspects of the "Order of the Menstrual Cycle."
2. LH and FSH jointly generate estradiol in the follicular phase of the menstrual cycle. As FSH is suppressed by inhibins, inhibins generate the day 11-13 peak estradiol using the dominant follicle theca and granulosa cells.
3. Growth of the follicle and the race to become the dominant follicle while initially supported by FSH, is promoted by IGF1 and IGF2, LH and inhibins.
4. A follicle which failed to grow into the dominant follicle can become an atretic follicle from the preceding menstrual cycle, and then compete with new follicles in the next menstrual cycle's follicle race.
5. Ovulation of a follicle is driven by proteases produced under the influence of LH or sulfate hCG.
6. The luteal phase of the menstrual cycle is marked by corpus luteum formation and LH or sulfated hCG-promoted progesterone production.

Chapter 7

Ovarian Cystic Disorders

There are numerous cancerous and benign forms of ovarian cyst. Here we examine the physiology of the most common forms of ovarian cyst; follicular cyst, corpus luteum cyst and polycystic ovary syndrome. It is noteworthy that all ovarian cysts can be avoided by taking birth control pills.

Follicular Cyst

A follicular cyst is a small fluid-filled sac that develops in a woman's ovaries. A follicular cyst can be as small as a pea, or larger than an orange. Most ovarian cysts are functional in nature, and harmless [1-4]. In the US, follicular cysts are found in nearly all premenopausal women. They occur most often during a woman's childbearing years.

A follicular cyst is an exaggeration of an event occurring before ovulation, promotion of follicular growth (Figure 7.1). This type of cyst forms when ovulation doesn't occur. Most commonly, ovulation is blocked by an insufficient luteinizing hormone (LH) and the time of the LH peak to promote the sequence of ovulation-related events. Alternatively, a follicular cyst can result from failure to ovulate due to excess production of FSH at the time of ovulation. When the follicle doesn't rupture or release its egg, it instead becomes a cyst. In each subsequent menstrual cycle, follicle stimulating hormone (FSH), inhibin and LH may promote the growth of the cyst as they normally promote the growth follicles (Figure 7.1). The oocyte remains active inside a follicular cyst. The cyst is thin-walled, lined by granulosa and theca cells, and filled with clear fluid. These cysts occasionally become palpable and cause concern. In general, as long as the cyst does not exceed the size of a tennis ball, or about 7 cm, it is unlikely to be a malignancy [1-4]. Nevertheless, any palpable cyst in a postmenopausal woman can be malignant. Functional fallopian cysts are the most common type of ovarian cyst. They usually disappear by themselves and seldom require treatment. Cysts that become abnormally large or last longer than a few months should be removed or examined to determine whether they are a sign of cancer [1-4].

Most follicular cysts disappear naturally in one to three months. Although they can rupture, follicular cysts rarely cause symptoms. They are benign and have no clear medical consequence. They may be diagnosed coincidentally during a pelvic examination in women who do not have any related symptoms. All women have follicular cysts at some point that generally go unnoticed [1-4].

Ultrasound is used to determine the best treatment strategy. The best treatment depends on a woman's age, the size of the cyst, and the cyst's appearance on ultrasound. Treatment may consist of observation, or if the follicular cyst is large it can be surgically removed with laparoscopy. Birth control pills offer little help in treating functional follicular cysts. Follicular cysts can interfere with fertility, making a person infertile. If a woman does not ovulate and does not produce a corpus luteum, it can in some cases block fertility, and may continue to block fertility as long as there is a follicular cyst each menstrual cycle [1-4].

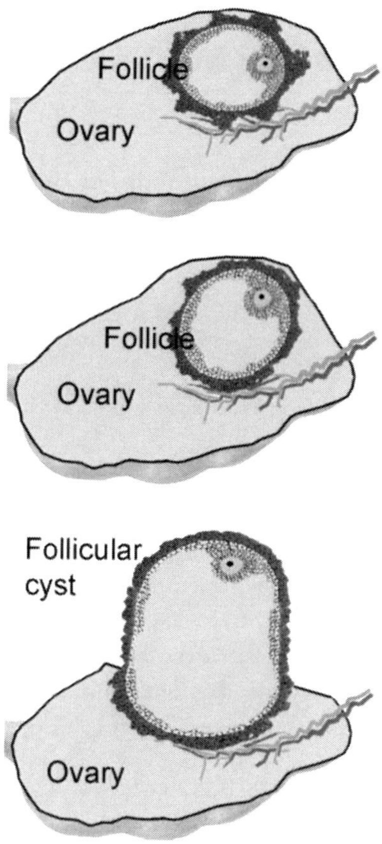

Figure 7.1. Growth of unovulated follicle into follicular cyst.

Corpus Luteum Cyst

Another type of functional cyst is known as a corpus luteum cyst. These occur less frequently than a follicular cyst, but can be more problematic. How can you tell if the cyst is corpus luteal or follicular? All is shown to be dependent on what is seen on the ultrasound and symptoms and signs the patient may be having. A missed period followed by spotting, one-sided pelvic pain and a pelvic examination which finds a tender ovarian mass suggest a corpus luteum cyst [5,6]. When a corpus luteum cyst ruptures, the bleeding and pain may necessitate urgent surgery. The surgery can be performed by laparoscopy.

A corpus luteal cyst occurs because a corpus luteum is not formed properly by LH. If the corpus luteum forms a sealed structure rather than an open structure, and contains some of the normally hemorrhaged blood from the follicle, a cyst is formed. Some corpus luteal cysts result in cases with sufficient LH to promote ovulation but insufficient to stimulate corpus luteum formation. A corpus luteal cyst produces progesterone like a corpus luteum. The progesterone can feed back and block gonadotropin releasing hormone (GnRH) production, blocking LH and FSH production and in turn causing infertility. Fertility drugs such as clomiphene citrate, an ovulation stimulant, can increase the chances of corpus luteal blockage or corpus luteal cysts. Corpus luteal cysts may grow as large as 4 inches in diameter. Cysts normally exist for up to 3 months and usually disappear with time or can be removed by laparoscopic surgery [5,6].

Corpus luteum cysts can occur in pregnancy, forming with the extended pregnancy corpus luteum (hCG extend the life of the corpus luteum to 6-7 weeks' gestation). Corpus luteum cysts are identified by sharp one-sided pelvic pain in early pregnancy and are confirmed by ultrasound, excluding the possibility of ectopic pregnancy by the demonstration of a fetal sac. If a corpus luteum cyst ruptures during pregnancy, leading to excessive hemorrhaging, laparoscopic surgery may be indicated. Normally corpus luteum cysts in pregnancy disappear by the second trimester of pregnancy [5,6].

Polycystic Ovary Syndrome

Polycystic ovary syndrome was first reported in 1935 by Stein and Levanthal (sometimes called Stein-Levanthal syndrome). Polycystic ovary syndrome is characterized by obesity, hirsuitism, infertility and oligomenorrhea. In polycystic ovary syndrome the entire ovary becomes filled with cysts (Figure 7.2) [7-10].

Under the influence of high levels of pulsatile LH and depressed levels of FSH polycystic ovary syndrome occurs. The low FSH prevents proper maturation of the follicle. Numerous follicles are inappropriately developed, becoming cysts with LH promotion, thus the polycystic appearance (Figure 7.2). As shown in Chapters 2 and 3, LH promotes androstenedione production by theca cells; FSH normally aromatizes androstenedione in granulosa cells. In polycystic ovary syndrome with the presence of LH or elevated LH and absence of FSH, excessive androstenedione and androgens (androstenedione is readily converted to testosterone) are produced and minimal estrogens are made. The high blood levels of androgens lead to hirsuitism. Without an estrogen peak no LH peak occurs and ovulation does not occur. Research suggests that the depression or deficiency of FSH is due to high inhibin production by granulosa cells, blocking pituitary FSH production. Polycystic ovary syndrome is particularly common in overweight women. The insulin resistance in these women leads to hyperinsulinemia which can further increase serum LH concentration and enhance further production of androgens [7-10].

Polycystic ovary syndrome is a common cause of infertility. With ovulation not occurring, a corpus luteum is not produced and no progesterone is produced. Follicles become cysts and grow with menstrual cycles until 2-4 inches.

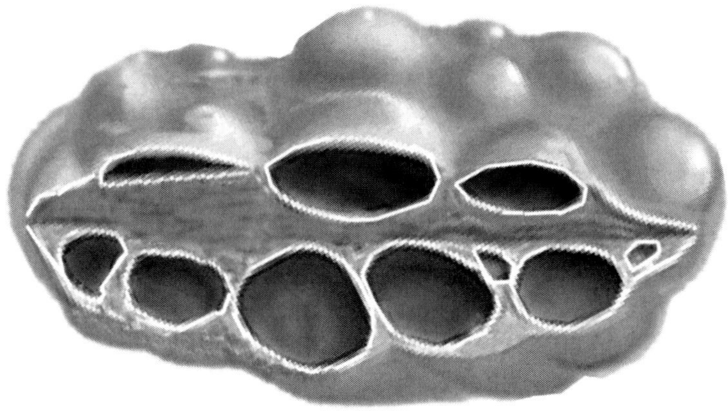

Figure 7.2. A polycystic ovary.

In polycystic ovary syndrome, 74% of cases complain of infertility, 69% of cases complain of hirsuitism, 66% of cases have ovarian enlargement due to the cysts, 41% of cases complain of obesity and 51% of cases have amenorrhea. Birth control pills inhibit GnRH, and so inhibit LH and stop excessive androgen production. Clomid (clomiphene citrate) promotes ovulation leading to the ovulation of cystic follicles. Laparascopic drilling surgery, making holes in the cyst, can dramatically help with ovarian androgen production. Normally, women are treated with Clomid and birth control pills first. If these do not help then laparoscopic drilling surgery is considered [7-10].

References

[1] Fang YM, Gomes J, Lysikiewicz A, Maulik D. Massive luteinized follicular cyst of pregnancy. *Obstet Gynecol* 2005;105:1218-1221.

[2] Garverick HA. Ovarian follicular cysts in dairy cows. *J Dairy Sci* 1997;80:995-1004.

[3] Stanley MW, Horwitz CA, Frable WJ. Cellular follicular cyst of the ovary: fluid cytology mimicking malignancy. *Diagn Cytopathol* 1991;7:48-52.

[4] Hamilton SA, Garverick HA, Keisler DH, Xu ZZ, Loos K, Youngquist RS, Salfen BE. Characterization of ovarian follicular cysts and associated endocrine profiles in dairy cows. *Biol Reprod* 1995;53:890-898.

[5] Choi HJ, Kim SH, Kim HC, MD, Park CM, Lee HK, Moon MH, MD, Jeong JY. Ruptured Corpus Luteal Cyst: CT Findings. *Korean J Radiol* 2003; 4:42-45.

[6] Jain M, Pujani M, Madan NK, Chadha R, Puri H. Congenital Ovarian Cyst: A Report of Two Cases. *J Lab Phys* 2012; 4: 63–65.

[7] Setji TL, Brown AJ. Polycystic ovary syndrome: diagnosis and treatment. *Am J Med* 2007;120:128-32.

[8] Agrawal R, Sharma S, Bekir J, Conway G, Bailey J, Balen AH, Prelevic G. Prevalence of polycystic ovaries and polycystic ovary syndrome in lesbian women compared with heterosexual women. *Fertil Steril* 2004;82:1352-1357.

[9] Liepa GU, Sengupta A, Karsies D. Polycystic ovary syndrome (PCOS) and other androgen excess-related conditions: can changes in dietary intake make a difference? *Nutr Clin Pract* 2008;23:63-71.

[10] 1Franks S. Polycystic ovary syndrome. *N Engl J Med* 1995;333:853-861.

Key Points

1. Follicular cysts derive from failure of the follicle to be ovulated. In each subsequent menstrual cycle a cyst grows with FSH, inhibin and LH promotion.
2. Follicular cysts normally self-resolve. If a cyst is exceptionally large it may be removed surgically with the laparoscope.
3. Corpus luteum cysts occur during corpus luteum formation. Corpus luteum cysts rupture and hemorrhage, leading to severe pain. This is an emergency and requires urgent laparoscopic surgery.
4. Corpus luteum cysts normally self-resolve or can be removed by laparoscopic surgery.
5. Corpus luteum cysts can occur with pregnancy. If sharp one-sided pelvic pain is detected a corpus luteum cyst should be investigated by ultrasound. If a cyst ruptures during pregnancy, laparoscopic surgery should be considered. Normally corpus luteum cysts during pregnancy self-resolve in the second trimester of pregnancy.
6. Polycystic ovary is caused by elevated LH in the presence of depressed FSH levels. This is probably due to overproduction of inhibin (inhibits pituitary production of FSH) by granulosa cells.
7. A polycystic ovary causes the overproduction of androgens leading to hirsuitism, and is a common cause for infertility.
8. A polycystic ovary is normally treated with birth control pills (will block LH) and clomiphene citrate (which will promote ovulation and the ovulation of cysts). If these do not help then laparoscopic treatment, drilling holes in cysts, is indicated.
9. It is noteworthy that all ovarian cysts are avoided when taking birth control pills.

Chapter 8

Contraception

Introduction

Contraception methods are a means to prevent sperm meeting an ovum, leading to pregnancy. Currently, there are barrier methods that literally block the meeting, and spermicides which destroy sperm. Ovulation timing tries to ensure that timing of the menstrual cycle prevents the sperm and egg from meeting. Coitus interruptus prevents sperm from entering the uterus, and sex hormone methods prevent an egg from ever being generated. Finally, male and female sterilization methods block sperm or egg release. Listed in Table 8.1 are efficiencies or failure rates of all these methods [1-12].

Based on the efficiencies (as shown in Table 8.1), the best method is the subdermal implant (Norplant and Jadelle) with 0.05% failure rate and no concern regarding typical use. The least efficient method is the female spermicide (18% failure rate for perfect use and 29% failure rate for typical use) [1-12]. What does typical use mean, versus perfect use? We give a few examples. Perfect use of a condom is a fresh condom put on perfectly, with appropriate withdrawal after ejaculation. Typical use may be to continue using the condom after ejaculation when it may become loose. Perfect use of a combined estrogen/progesterone pill is to take the pill every morning at 8 am, and never miss a pill. In typical use, the time of taking the pill varies, and missing a pill occasionally occurs. Let us look at the methods in detail.

Barrier Methods

Male Condom

The male condom is normally made of latex (polyurethane condoms are available for those with latex allergy), and is lubricated for comfort; it covers the penis firmly. The condom must be removed after ejaculation and before the erection ends to prevent sperm leakage. Condoms protect against sexually transmitted diseases (STDs), including HIV.

Table 8.1. Efficiency of contraception methods (as published by Trussell J, in Hatcher RA (ed) Contraceptive technology (19th revision), Ardent Media, New York, 2007)

Method	Type of contraceptive	Failure rate Typical use	Failure rate Perfect use
Subdermal implant of progestogen, 5 years' duration	Sex hormone methods	0.05%	0.05%
Female intrauterine device	Barrier method	0.8%	0.6%
Injected progestogen, 2-3 months' duration	Sex hormone methods	3%	0.3%
Female cervical cap plus spermicide	Barrier method	8%	?
Female combined estrogen/progestogen pill	Sex hormone methods	8%	0.3%
Female progestogen only pill	Sex hormone methods	8%	0.3%
Female estrogen/progestogen patch	Sex hormone methods	8%	0.3%
Male condom	Barrier method	15%	2%
Female over-the-counter LH peak test	Ovulation timing	15%	3%
Female diaphragm and spermicide	Barrier method	16%	6%
Female condom	Barrier method	21%	5%
Female basal temperature	Ovulation timing	25%	3%
Coitus interruptus	Coitus interruptus	27%	4%
Female spermicide	Spermicide	29%	18%
Male vasectomy	Sterilization	0.15%	0.1%
Female tubal ligation	Sterilization	0.5%	0.5%
No contraception		85%	85%

Female Cervical Cap

The female cervical cap is a small, deep rubber cap that fits tightly over the cervix to prevent sperm from entering. It is used with a spermicide gel. When a woman pushes the cap up her vagina and over the cervix before having intercourse, it must be left in place for at least 6 hours afterwards. A cervical cap protects a woman against pregnancy and some STDs. It does not protect against AIDS or the other STDs that are caused by viruses.

Female Condom

The female condom is larger and looser than a male condom. The closed end fits over the cervix, inside the vagina. The open end hangs slightly outside and protects the lips of the vagina. Because it is made of polyurethane, it becomes very soft and flexible when it is in place. It protects the woman from STCs and AIDS. Men generally prefer female condoms over male condoms because they do not have to withdraw as soon as they have ejaculated.

Female Diaphragm

The female diaphragm looks like a rubber cap with a flexible rim. It is always used with a spermicide gel. It is designed to fit over the cervix to prevent sperm from entering. It is put in place immediately before intercourse. It protects against some STDs, but not all. It has not been shown to protect against HIV. A diaphragm must be left in place for at least 6 hours after intercourse.

Female Intrauterine Device

The intrauterine device (IUD) is a small, T-shaped piece of plastic that is placed in a woman's uterus by a physician or nurse. Not all women can use an IUD. If a woman has had an infection like gonorrhea or chlamydia, she may not be able to use an IUD. The IUD is best for women who are in long-term, monogamous relationships. The intrauterine device does not protect against STDs or HIV.

Spermicide

Spermicides come in several different forms; as creams, as gels, as a foam, as a film, and suppositories. Most spermicides contain nonoxynol-9, a chemical that kills sperm. Spermicides can be used alone but are more effective when used with another method of birth control, such as a male or female condom, cervical cap or diaphragm. Spermicides immobilize and kill the sperm before they are able to act on an egg. The spermicide is deep in the vagina, close to the cervix. Spermicides must be used at least 15 minutes before sex so they have enough time to dissolve and spread. They do not offer protection against sexually transmitted diseases.

Ovulation Timing and Coitus Interruptus

Female Ovulation Timing

Women use ovulation timing methods such as basal temperature and over-the-counter ovulation detectors to recognize changes in their bodies that indicate the most fertile phase of the menstrual cycle. For these methods the male partner has to be willing to avoid intercourse during these days. For the basal temperature approach to work, women who become very familiar with their body's changes, having followed their temperature daily for multiple menstrual cycles (daily temperature 96-98 preovulation and 97-99 after ovulation) can be successful in using this method to avoid pregnancy. The rule is: no intercourse for the week following ovulation. Today many woman use over-the-counter luteinizing hormone (LH) peak detectors as indicators of ovulation and the times to avoid intercourse. These have the advantage of detecting impending ovulation one day early. Ovulation timing methods do not prevent against STDs or HIV.

Male Coitus Interruptus

In this method a man withdraws from the vagina when he feels he is going to ejaculate. The problem with this method is that it diminishes the man's opportunity to have an orgasm. The man then ejaculates outside the woman's body. Withdrawal has a high failure rate, 4% perfect and 27% typical. It is used mostly by married couples who want to space their children. Withdrawal does not protect against STDs or HIV.

Sex Hormone Methods

Sex hormone methods rely on estrogen to inhibit gonadotropin releasing hormone (GnRH) production by the hypothalamus using the feedback pathways. The body also uses the estrogen and progesterone administered to replace the natural hormones made by the ovary. This permits normal development of the endometrial lining of the uterus, and menses once each month. Sex hormone methods commonly use commercial hormone antagonists, such as ethinyl estradiol as an estrogen and norethisterone as a progestogen.

The Estrogen/Progestogen Combined Pill

Combined birth control pills are taken by women. Each pill contains an estrogen and a progestogen. It is essential that the pill is taken every day about the same time. The pill does not protect a person against STDs or HIV. One package of pills will last a person one month. The last seven pills are a placebo, and the person will have menses every month. Contraceptive pills can have mild side effects such as gaining a few pounds, nausea, headaches, breast tenderness, and acne.

The Progestogen only Pill

The progestogen only pill may have less problems with side effects than the combination pill. It is essential that the pill is taken every day about the same time. The pill does not protect a person against STDs or HIV. One package of pills will last a person one month. The last seven pills are a placebo, and a person will have menses every month.

The Estrogen/Progestogen Patch

A contraceptive patch is like a square band-aid. It is applied to the abdomen, buttocks, or upper arm. The patch is changed each week for a schedule of 3 weeks on and 1 week off (like the 21 days of sex steroids and 7 days of placebo with pills). The contraceptive patch works by slowly releasing a combination of estrogen and progestogen through the skin. The patch does not protect against STDs or HIV.

The Injected Progestogen

Depo-Provera as a progesterone agonist is given as an injection every 2-3 months to prevent pregnancy. Depo-Provera does not protect against STDs or HIV. The most common side effect is a change in menses. Eventually some women have no periods at all. If a person stops having the injections the menses will start again.

The Subdermal Implant of Progestogen

This is a form of contraception developed by the Population Council. This progestogen only contraceptive is implanted once and worn for up to five years. Norplant and Jadelle are made up of six tiny silicone rods that contain a progestogen. These rods are implanted under the skin of the upper arm for as long as five years. The implant procedure can be done in the physician's office and takes about 10 minutes. Norplant and Jadelle become effective within 24 hours of implantation, when progestogen is slowly released into the body. The progestogen works to thicken the cervical mucus, thereby creating a barrier for sperm. As shown in Table 8.1, this has proven to be the most effective of all contraceptive methods.

Sterilization

When all other methods are excluded or not possible, sterilization may be considered. Often when a married couple is finished having babies one partner may agree to surgical sterilization. Unfortunately, even sterilization is not perfect. When a female receives tubal ligation, for instance, the tied tube can in some cases leak, permitting sperm to pass [1-12].

Male Vasectomy

A vasectomy is considered a permanent method of birth control. A vasectomy prevents the release of sperm when a man ejaculates. During a vasectomy, the vas deferens from each testicle is clamped or cut. The testicles continue to produce sperm, but the sperm are reabsorbed by the body. Because the tubes are blocked before the seminal vesicles and prostate, a man still ejaculates about the same amount of fluid. It usually takes several months after a vasectomy for all remaining sperm to be ejaculated or reabsorbed. A patient must use another method of birth control until they have a semen sample tested and it shows a zero sperm count. No-scalpel vasectomies are techniques that use a small clamp with pointed ends rather than a scalpel. The clamp is poked through the skin of the scrotum and then opened. This procedure does not prevent STDs or HIV.

Female Tubal Ligation

Tubal ligation is a surgical sterilization technique for women that closes the fallopian tubes stopping the egg from traveling to the uterus. In a tubal ligation, fallopian tubes are cut or blocked with clips. The surgery is effective immediately. The surgery can be done by laparoscopy using a small incision below the navel. Tubal ligation does not prevent against STDs or HIV.

Advising Patients Regarding Contraception

If asked for a contraception recommendation one must take into consideration, from your knowledge of the person, how well it will be used. If you are considering a pill, how reliably will this person take the pill, every day at 8am? If you are thinking about a barrier method, how appropriately and correctly will it be used [1-12]? You must also consider, if it is for a single person, how effective a device or method they need. If it is a married couple, could they have a baby if the contraception failed? There are many things that have to be carefully considered before giving advice [1-12].

References

[1] Peralta O, Diaz S, Croxatto H. Subdermal contraceptive implants. *J Steroid Biochem Mol Biol* 1995;53:223-226.

[2] Morgan KW. The intrauterine device: rethinking old paradigms. *J Midwifery Womens Health* 2006;51:464-470.

[3] Sitruk-Ware R. New progestogens for contraceptive use. *Hum Reprod Update* 2006; 12:169-178.

[4] Fairbanks B, Scharfman B. The cervical cap: past and current experience. *Women Health* 1980;5:61-80.

[5] Gillmer MD. Progestrogen potency in oral contraceptive pills. *Am J Obstet Gynecol* 1987;157:1048-1052.

[6] Vigna GB, Donegà P, Zanca R, Barban A, Passaro A, Pansini F, Bonaccorsi G, Mollica G, Fellin R. Simvastatin, transdermal patch, and oral estrogen-progestrogen preparation in early-postmenopausal hypercholesterolemic women: a randomized, placebo-controlled clinical trial. *Metabol* 2002;51:1463-1470.

[7] Duerr A, Gallo MF, Warner L, Jamieson DJ, Kulczycki A, Macaluso M. Assessing male condom failure and incorrect use. *Sex Transm Dis* 2011;38:580-586.

[8] Ferreira AE, Araújo MJ, Regina CH, Diniz SG, Faúndes A. Effectiveness of the diaphragm, used continuously, without spermicide. *Contraception* 1993;48:29-35.

[9] Witte SS, el-Bassel N, Wada T, Gray O, Wallace J. Acceptability of female condom use among women exchanging street sex in New York City. *Int J STD AIDS* 1999;10:162-168.

[10] Bauman JE. Basal body temperature: unreliable method of ovulation detection. *Fertil Steril* 1981;36:729-733.

[11] Doherty IA, Stuart GS. Coitus interruptus is not contraception. *Sex Transm Dis.* 2011; 38:356.

[12] Raymond E, Alvarado G, Ledesma L, Diaz S, Bassol S, Morales E, Fernandez V, Carlos G. *Acceptability of two spermicides in five countries. Contraception.* 1999;60:45-50.

Key Points

1. There are numerous methods of contraception that can be generally described as barrier methods, spermicide, ovulation timing, coitus interruptus, sex hormone methods and sterilization.
2. By far the most generally effective contraceptives are the sex hormone methods, sterilization and the female intrauterine device. Barrier methods can work but generally have high failure rates. Ovulation timing methods and coitus interruptus work but with high risk rates.
3. Sex hormone methods can be very effective if used correctly. A patient has to train themselves into taking one pill at the same time every day without forgetting. If this is not possible, injected progestogen every 2-3 months and subdermal implants are possibilities.

The Testes and Male Reproduction

Chapter 9

Male Steroidogenesis

Steroidogenesis

We now consider the critical cells of the testis, Figure 9.1. The Leydig cells are the site of action of luteinizing hormone (LH) and the Sertoli cells are the site of action of follicle stimulating hormone (FSH). LH is the pituitary hormone that promotes steroidogenesis in men, testosterone, super testosterone or dihydrotestosterone, and estradiol. Dihydrotestosterone is made in Sertoli cells (Figure 9.1).

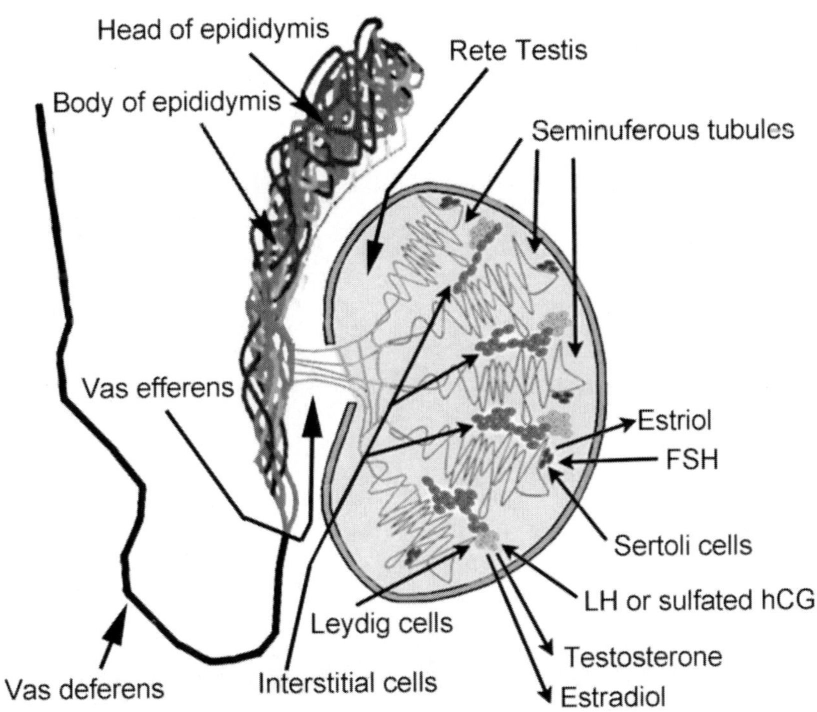

Figure 9.1. The testis.

As discussed in Chapter 3, the root molecule for all sex steroids is cholesterol, a 27 carbon steroid. Cholesterol is produced from Acetyl CoA as discussed in Chapter 4. Cholesterol is degraded by cholesterol side chain cleavage enzyme to make pregnenolone, a 21 carbon steroid. It is degraded further to make androgens like androstenedione and testosterone which are 19 carbon steroids. Estrogens are 18 carbon aromatic steroids (Chapter 4) [1-3].

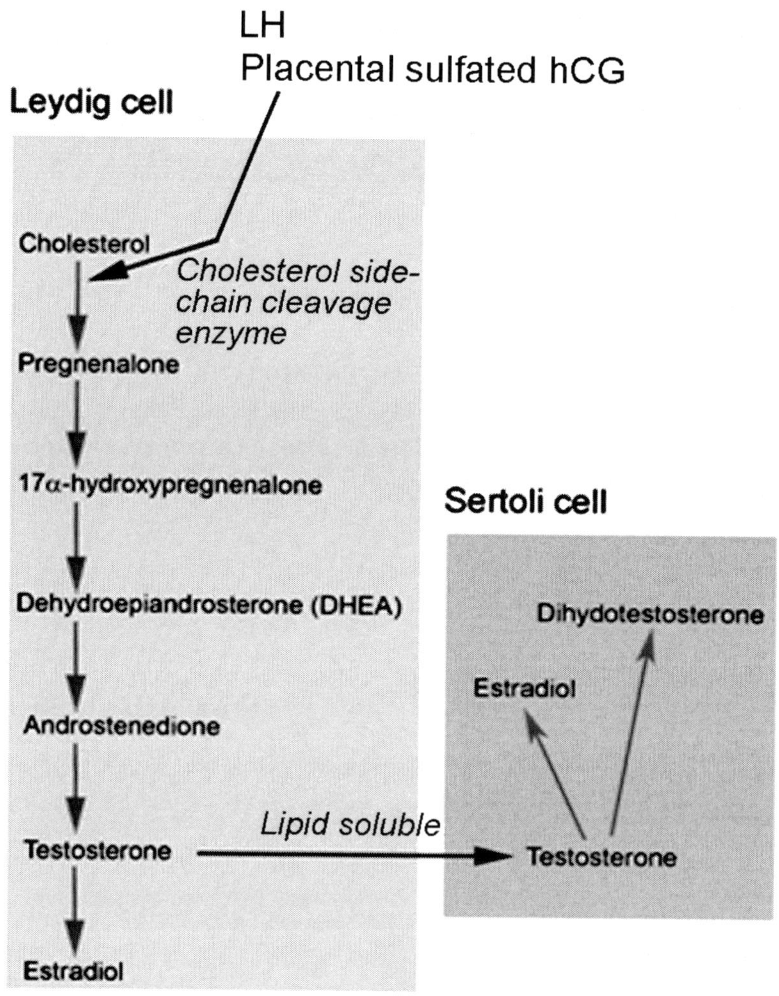

Figure 9.2. Steroidogenesis in the postpubertal male.

Gonadotropin releasing hormone (GnRH) is releases in pulses by the hypothalamus as discussed Chapters 3. LH and FSH are releasing from pituitary gonadotrope cells in response to GnRH pulses (see Chapter 3). LH directly promotes cholesterol side chain cleavage enzyme in Leydig cells, converting cholesterol to pregnenolone (Figure 9.2). The pregnenolone is converted to androstenedione like in theca cells in women (see Chapter 4), and then to testosterone (Figure 9.2). The testosterone can be aromatized directly in the Leydig cell to make estradiol. Testosterone enters the blood from this point and gets transferred to the testis seminiferous tubules. Some testosterone gets transferred to the Sertoli cells (see Figure 9.2), where it undergoes reduction to make the more active androgen dihydrotestosterone and is aromatized to estradiol. Testosterone feeds back to the hypothalamus modulating GnRH pulses. The major difference between steroidogenesis in the male and female gonads is that testosterone production is continuous in the postpubertal male and not cyclic with a follicular, ovulatory and luteal phase as steroids are in the postpubertal woman [1-3].

Table 9.1. Examining total levels of androgens and estrogens in male blood

Steroid	Serum concentration (ng/ml)
Testosterone	2.6 – 10
Dihydrotestosterone	0.25 – 0.75
Androstenedione	0.5 – 2.5
Estradiol	0.01 – 0.05

Functions of Sex Steroids in Men

As shown in Table 9.1, testosterone is the principal steroid produced by the testes on a constant, non-cyclic, basis.

Androgens in Adults

Testosterone, supplemented by dihydrotestosterone, has clear functions in the adult. Firstly, testosterone promotes sperm development in seminiferous tubules (see Chapter 10) [4-6]. Secondly, testosterone is the substrate for synthesis of the more potent androgen dihydrotestosterone, and for aromatization to estriol. Thirdly, testosterone controls secondary sexual characteristics in males [7-9]. Testosterone increases bone mass and muscular masses and hair growth. As illustrated in Figure 9.3, testosterone acts on an internal testosterone receptor in cells to promote nuclear action.

Fourthly, testosterone acts on libido development and the promotion of penile erection [10-12]. As described in Chapter 13, testosterone can cross the blood-brain barrier. It acts on a receptor (Figure 9.3) in the sexual dimorphic nucleus in the preoptic area of the hypothalamus [10-12]. This sexual dimorphic nucleus and the limbic system of the brain controls libido and penile erection [13-15]. Fifthly, testosterone acts on other areas of the brain, promoting adult male mental and physical energy [16]. Questionable research suggests that it may also have a role in the maintenance of cardiovascular health, and in risk-taking.

Prenatal Role of Androgens

Prenatally testosterone is important in genital virilization, development of the prostate and seminal vesicles and in gender identity. In the male fetus, testosterone promotes the differentiation of the Wolffian duct to form an epididymis and vas deferens.

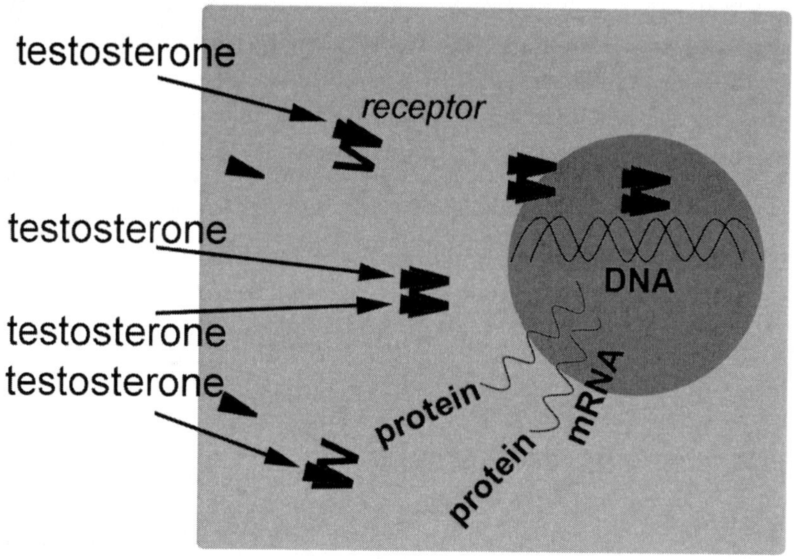

Figure 9.3. Testosterone action on cells.

Pubertal of Androgens

During puberty testosterone promotes enlargement of the sebaceous glands, phallic enlargement, promotes male libido, increases facial hair, chest hair, leg hair, axillary hair and growth of the jaw [17,18].

Function of Estradiol in Adult Men

The function of estradiol formed normally in men is far from certain. Research evidence suggests that estradiol has a role in growth of the penis, development of testicles, growth of hair, deepening voice in men, and maturations of sperm [19-21]. These are all curious research findings. More research is needed to confirm the exact functions of estradiol in men.

References

[1] Mitamura R, Yano K, Suzuki N, Ito Y, Makita Y, Okuno A. Diurnal rhythms of luteinizing hormone, follicle-stimulating hormone, and testosterone secretion before the onset of male puberty. *J Clin Endocrinol Metab* 1999;84:29-37.

[2] Spratt DI, O'Dea LS, Schoenfeld D, Butler J, Rao PN, Crowley WF Jr. Neuroendocrine-gonadal axis in men: frequent sampling of LH, FSH, and testosterone. *Am J Physiol* 1988; 254:E658-E666.

[3] Ruiz E, Osorio A, Torres JM, Ortega E. Evidence of different actions of testosterone, estradiol, FSH, and LH on the growth axis. *Endocr Res* 2001;27:25-33.

[4] Gui YL, He CH, Amory JK, Bremner WJ, Zheng EX, Yang J, Yang PJ, Gao ES. Male hormonal contraception: suppression of spermatogenesis by injectable testosterone undecanoate alone or with levonorgestrel implants in Chinese men. *J Androl* 2004;25:720-727.

[5] McLachlan RI, Wreford NG, Meachem SJ, De Kretser DM, Robertson DM. Effects of testosterone on spermatogenic cell populations in the adult rat. *Biol Reprod* 1994;51:945-955.

[6] Meistrich ML, Shetty G. Suppression of testosterone stimulates recovery of spermatogenesis after cancer treatment. *Int J Androl* 2003;26:141-146.

[7] Isidori AM, Giannetta E, Gianfrilli D, Greco EA, Bonifacio V, Aversa A, Isidori A, Fabbri A, Lenzi A. Effects of testosterone on sexual function in men: results of a meta-analysis. *Clin Endocrinol* 2005;63:381-394.

[8] Gooren LJ. Androgen levels and sex functions in testosterone-treated hypogonadal men. *Arch Sex Behav* 1987;16:463-473.

[9] Winters SJ, Brufsky A, Weissfeld J, Trump DL, Dyky MA, Hadeed V. Testosterone, sex hormone-binding globulin, and body composition in young adult African American and Caucasian men. *Metabol* 2001;50:1242-1247.

[10] van Anders SM. Testosterone and sexual desire in healthy women and men. *Arch Sex Behav* 2012;41:1471-1484.

[11] Boloña ER, Uraga MV, Haddad RM, Tracz MJ, Sideras K, Kennedy CC, Caples SM, Erwin PJ, Montori VM. Testosterone use in men with sexual dysfunction: a systematic review and meta-analysis of randomized placebo-controlled trials. *Mayo Clin Proc* 2007;82:20-28.

[12] Gonzales GF, Córdova A, Vega K, Chung A, Villena A, Góñez C, Castillo S. Effect of Lepidium meyenii (MACA) on sexual desire and its absent relationship with serum testosterone levels in adult healthy men. *Andrologia* 2002;34:367-372.

[13] Mikhail N. Does testosterone have a role in erectile function? *Am J Med* 2006; 119:373-382.

[14] Blute M, Hakimian P, Kashanian J, Shteynshluyger A, Lee M, Shabsigh R. Erectile dysfunction and testosterone deficiency. *Front Horm Res* 2009;37:108-122.

[15] Martínez-Jabaloyas JM, Queipo-Zaragozá A, Pastor-Hernández F, Gil-Salom M, Chuan-Nuez P. Testosterone levels in men with erectile dysfunction. *BJU Int* 2006; 97:1278-1283.

[16] Hickson M. *Malnutrition and ageing.* http://www.ncbi.nlm.nih.gov/pmc/articles/PMC2563720/

[17] Kulin HE, Finkelstein JW, D'Arcangelo MR, Susman EJ, Chinchilli V, Kunselman S, Schwab J, Demers L, Lookingbill G. Diversity of pubertal testosterone changes in boys with constitutional delay in growth and/or adolescence. *J Pediatr Endocrinol Metab* 1997; 10:395-400.

[18] Wilson DM, Kei J, Hintz RL, Rosenfeld RG. Effects of testosterone therapy for pubertal delay. *Am J Dis Child* 1988;142:96-99.

[19] Vermeulen A, Kaufman JM, Goemaere S, van Pottelberg I. Estradiol in elderly men. *Aging Male* 2002;5:98-102.

[20] Carani C, Qin K, Simoni M, Faustini-Fustini M, Serpente S, Boyd J, Korach KS, Simpson ER. Effect of testosterone and estradiol in a man with aromatase deficiency. *N Engl J Med* 1997;337:91-95. Schneider G, Kirschner MA, Berkowitz

R, Ertel NH. Increased estrogen production in obese men. *J Clin Endocrinol Metab* 1979;48:633-638.

Key Points

1. Testosterone and estradiol are made from cholesterol in Leydig cells. Leydig cells are directly promoted by pituitary LH.
2. Testosterone can make its way to Sertoli cells. Sertoli cells may produce dihydrotestosterone and estradiol opular from the testosterone.
3. Testosterone has multiple functions in adult men; promotion of sperm development in seminiferous tubules, promotion of secondary sexual characteristics, increased bone and muscular masses, and hair growth. Testosterone controls libido development and promotion of penile erection in men. It also affects adult males' mental and physical energy. Questionable research suggests that it may have a role in the maintenance of cardiovascular health, and in risk-taking.
4. The estradiol made in the testis has several uncertain actions. It promotes growth of the penis, development of testicles, growth of the hair in men, deepening of the voice in men and maturations of sperm.

Chapter 10

Sperm Production and Seminal Fluids

Introduction

This chapter is divided into multiple sections; firstly, spermatogenesis or the complex mechanism by which germ cells become sperm cells is examined. Spermatogenesis is dealt with in three stages; mitotic proliferation, meiotic division and cytodifferentiation and packaging of sperm cells. All told, a massive amount of sperm is generated; approximately 300 to 600 spermatozoa are made per gram of testis per second, or multiple millions of sperm cells per day. Secondly, seminal fluids are considered, which are ejaculated along with the sperm.

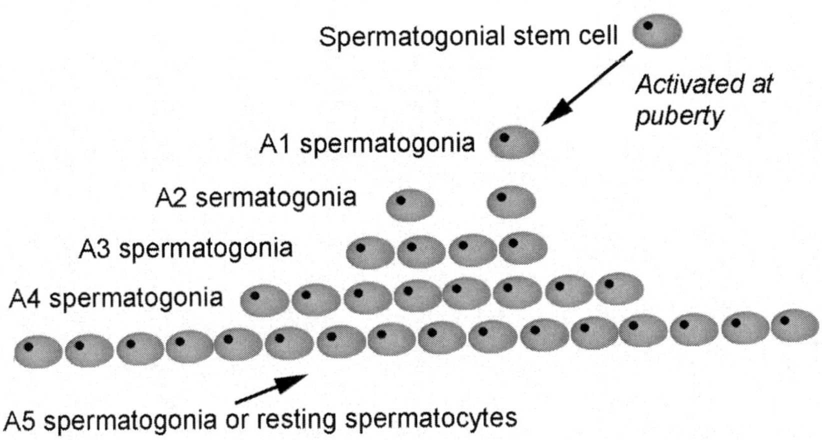

Figure 10.1. Cloning (mitotic proliferation) of spermatogonia.

Spermatogenesis 1: Mitotic Proliferation

The germ cells of the immature testis are the root cells in the production of sperm. These germ cells become activated at puberty. These are the spermatogonial stem cells. With activation these cells become A1 spermatogonia. Over 36-48 hours these cells undergo multiple divisions or cloning steps, multiplying these cells many times over. If cells undergo 6 divisions, for instance, each cell becomes 2^6 cells or is multiplied 64-fold (Figure 10.1). After 4-5 divisions the final clones become resting primary spermatocytes (Figure 10.1) [1-3].

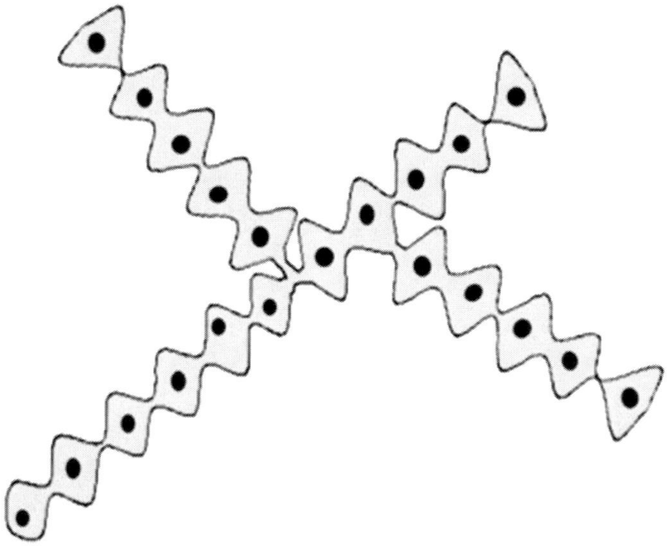

Figure 10.2. Spermatogonia syncytium.

This mitotic division or cloning occurs in the basal compartment of the testicular seminiferous tubules (Figure 10.4). During this rapid cloning process nuclear division is always completed, but cytoplasmic division remains incomplete. As such, all spermatogonia remain linked together through their cytoplasm, joined by cytoplasmic bridges. This makes a spermatogonial syncytium or spermatogonia strings (see Figure 10.2)[1-3].

Spermatogenesis 2: Meiotic Division

The resting primary spermatocytes push their way into the aluminar compartment of the seminiferous tubules (Figure 10.4). These cells undergo both stages (first meiotic division and second meiotic division) of meiosis (Figure 10.3). All 23 chromosome pairs undergo meiosis. Each diploid cell with 23 pairs of chromosomes becomes during meiosis 4 haploid cells ready for use in sperm and for combining with haploid chromosomes in the egg (Figure 10.3). In the process of meiosis, each pair of chromosomes is first duplicated (generating 4 chromatids) in prophase 1-leptotene (Figure 10.3), then tied together in prophase 1-zygotene (Figure 10.3), and then undergoes interchange of genes between all 4 chromatids or "chiasmata," in prophase 1-diakinesis. Then chromatids are pulled apart in anaphase 1 to make two cells in late telophase 1 (Figure 10.3). In anaphase 2, all 4 chromatids are completely separated and make 4 cells each containing a single chromatid set, telophase 2 [4-6].

The product of meiosis is "early round spermatids." It can be calculated that if a spermatogonia underwent 6 stages of duplication or cloning, it would generate 64 primary spermatocytes; after entering meiosis this would generate 256 early round spermatids. Considering losses due to failures, the actual number may be much lower than this. All these spermatids remain linked like a syncytium, as illustrated in Figure 10.2. The round spermatids become separated [4-6].

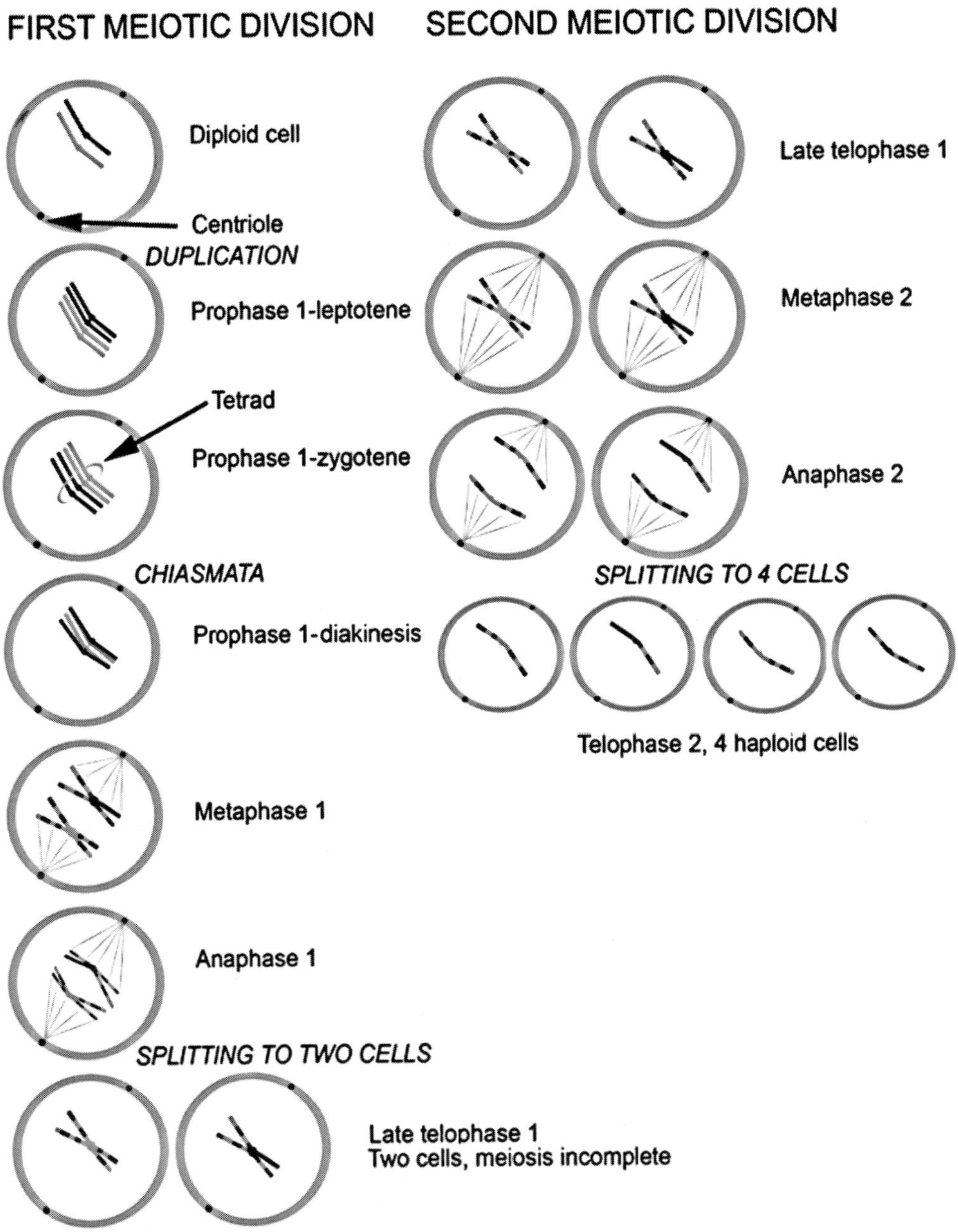

Figure 10.3. The two stages of meiosis. The example cells have one pair of chromosomes; in reality, 23 diploid chromosomes undergo meiosis to make haploid cells.

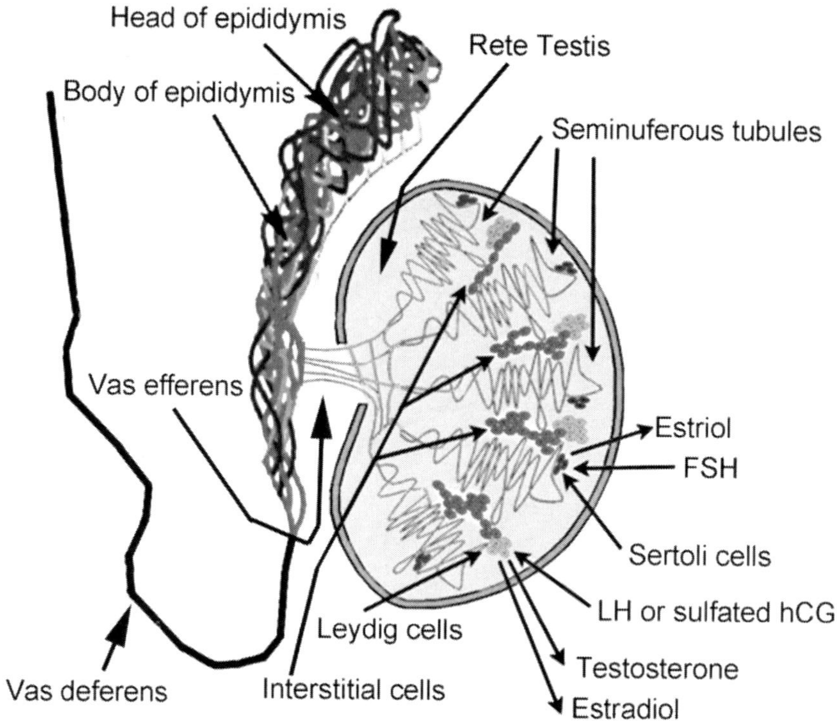

Figure 10.4 The testis.

Spermatogenesis 3: Cytodifferentiation and Packaging of Sperm Cells

The most complex stage of sperm formation is the cytoplasmic differentiation and remodeling. This is performed at the seminiferous tubule/Sertoli cell interface (Figure 10.4). Here, round spermatids are reshaped and a tail is added to the spermatozoon propulsion. Firstly, out of glycoprotein rich granules which accumulate in the golgi apparatus, an acrosome granule forms growing over the nucleus forming a cap-like structure (see Figure 10.5 panel A and B). A single fiber flagellum or tail is formed that emanates from the acrosome and nucleus. The cytoplasm then becomes very squeezed and elongated. A neck or connecting piece is formed by the cytoplasm, the nucleus and acrosome become flattened (Figure 10.5 panel C). Nine fibers then form a long tail, forming the spermatozoon. Mitochondria accumulate in the middle piece as a power center for tail propulsion. While mitosis or cloning occurs very quickly, these stages of cytodifferentiation and packaging of sperm cells are slower, taking approximately 45-50 days [7-9].

The flagella are filled with dense fibers, which move with energy (ATP) generated in the mitochondria, permitting spermatozoa propulsion. A mature spermatozoon is shown in Figure 10.5 panel D. It distinctly has a head, a middle piece and a trail or flagella. Rounds of spermatogenesis are initiated at constant time intervals in males [7-9].

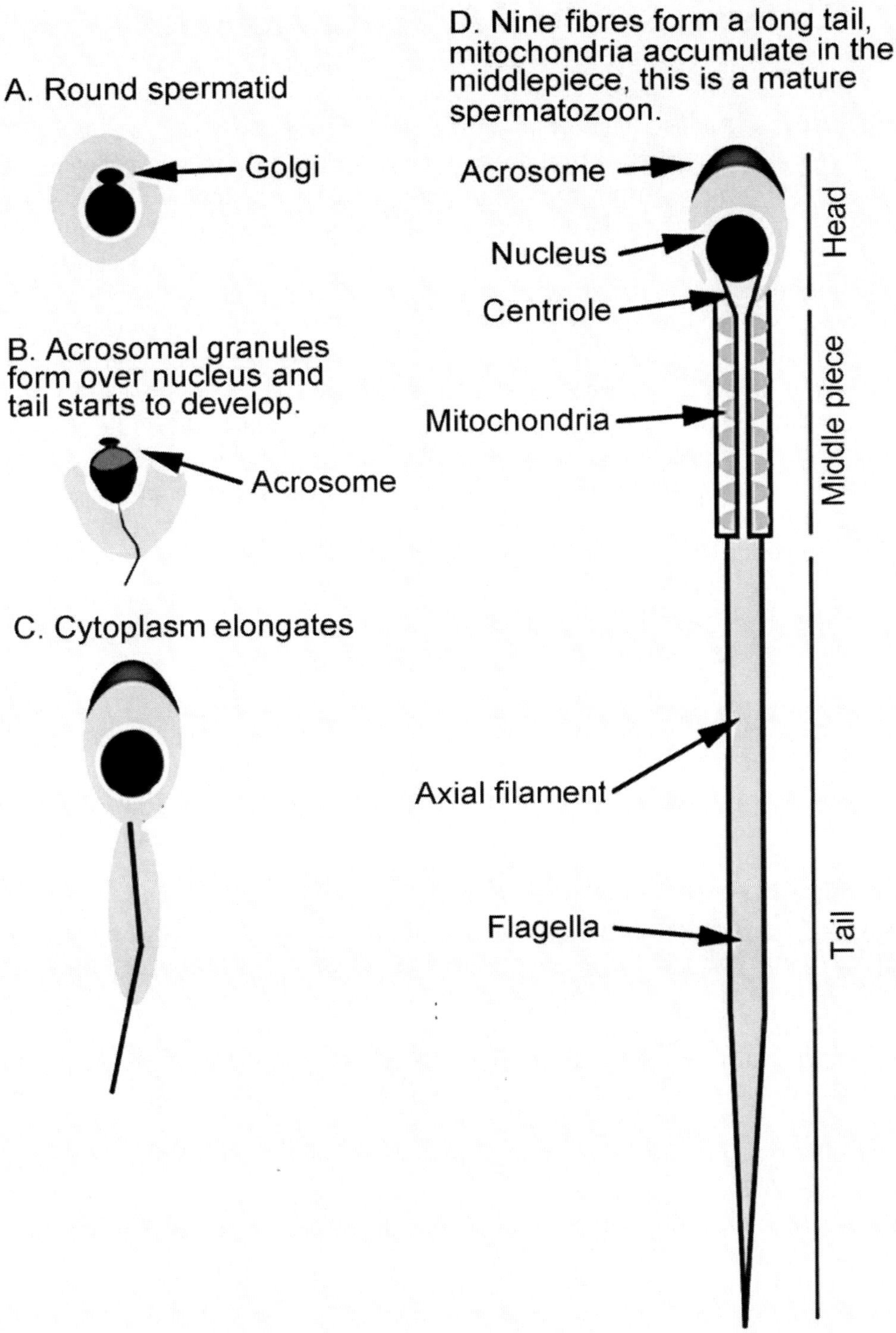

Figure 10.5. Cytodifferentiation of spermatids to form spermatozoon.

Endocrine Control of Spermatogenesis

Spermatogenesis commences at puberty, when testosterone levels rise. As testosterone levels rise, spermatogenesis commences. Testosterone is critical to spermatogenesis [10-12]. In the absence of testosterone spermatogenesis only proceeds as far as the prophase 1-leptotene stage of meiosis (Figure 10.3). Hypophysectomy (or the removal of the pituitary gland) leads to an absence of luteinizing hormone (LH). With the absence of LH Leydig cells stop producing testosterone and spermatogenesis comes to a halt. In this respect, LH is as critical to spermatogenesis as testosterone [10-12].

The role of FSH in men is less certain. FSH promotes androgen binding protein which is critical to testosterone steroidogenesis in men [10-12]. For that function it is mandatory. FSH also promotes growth of testosterone receptors on Sertoli cells and seminiferous tubules; this is also important. The role of FSH in spermatogenesis is less certain. FSH, seemingly in males, is mandatory for regaining full fertility following hypophysectomy. FSH seemingly both regulates the sperm production rate and promotes spermatogenesis in the seminiferous tubules. LH may also promote spermatogenesis. Optimally the hypophysectomized male should receive FSH and human chorionic gonadotropin or LH [10-12].

Maturation of Spermatozoa

Spermatozoa are released from Sertoli cells into a saline fluid and then washed towards the rete testis (Figure 10.4). As the fluid passes through the rete testis the composition of the fluid changes; it becomes oxygen-rich (needed to power middle piece mitochondria) and contains serum albumin. The spermatozoa are then washed into the vas efferens and into the epididymis (Figure 10.4). In the epididymis fluid is adsorbed and spermatozoa concentrated 100-fold. The epididymis then adds secretory products including fructose, carnitine, and glycoproteins. The glycoproteins coat the surface of the spermatozoa. Passage through the epididymis takes 6-12 days and affects spermatozoa behavior profoundly. Spermatozoa in the epididymis have acquired what is needed to swim progressively by being supplied with nutrients, including fructose as sugar fuel, and by spermatozoa being coated with glycoprotein, or coated with charge sugars (sialic acid). This whole process of activation of spermatozoa is crucially dependent upon stimulation of the epididymis by testosterone [13-15].

In humans the epididymis can store sperm for 1-3 days. After the epididymis spermatozoa enter the vas deferens (Figure 10.4). The normal vas deferens serves as a storage compartment for spermatozoa. In the absence of ejaculation spermatozoa seep into the urethra and are washed away [13-15].

Seminal Fluids

After the epididymis spermatozoa enter the vas deferens (Figure 10.4) where they can be stored. Ejaculated spermatozoa are carried to the female tract in seminal plasma. The combination of spermatozoa and seminal plasma are called semen. The seminal plasma provides nutritional factors such as fructose and sorbitol. It also provides an alkaline buffering capacity to neutralize the acidic vagina. Seminal plasma contains leucocytes to assist in sperm fertility [16-22].

The vas deferens first delivers the spermatozoa to the seminal vesicles (Figure 10.6). From the seminal vesicles the sperm passes into the prostate gland, and then through the Cowper's gland before entering the urethra and being ejaculated (Figure 10.6). In the seminal vesicles most of the seminal plasma is made. A protein called lipofuscin from dead epithelial cells gives the semen a yellowish color (Figure 10.7). The seminal vesicles supply the semen with fructose and sorbitol as fuel, and an alkaline buffer to cope with the acidity of the vagina (Figure 10.7) [16-22].

In the prostate gland, semen receive citric acid at a calcium cheater. The semen is supplied with 1% proteolytic enzymes to burn the way of spermatozoa into ova. The semen also receive in the prostate an alkaline phosphatase to cleave glycerylphosphorylcholine for use in phospholid metabolism (Figure 10.7) [16-22].

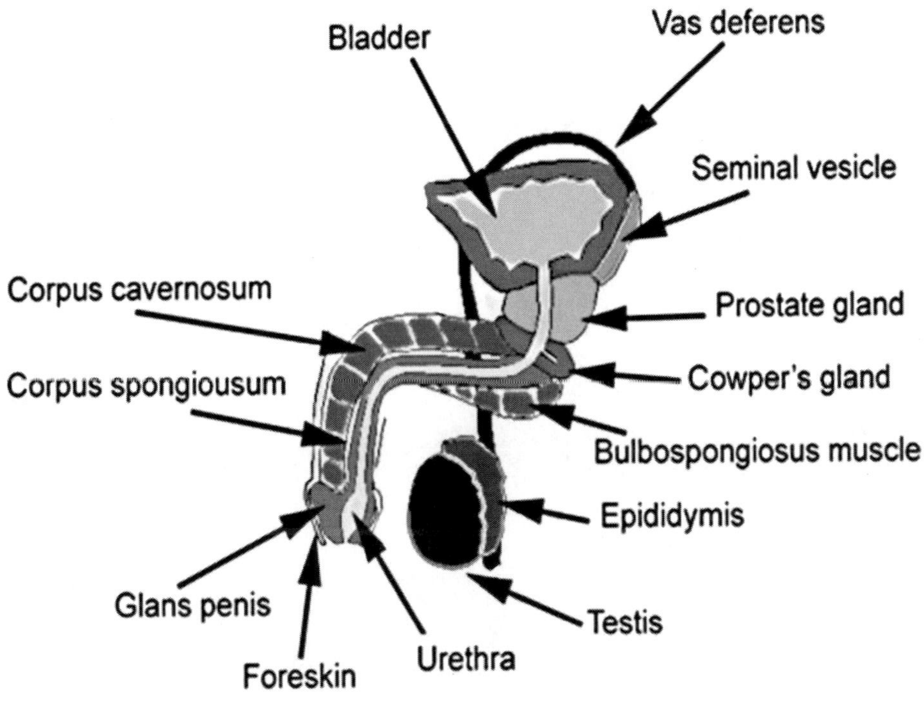

Figure 10.6. Male reproductive anatomy.

The Cowper's gland provides the semen with a mucus lubricant that clears the flow of semen through the urethra. The viscous mucus made in Cowper's gland is the principal component of the pre-ejaculate in men (Figure 10.7) [16-22].

The Ingredient of Semen

1. Testis	The sperm, ~15 million cells per milliliter
2. Seminal vesicle	Lipofuscin, the yellow coloring of semen Fuctose, an energy source or fuel Sorbitol, an energy source or fuel
3. Prostate gland	Citric acid, a Ca^{++} chelator Proteolytic enzymes, 1% w/w, to burn entrance into ovum. Alkaline phosphatase, to cleave gycerylph-osphorylcholine for lipid metabolism.
4. Cowper's gland	Mucus lubricant, to clear flow through urethra (principal ingredient of semen).

Figure 10.7. The ingredients of semen.

References

[1] Barry KA, Schultz KM, Payne CJ, McGarry TJ. Geminin is required for mitotic proliferation of spermatogonia. *Dev Biol* 2012;371:35-46.

[2] d'Istria M, Palmiero C, Serino I, Izzo G, Minucci S. Inhibition of the basal and oestradiol-stimulated mitotic activity of primary spermatogonia by melatonin in the testis of the frog, Rana esculenta, in vivo and in vitro. *Reproduction* 2003;126:83-90.

[3] Griswold MD. The central role of Sertoli cells in spermatogenesis. *Semin Cell Dev Biol* 1998;9:411-416.

[4] Chihara M, Ikebuchi R, Otsuka S, Ichii O, Hashimoto Y, Suzuki A, Saga Y, Kon Y. Mice stage-specific claudin 3 expression regulates progression of meiosis in early stage spermatocytes. *Biol Reprod* 2013;89:3.

[5] Handel MA, Caldwell KA, Wiltshire T. Culture of pachytene spermatocytes for analysis of meiosis. *Dev Genet* 1995;16:128-139.

[6] Parvinen M, Wright WW, Phillips DM, Mather JP, Musto NA, Bardin CW. Spermatogenesis in vitro: completion of meiosis and early spermiogenesis. *Endocrinol* 1983;112:1150-1152.

[7] Nunes ET, Braga AA, dos Santos DC, Camargo-Mathias MI. *Micron* 2010;41:585-591.

[8] Jan SZ, Hamer G, Repping S, de Rooij DG, van Pelt AM, Vormer TL. Molecular control of rodent spermatogenesis. *Biochim Biophys Acta* 2012;1822:1838-1850.

[9] Anderson WA, Weissman A, Ellis RA. Cytodifferentiation during spermiogenesis in Lumbricus terrestris. *J Cell Biol* 1967;32:11-26.

[10] Matsumoto AM, Bremner WJ. Endocrine control of human spermatogenesis. *J Steroid Biochem 1989*;33:789-790.

[11] Courot M, Ortavant R. Endocrine control of spermatogenesis in the ram. *J Reprod Fertil Suppl.* 1981;30:47-60.

[12] Matsumoto AM, Bremner WJ. Endocrinology of the hypothalamic-pituitary-testicular axis with particular reference to the hormonal control of spermatogenesis. *Baillieres Clin Endocrinol Metab* 1987;1:71-87.

[13] Schimenti KJ, Feuer SK, Griffin LB, Graham NR, Bovet CA, Hartford S, Pendola J, Lessard C, Schimenti JC, Ward JO. AKAP9 is essential for spermatogenesis and sertoli cell maturation in mice. *Genetics* 2013;194:447-457.

[14] Meo SA, Arif M, Rashied S, Khan MM, Vohra MS, Usmani AM, Imran MB, Al-Drees AM. Hypospermatogenesis and spermatozoa maturation arrest in rats induced by mobile phone radiation. *J Coll Physicians Surg Pak* 2011;21:262-265.

[15] Poulakis V, Ferakis N, de Vries R, Witzsch U, Becht E. Induction of spermatogenesis in men with azoospermia or severe oligoteratoasthenospermia after antegrade internal spermatic vein sclerotherapy for the treatment of varicocele. *Asian J Androl* 2006;8:613-619.

[16] Robert M, Gagnon C. Sperm motility inhibitor from human seminal plasma: presence of a precursor molecule in seminal vesicle fluid and its molecular processing after ejaculation. *Int J Androl* 1994;17:232-240.

[17] Gonzales GF, Kortebani G, Mazzolli AB. Leukocytospermia and function of the seminal vesicles on seminal quality. *Fertil Steril* 1992 May;57:1058-1065.

[18] Ahlgren G, Rannevik G, Lilja H. Impaired secretory function of the prostate in men with oligo-asthenozoospermia. *J Androl* 1995;16:491-498.

[19] Huggins C, Neal W. Coagulation and liquefaction of semen: proteolytic enzymes and citrate in prostatic fluid. *J Exp Med* 1942;76:527-541.

[20] Zukerman Z, Weiss DB, Orvieto R. Does preejaculatory penile secretion originating from Cowper's gland contain sperm? *J Assist Reprod Genet* 2003;20:157-159.

[21] Hart RG, Greenstein JS. A newly discovered role for Cowper's gland secretion in rodent semen coagulation. *J Reprod Fertil* 1968;17:87-94.

[22] Production of semen. http://faculty.stcc.edu/AandP/AP/AP2pages/reprod/makingsemen.htm

Key Points

1. The germ cells of the immature testis are the root cells in the production of sperm. These germ cells become activated at puberty. These are the spermatogonial stem cell. With activation these cells become A1 spermatogonia.
2. Over 36-48 hours these cells undergo multiple divisions or cloning steps, multiplying these cells many times over. If cells undergo 6 divisions, for instance, each cell

becomes 2^6 cells or is multiplied 64-fold. After 4-5 divisions the final clones become resting primary spermatocytes.

3. Resting primary spermatocytes undergo both stages of meiosis (Figure 9.3). All 23 chromosome pairs undergo meiosis. Each diploid cell with 23 pairs of chromosomes becomes during meiosis 4 haploid cells ready for use in sperm and for combining with haploid chromosomes from the egg.
4. The most complex stage of sperm formation is the cytoplasmic differentiation and remodeling. This is performed at the seminiferous tubule/Sertoli cell interface (Figure 9.4). Here, round spermatids are reshaped and a tail is added to give the spermatozoon propulsion.
5. Testosterone is critical to spermatogenesis. In the absence of testosterone spermatogenesis only proceeds as far as the prophase 1-leptotene stage of meiosis. Removal of the pituitary gland leads to an absence of luteinizing hormone (LH). With the absence of LH Leydig cells stop producing testosterone and spermatogenesis comes to a halt. In this respect, LH is as critical to spermatogenesis as testosterone.
6. Spermatozoa are released from Sertoli cells into a saline fluid and then washed towards the rete testis. As the fluid passes through the rete testis it becomes oxygen-rich (needed to power middle piece mitochondria). The spermatozoa are then washed into the vas efferens and into the epididymis (Figure 9.4). In the epididymis fluid is adsorbed and spermatozoa concentrated 100-fold. The epididymis then adds critical secretory products including fructose, carnitine, and glycoproteins.
7. After the epididymis spermatozoa enter the vas deferens. The normal vas deferens serves as a storage compartment for spermatozoa. Ejaculated spermatozoa are carried to the female tract in seminal plasma. The combination of spermatozoa and seminal plasma are called semen. The seminal plasma provides nutritional factors such as fructose and sorbitol, an alkaline buffer and lubricant to sperm.

Chapter 11

Erection and Ejaculation

Erection

Erection can be promoted by psychological stimuli, by visual cues and by erotic imagery. These neurological sensations are developed in the paraventricular shaft nucleus of the hypothalamus of the brain [1,2]. The paraventricular shaft nucleus sends a signal through the central and peripheral autonomic nervous system to the corpus cavernosum and corpus spongiosum of the penis. Also, a tactile stimulation of the penis and surrounding area can cause erection of the penis; they signal the paraventricular shaft nucleus and in turn signal the genitalia. Research indicates that activation of the paraventricular shaft nucleus occurs by dopamine and its agonists, excitatory amino acids (N-methyl-D-aspartic acid) or oxytocin itself, or by electrical stimulation leading to penile erection.

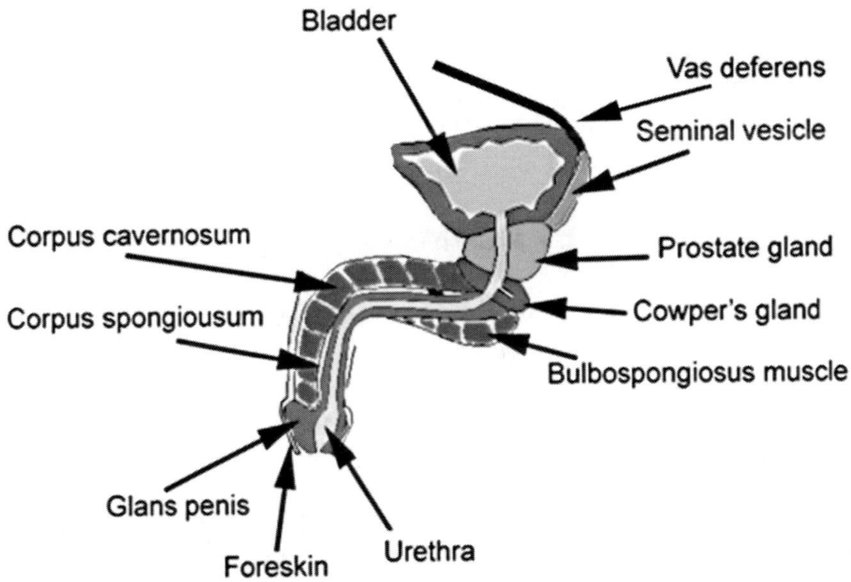

Figure 11.1. Anatomy of male reproductive system.

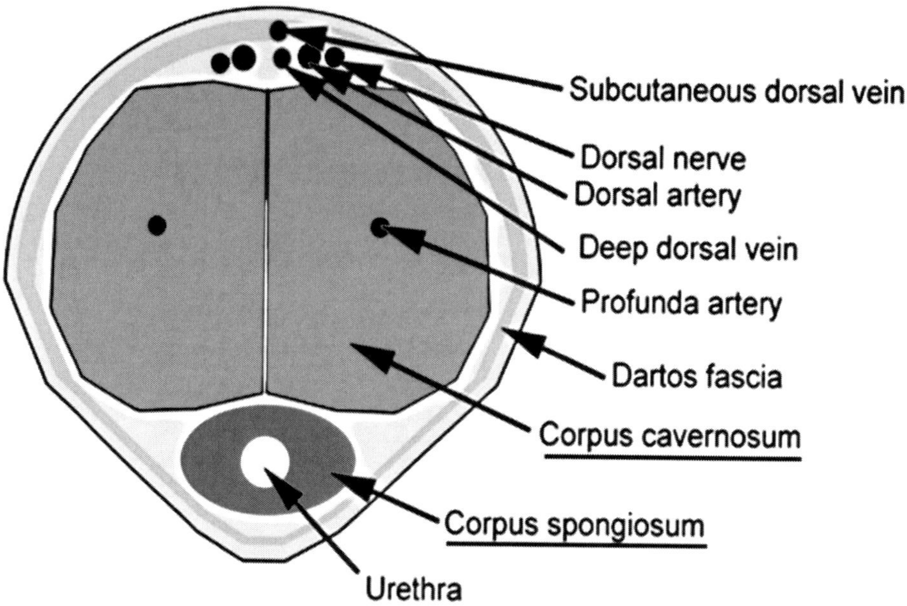

Figure 11.2. Transverse cut through shaft of penis.

The two corpus cavernosa provide most of the erection of the penis (see Figures 11.1 and 11.2). Erection is aided by the corpus spongiosum (see Figures 11.1 and 11.2). Examining how a flaccid penis becomes fully erect; the nerve signal from the paraventricular shaft nucleus is received by parasympathetic and sympathetic nerves on the smooth muscle surrounding the internal pudendal artery and left and right profunda arteries feeding the penis. The smooth muscles contract on the arteries causing dilation and an increased blood flow to the two corpus cavernosa and corpus spongiosum of the penis (Figure 11.2). Additionally the arteriovenous shunts direct blood to the corpus cavernosa. The events change the corpus cavernosa from low volume, low pressure chambers into high volume, high pressure chambers, erecting the penis. The corpus spongiosum increases in pressure in a similar fashion. Its slightly lower pressure protects the urethra from the pressures of erection.

Ejaculation

As ejaculation approaches, the pressures in the corpus cavernosa and corpus spongiosum, or the extent of erection, increases further. Firstly, the scrotal skin contracts due to the contraction of the dartos muscle. With further stimulation a sequence of contraction occurs; the muscle of the prostate, vas deferens and seminal vesicles expel the spermatozoa and seminal plasma together into the urethra. This is the result of a hypothalamus paraventricular nucleus shaft sympathetic nervous system reaction [3-6]. Expulsion of the seminal plasma-spermatozoa mix or semen, or ejaculation, is achieved by coordinated contraction of the smooth muscles lining the urethra, the bulbocavernous muscles, and multiple muscles of the pelvic floor.

At ejaculation the cardiovascular system changes; muscle spasms occur, together with hyperventilation [7,8]. The orgasm that can occur is associated with sexual tension and arousal. These are suddenly released, leading to an intense sensation of pleasure. Significant brain dopamine release occurs; endorphin release along with the release of posterior pituitary oxytocin. This together creates the intense sensation of pleasure. Males commonly feel tired after intercourse and want to go to sleep. This is because of the amount of exercise involved in intercourse and the release of endorphins during intercourse, which leads to sleep.

References

[1] Argiolas A, Melis MR. Central control of penile erection: role of the paraventricular nucleus of the hypothalamus. *Prog Neurobiol* 2005;76:1-21.

[2] Chen KK, Chang LS. Involvement of L-arginine/nitric oxide pathway at the paraventricular nucleus of hypothalamus in central neural regulation of penile erection in the rat. *Nature* 2002;14:139-145.

[3] Ackerman AE, Lange GM, Clemens LG. Effects of paraventricular lesions on sex behavior and seminal emission in male rats. *Physiol Behav* 1997;63:49-53.

[4] Eaton RC, Markowski VP, Lumley LA, Thompson JT, Moses J, Hull EM. D2 receptors in the paraventricular nucleus regulate genital responses and copulation in male rats. *Pharmacol Biochem Behav* 1991;39:177-181.

[5] Luiten PG, Horst GJ, Karst H, Steffens AB. The course of paraventricular hypothalamic efferents to autonomic structures in medulla and spinal cord. *Brain Res* 1985;329:374-378.

[6] Goldstein I. The Central Mechanisms of Sexual Function. http://www.bumc.bu.edu/sexualmedicine/publications/the-central-mechanisms-of-sexual-function/

[7] Hatzimouratidis K, Amar E, Eardley I, Giuliano F, Hatzichristou D, Montorsi F, Vardi Y, Wespes E. Guidelines on male sexual dysfunction: erectile dysfunction and premature ejaculation. *Eur Urol.* 2010 May;57:804-814.

[8] Ekland MB, Krassioukov AV, McBride KE, Elliott SL. Incidence of autonomic dysreflexia and silent autonomic dysreflexia in men with spinal cord injury undergoing sperm retrieval: implications for clinical practice. *J Spinal Cord Med* 2008;31:33-39.

Key Points

1. The two corpus cavernosa provide most of the erection of the penis. Erection is aided by the corpus spongiosum. Examining how a flaccid penis becomes fully erect; the nerve signal from the limbic system is received by parasympathetic and sympathetic nerves on the smooth muscle surrounding the internal pudendal artery and left and right profunda arteries feeding the penis. The smooth muscles contract on the arteries causing dilation and an increased blood flow to the two corpus cavernosa and corpus spongiosum of the penis
2. As ejaculation approaches, the pressures in the corpus cavernosa and corpus spongiosum, or the extent of erection, increase further. Firstly, the scrotal skin

contracts due to contraction of the dartos muscle. With further stimulation a sequence of contraction occurs; the muscle of the prostate, vas deferens and seminal vesicles expel the spermatozoa and seminal plasma together into the urethra. This is the result of a sympathetic nervous system reaction. Expulsion of the seminal plasma-spermatozoa mix or semen, or ejaculation, is achieved by coordinated contraction of the smooth muscles lining the urethra, the bulbocavernous muscles, and multiple muscles of the pelvic floor.

Chapter 12

Coitus

Sex

Animal species are specialized into male and female. Each is a gender or each is a sex. Sexual reproduction involves the mixing of genetic traits, specialized cells known as gametes, from each parent or each gender. Gametes can be asymmetric such that two sex-specific types of gametes exist. The male gametes or spermatozoon are small, motile, and designed to transport their genetic information over a distance, while the female gametes, the ova, are large, non-motile and contain the ingredients needed for the development of the organism. The male gamete carries an X or Y haploid half-set of chromosomes, while the female gamete carries an X or X haploid half-set of chromosomes.

The combination of gamete haploid sets at fertilization, X and Y, produces a male organism, while the combination of haploid sets, X and X, generates a female organism. Major physical differences are associated with the different sexes of an organism; these sexual dimorphisms reflect the different reproductive pressures the sexes experience.

Both males and females have distinct regions of the brain associated with sexual reactions. In females, the sexual dimorphic nucleus of the hypothalamus responds to stimulation by androgens and controls sexual libido. The amygdala of the temporal lobe responds directly to visual sexual stimulation in the female. In men, testosterone and the sexual dimorphic nucleus of the hypothalamus controls sexual libido. Meanwhile, the paraventricular nucleus of the hypothalamus and sympathetic nervous system controls penis erection and penis ejaculation. The amygdala of the temporal lobe is also important in controlling male sexual visual stimulation.

What is sex? Is it gender, is it sexual interaction or is it a combination thereof? The English language dictionary considers both definitions valid. From a scientific perspective it is all the complex biological processes by which a woman makes ova and a man makes spermatozoa, how spermatozoa and ova meet, and how humans generate a pregnancy.

Sexual reproduction evolved about one billion years ago as an ingenious means of creating sexual dimorphism and hyper-prolific organisms. The reason for the initial evolution of sex is considered to be a means to generate wide variation among offspring, or a means to inject into every organism the genes of two separate and independent parents.

Sex, Medical Problems

There is a wide mixture of common male sexual probems. Help should be sought from a sex clinic, a sex specialist or a urologist. One such problem is erectile dysfunction, or failure of erection, most commonly due to medications taken. This may affect 1 in 10 men. It may be aided by simple over-the-counter medication like Viagra and Cialis. Other problems include premature ejaculation. This occurs when a man experiences orgasms and expels semen soon after sexual activity and with minimal penile stimulation. This requires the help of a sex specialist to find means of controlling ejaculation. Another problem is delayed ejaculation or retarded ejaculation, or inability to ejaculate. This affects about 8% of men, and is commonly due to pituitary or thyroid problems or psychological factors. Commonly, masturbation may cause delayed ejaculation, with the development of masturbation criterion for ejaculation. Many of these problems can be helped by a sex specialist or sex clinic.

Other problems include retrograde ejaculation, in which a man ejaculates sperm backwards into the bladder rather than out of the penis. This can result from hypertension, drug use and prostate medications. In these cases semen can be detected in a man's urine. To finish, there is no question that good sex, with the penis ejaculating deep into the vagina, has the highest likelihood of generating a pregnancy.

Intercourse problems do not stop with the male. The female may have vaginitis limiting intercourse, as described in Chapter 31. This can be bacterial vaginosis, yeast infection, or trichomoniasis, a parasite infection. The general symptom is a vaginal discharge, odorous discharge, itching and painful intercourse. Other female problems include failure of the ovum cortical granules to prevent polyspermic fertilization. The result can be partial hydatidiform mole (see Chapter 18), or failure of meiosis which can also lead to a hydatidiform mole (see Chapter 18) or genetic abnormality (see Chapter 26).

References

[1] Stanislavov R, Nikolova V. Treatment of erectile dysfunction with pycnogenol and L-arginine. *J Sex Marital Ther* 2003;29:207-213.

[2] Csoka AB, Bahrick A, Mehtonen OP. Persistent sexual dysfunction after discontinuation of selective serotonin reuptake inhibitors. *J Sex Med* 2008;5:227-233.

[3] Choi HK, Seong DH, Rha KH. Clinical efficacy of Korean red ginseng for erectile dysfunction. *Int J Impot Res* 1995;7:181-186.

[4] Aversa A, Rossi F, Francomano D, Bruzziches R, Bertone C, Santiemma V, Spera G. Early endothelial dysfunction as a marker of vasculogenic erectile dysfunction in young habitual cannabis users. *Int J Impot Res* 2008;20:566-573.

[5] Erectile dysfunction. http://www.nlm.nih.gov/medlineplus/erectiledysfunction.html

[6] Richardson D, Nalabanda A, Goldmeier D. Retarded ejaculation - a review. *Int J STD AIDS* 2006;17:143-150.

Key Points

1. Sex evolved as a means of generating wide variation among offspring.
2. Problems with injecting sperm in a woman's vagina range from male erectile dysfunction to premature ejaculation, to delayed or retarded ejaculation, to retrograde ejaculation.

Conception, Sex and Fertility

Chapter 13

Sex and the Brain

Introduction

We have noted so far how steroids - most notably testosterone, a mostly unconjugated steroid not bound by proteins - stimulate libido in male and female brains. As noted previously (Chapter 9), it acts on the sexual dimorphic nucleus in the preoptic area of the hypothalamus.

As also noted (Chapter 11), males use the paraventricular shaft nucleus in the hypothalamus to control erection, or a further sexual stimulus. Stimuli able to promote sexual interaction affect us all day long. Yet only occasionally does sexual interaction occur. In humans, social factors, attraction factors and desire factors of the brain control when these sexual stimuli should be active. Here we examine what is known about sexual interaction, steroids and brain nuclei in humans.

Action of Steroid Hormones on Men

Testosterone is the key hormone in men; it controls sexual libido, being "turned on," and many sexual sensations. Testosterone is also important to permit nocturnal erections to occur. If a man is castrated or has the pituitary gland removed he will stop producing testosterone. While disappearance of testosterone in plasma can be shown just hours after castration, sexual sensation will disappear slowly over months. Testosterone therapy has been used successfully to treat hypogonadal or agonadal men.

Testosterone controlled sexual libido has been shown to be due to how testosterone crosses the blood-brain barrier, and modulates the sexual dimorphic nucleus in the preoptic area of the hypothalamus of the brain (Figure 13.1).

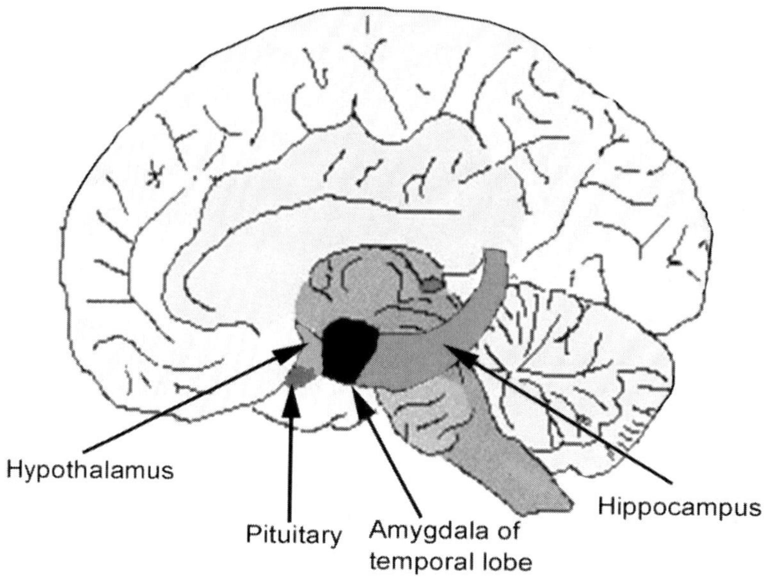

Figure 13.1. Human brain showing hypothalamus and temporal lobe amygdale.

Action of Steroid Hormone on Women

Just as men lose libido and sexuality upon the loss of testosterone, a woman largely loses most of her libido and sexuality after a bilateral oophorectomy or upon menopause. This can be fully recovered by administering testosterone.

Recent research shows that testosterone may be the principal controller of libido and sexuality in women. Research suggests that testosterone and its weak counterpart androstenedione may actually be the controlling agents in women. It is recommended today that testosterone be given to women with a lack of sexuality due to menopause or oophorectomy.

Testosterone in women, like testosterone in men, modulates the sexual dimorphic nucleus in the preoptic area of the hypothalamus of the brain (Figure 13.1). Women have much lower circulating concentrations of testosterone than men (Normal concentrations are 3190 – 9560 pg/ml in postpuberty men and have a mean of 225 pg/ml in postpuberty women). Clearly the lower concentrations in women elicit a feminine sexual reaction.

Role of Sexually Dimorphic Nucleus in Preoptic Area of Hypothalamus

An area of the brain has been clearly associated with libido and sexuality; this is the sexually dimorphic nucleus in the preoptic area of the hypothalamus (see Figure 13.1).

The figure shows the pituitary gland and the associated hypothalamus directly above it.

For orientation, the hypothalamus is at the bottom of the brain.

As demonstrated, the sexually dimorphic nucleus in the preoptic area of the hypothalamus is an area rich in androgen receptors. In a castrated primate, implantation of testosterone into the sexually dimorphic nucleus in the preoptic area of the hypothalamus restores libido and sexuality. Research suggests that ß-endorphins and dopamine may be released by the sexually dimorphic nucleus in the preoptic area of the hypothalamus, and may explain the neural mechanisms underlying sexual behavior. It is noteworthy that the volume of the sexual region of the sexually dimorphic nucleus in the preoptic area of the hypothalamus is larger in volume in males compared to females. The large size may be due to the higher concentration of testosterone levels in males than in females. No size relationship has been demonstrated in homosexual males and females.

In summary, androgens are the principal stimulator of libido and sexuality in males and females. Androgens act on the brain, on the sexually dimorphic nucleus in the preoptic area of the hypothalamus, promoting libido and sexuality. Upon menopause, when a women loses the source of estrogens, she can lose libido and sexuality. This can be reversed with estrogen or testosterone treatment. The pathway of estrogen controlled libido and sexuality in females is unclear.

Role of Paraventricular Shaft Nucleus

The sexually dimorphic nucleus in the preoptic area of the hypothalamus may control human libido, but it is not the only sexually active area of the brain. The paraventricular shaft nucleus in the hypothalamus of the brain controls male erection in response to sexual attraction (Figure 13.1). It also controls ejaculation as part of the erection process. It appears that the sexually dimorphic nucleus works jointly with the paraventricular shaft nucleus. The sexually dimorphic nucleus absorbs the attraction and libido response. Then the paraventricular nucleus causes an erection.

Role of Amygdala in Temporal Lobe

The amygdala in the temporal lobe is approximately the size of an almond (Figure 13.1). Multiple studies using MRI technology show that the amygdala of the temporal lobe of the brain is also involved in human sexual responses. When men are shown pornographic pictures of naked women, or are stimulated by naked women, significant activity can be demonstrated in the amygdala region. Similarly, when women are shown pictures of naked men, or are stimulated by naked men, activity can be demonstrated in the amygdala. It appears that the amygdala is the region of the brain that responds to visual sexual stimulation. This is not surprising since the amygdala is a region that deals with powerful emotions.

Research shows that significantly greater activity can be detected in men's amygdala, in response to the stimulus of naked women, than in women's amygdala in response to naked men. This is consistent with psychological findings, that men are generally more interested in and responsive to visual sexually arousing stimuli than are women.

References

[1] Boloña ER, Uraga MV, Haddad RM, Tracz MJ, Sideras K, Kennedy CC, Caples SM, Erwin PJ, Montori VM. Testosterone use in men with sexual dysfunction: a systematic review and meta-analysis of randomized placebo-controlled trials. *Mayo Clin Proc* 2007;82:20-28.

[2] Low testosterone. http://www.nlm.nih.gov/medlineplus/tutorials/lowtestosterone/ ur189103.pdf

[3] A Jiang M, Xin J, Zou Q, Shen JW. Research on the relationship between ejaculation and serum testosterone level in men. *J Zhejiang Univ Sci* 2003;4:236-240.

[4] van Anders SM. Testosterone and sexual desire in healthy women and men. *Arch Sex Behav* 2012;41:1471-1484.

[5] Burger HG, Papalia MA. A clinical update on female androgen insufficiency - testosterone testing and treatment in women presenting with low sexual desire. *Sex Health* 2006;3:73-78.

[6] Shifren JL, Braunstein GD, Simon JA, Casson PR, Buster JE, Redmond GP, Burki RE, Ginsburg ES, Rosen RC, Leiblum SR, Caramelli KE, Mazer NA. Transdermal testosterone treatment in women with impaired sexual function after oophorectomy. *N Engl J Med* 2000;343:682-688.

[7] Döhler KD, Srivastava SS, Shryne JE, Jarzab B, Sipos A, Gorski RA. Differentiation of the sexually dimorphic nucleus in the preoptic area of the rat brain is inhibited by postnatal treatment with an estrogen antagonist. *Neuroendocrinol* 1984;38:297-301.

[8] Gorski RA, Harlan RE, Jacobson CD, Shryne JE, Southam AM. Evidence for the existence of a sexually dimorphic nucleus in the preoptic area of the rat. *J Comp Neurol* 1980;193:529-539.

[9] Argiolas A, Melis MR. Central control of penile erection: role of the paraventricular nucleus of the hypothalamus. *Prog Neurobiol* 2005;76:1-21.

[10] Chen KK, Chan JY, Chang LS. Dopaminergic neurotransmission at the paraventricular nucleus of hypothalamus in central regulation of penile erection in the rat. *J Urol* 1999;162:237-242.

[11] Hamann S, Herman RA, Nolan CL, Wallen K. Men and women differ in amygdala response to visual sexual stimuli. *Nat Neurosci* 2004;7:411-416.

[12] Cahill L, Haier RJ, White NS, Fallon J, Kilpatrick L, Lawrence C, Potkin SG, Alkire MT. Sex-related difference in amygdala activity during emotionally influenced memory storage. *Neurobiol Learn Mem* 2001;75:1-9.

Key Points

1. Testosterone promotes sexual libido and sexuality in men. An androgen (testosterone or androstenedione) or estradiol controls sexual libido and sexuality in women.

2. Androgens act on receptors in the sexually dimorphic nucleus in the preoptic area of the hypothalamus in the brain to promote sexual libido and sexuality in men and women.
3. The amygdala of the temporal lobe responds to visual sexual signals, as does the paraventricular shaft nucleus in men which controls erection of the penis and ejaculation.

Chapter 14

Fertility and Infertility

Introduction

In this chapter, the fertility of an individual or couple is defined as the ease of becoming pregnant. The fertility rate of the population is defined as the number of births per woman. Fecundability is defined as the chances of a women becoming pregnant in any menstrual cycle.

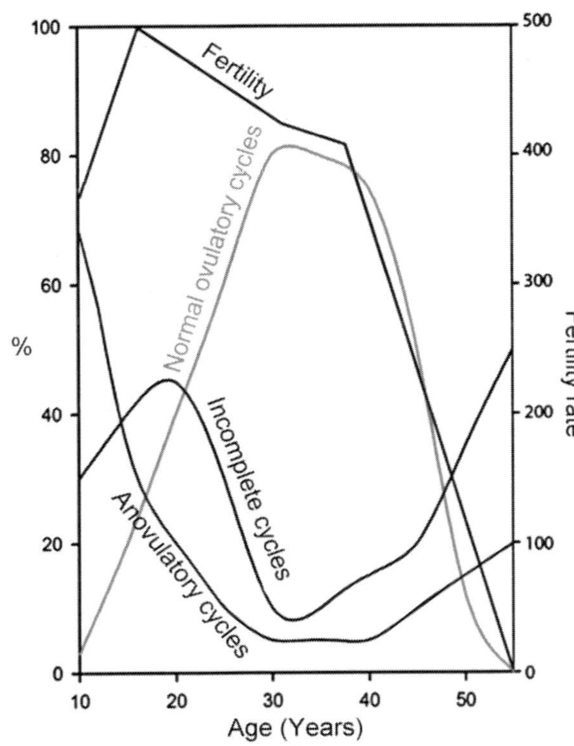

Figure 14.1. Normality of menstrual cycles and ovulation in females with age.

Fecundity is the probability of achieving a live birth in any one menstrual cycle. Fecundity and fecundability both decrease over time. Statistically, as long as a young couple are in their twenties and are having frequent intercourse, the odds of achieving pregnancy in any one menstrual cycle is 20-25% (Figure 14.1). After 12 months without using contraception, approximately 50% of couples will conceive. If a couple does not conceive by this point, then infertility is likely. Eighty-five percent of infertile couples who undergo treatment can expect to have a child.

Conception requires a series of events to occur perfectly: 1. Ovulation of a valid oocyte; 2. Production of valid spermatozoa; 3. Successful capacitation and acrosome reaction of spermatozoa (see Chapter 16); 4. Association of spermatozoa and the oocyte and subsequent fertilization; 5. Generation of a viable embryo; 6. Transport of the embryo into the uterine cavity; 7. Successful implantation of the blastocyst into the decidua. Overall, infertility affects 15% of reproductive age couples in the United States. Of these, female factors are responsible for 65% of cases, male factors for 35% of cases.

Female Fertility

In women fertility varies greatly with age (Figure 14.1). Menstrual cycles may start as early as 12 years of age with menarche. However, the majority of menstrual cycles from 12 years of age to approximately 15 years of age may be inactive or anovulatory menstrual cycles (Figure 14.1).

As shown in Figure 14.1, fertility or the ease of becoming pregnant is highest in women in their early twenties. At this time women are producing the best quality or most fertile eggs and are ovulating almost every menstrual cycle. As women age, in their thirties, they may have the most normal menstrual cycles (Figure 13.1), but their fertility will have dropped significantly. Today, few women purposely get pregnant at 20 years of age, when their fertility is highest (Figure 14.1). Increasing numbers of women are purposely achieving pregnancy in their thirties, or at a time when their fertility is lower. Fertility and fecundability drop dramatically after age 40 (Figure 14.1). This age is marked by decreased fertility, and increased incidence of irregular menstrual cycles with a short luteal phase (Figure 14.1). After age 45, fertility is very low, menstrual cycles can become very irregular, and women are subject to a higher incidence of anovulatory menstrual cycles. If such a woman achieves pregnancy, the risk of a genetically abnormal pregnancy such as trisomy 21 or Down syndrome pregnancy is at its highest. The risk of spontaneous abortion or miscarried pregnancy is also at its highest. At age 45 a woman is normally entering perimenopause, marked by irregular menstrual cycles or oligomenorrhea (see Chapter 29). Perimenopause is marked by high FSH (>30 mIU/ml) due to poor steroid feedback to the hypothalamus, high LH and detectable hCG (>2 mIU/ml).

After age 45, women can still get pregnant, if an egg is donated, and may carry a pregnancy until term. The issues of perimenopause and menopause are dealt with in Chapter 29. In summary, it is most ideal if a woman tries to achieve pregnancy in her twenties, when she has the most fertile eggs and is ovulating almost every menstrual cycle. It is ideal from the perspective of fertility, in that it will be the easiest time to achieve pregnancy. It is also ideal from the perspective of pregnancy, with lower chances of a failing pregnancy or a trisomy or genetically abnormal pregnancy (Chapter 26).

Female Infertility

It is important to realize that infertility may be due to a mixture of factors in any one woman, or in men and women. To evaluate infertility a careful history needs to be taken. You need to consider other factors that may be involved, such as medical disorders, the medication a woman takes, sexual dysfunction, tobacco use and drug use.

A history of regular menses suggests ovulatory cycle problems as a source of infertility. Many women may experience characteristic symptoms associated with ovulation and the formation of a corpus luteum and production of progesterone. These include pelvic discomfort during the latter half of the menstrual cycle, fullness and tenderness of the breasts, decreased vaginal secretions, abdominal bloating and slight increase in weight during the latter half of the menstrual cycle. The symptoms are rarely found in anovulatory women. Two tests prove that ovulation is occurring; one is the basal body temperature test, showing an increase in body temperature by 0.6° F during progesterone production in the luteal phase of the menstrual cycle. Second, there is serum luteinizing hormone (LH) or home urine LH tests showing that the LH peak occurred immediately prior to ovulation.

A common cause of ovulatory dysfunction in reproductive age women is polycystic ovary syndrome (PCOS) and follicular and luteal cysts (see Chapter 7). Women with these cystic disorders generally present with oligomenorrhea, and women with PCOS present with hyperandrogenism. Furthermore, some infertile women present with primary amenorrhea, or lack of a menstrual cycle. Causes of primary amenorrhea include pregnancy and neuroendocrine failure. Neuroendocrine failure may be from failure of the pituitary to produce human chorionic gonadotropin (hCG), LH and follicle stimulating hormone (FSH), due to a gonadotropinoma, the most common form of pituitary tumor or microadenoma. Alternatively, it may be from failure of the hypothalamus to produce pulsed gonadotropin releasing hormone (GnRH), due to hypothalamic dysfunction, caused by stress, or hypothalamic tumor. Primary amenorrhea may be the consequence of a genetic abnormality, such as Turner's syndrome (see Chapters 15 and 26), or from SRY genetic abnormalities such as $46,XX^{SRY}$ or $46,XY^{-SRY}$ (see Chapters 14 and 25), or due to the absence of genitalia as observed with testicular feminizing syndrome.

The pelvic anatomy should be assessed in an infertility evaluation. Uterine anatomic abnormalities are rare and are not common causes of infertility. The fallopian tubes need to be evaluated by laparoscopy or hysterosalpingography. Pelvic adhesions occur, preventing the oocyte or fertilized oocyte from entering the uterus. Pelvic adhesions primarily occur due to pelvic inflammatory disease or endometriosis (see Chapter 31). The sequelae of any of the processes can include fallopian tube scarring or obstructions, which can cause infertility.

Treatments for female infertility include ovulation stimulation using clomiphene citrate. Clomiphene citrate is an estrogen receptor inhibitor. It limits estrogen feedback to the hypothalamus leading to enlarged GnRH pulses. The enlarged GnRH pulses cause an hCG and LH peak which promotes ovulation and ovulation-related processes. Ultrasound can show the presence of a dominant follicle or Graafian follicle in a woman around day 11-12 of a menstrual cycle. hCG can then be administered by subcutaneous injection and cause ovulation. In some cases exogenous gonadotropin are administered, or controlled ovarian hyperstimulation. Purified human menopausal gonadotropins or a combination of placental hCG or LH, and FSH is administered to push the ovary through a complete menstrual cycle.

Intrauterine insemination is needed in some infertility cases. Assisted reproductive technologies can be considered; most notably, in vitro fertilization. This can bypass obstructed fallopian tubes in an infertile woman.

Male Fertility

Spermatozoa can be produced by men whether they are young or old, extending into their eighties. Erectile dysfunction, loss of libido and failure to achieve to orgasm occur commonly in men as they climb through their 40s, 50s, 60s and 70s. The use of Viagra and other popular drugs can improve erectile dysfunction in men with a solid libido. Testosterone normally remains elevated in men from their teens to their twenties and on to their eighties. As discussed in the previous chapter, testosterone maintains libido and sexuality through its actions with the sexually dimorphic nucleus of the hypothalamus.

Numerous studies show, however, that sperm count and sperm motility decline approximately two-fold with age, from <35 years age to >55 years age. With this decline comes a significant drop in fertility. Older men's sperm also has a higher risk of genetic abnormality generating Apert syndrome (skull malformations coming from the premature fusion of the skull bones) and approximately 20 other genetic abnormalities. All told, men may not enter menopause, and have consistent testosterone blood levels throughout their lives. Men may develop erectile dysfunction, loss of libido and failure to achieve an orgasm with advancing age. However, spermatozoa, although produced from puberty until late in life, do go downhill with age. Male fertility declines with age.

Male Infertility

Male infertility is quite common. As such, it is important to perform a masturbated semen analysis on the partner at the same time as the female is being evaluated. The standard semen analysis evaluates the quantity of spermatozoa and the quality or motility of spermatozoa.

Table 14.1 shows the common causes of abnormal semen in a semen analysis. Abnormalities of spermatogenesis are a major cause of male infertility. Unlike oocytes, which undergo development in a cyclic manner, spermatozoa are being produced constantly by the testis. Further evaluation of the infertile male may include endocrine analysis and genetic testing. Endocrine evaluation should examine LH, FSH and testosterone. Genetic testing is indicated in men with azoospermia or no spermatozoa. The most common genetic abnormalities include gene mutations in the cystic fibrosis transmembrane regulator, and sex chromosome abnormalities or microdeletions.

Table 14.1. Cause of abnormal semen analysis

Semen analysis finding	Cause
Small semen volume	Ejaculatory dysfunction
	Hypogonadism
Acidic semen	Ejaculatory duct obstruction
	Congenital absence of vas deferens or seminal vesicles
Azoospermia (no spermatozoa) or	Endocrine disorder
Oligospermia (low sperm count)	Genetic disorder
	Variocele
	Cryptorchidism
	Infection
	Medications
	Genital tract obstruction
Decreased motility	Partial genital tract obstruction
	Prolonged abstinence
	Sperm structural defect
Abnormal morphology	Varicocele
	Genetic disorder
	Infection
	Medications

References

[1] Ho KY, Evans WS, Blizzard RM, Veldhuis JD, Merriam GR, Samojlik E, Furlanetto R, Rogol AD, Kaiser DL, Thorner MO. Effects of sex and age on the 24-hour profile of growth hormone secretion in man: importance of endogenous estradiol concentrations. *J Clin Endocrinol Metab* 1987;64:51-58.

[2] Pakkenberg B, Gundersen HJ. Neocortical neuron number in humans: effect of sex and age. *J Comp Neurol* 1997;384:312-320.

[3] Dunson DB, Baird DD, Colombo B. Increased infertility with age in men and women. *Obstet Gynecol.* 2004;103:51-56.

[4] Liu K, Case AJ, Cheung AP, Sierra S, AlAsiri S, Carranza-Mamane B, Case A, Dwyer C, Graham J, Havelock J, Hemmings R, Lee F, Liu K, Murdock W, Senikas V,Vause TD, Wong BC. Advanced reproductive age and fertility. *Obstet Gynaecol Can* 2011; 33:1165-1175.

[5] Pasquali R, Patton L, Gambineri A. Obesity and infertility. *Curr Opin Endocrinol Diabetes Obes* 2007;14:482-487.

[6] Joffe M, Li Z. Male and female factors in fertility. *Am J Epidemiol* 1994;140:921-929.

[7] Crosnoe LE, Kim ED. Impact of age on male fertility. *Curr Opin Obstet Gynecol* 2013; 25:181-185.

[8] Frank O, Bianchi PG, Campana A. The end of fertility: age, fecundity and fecundability in women. *J Biosoc Sci* 1994;26:349-368.

[9] Dunson DB, Colombo B, Baird DD. Changes with age in the level and duration of fertility in the menstrual cycle. *Hum Reprod* 2002;17:1399-1403.

[10] Chart: The effect of age on fertility. http://www.babycenter.com/0_chart-the-effect-of-age-on-fertility_6155.bc

Key Points

1. Female fertility is very dependent upon age. A female is most fertile in her 20s, and may enter perimenopause in her 40s.
2. PCOS or ovarian cysts are a common cause of infertility in women. Fallopian tube anatomy needs to be evaluated by laparoscopy. Pelvis adhesions or obstructions cause infertility.
3. Clomiphene citrate is a useful method for promoting ovulation. hCG injection can directly promote ovulation. In vitro fertilization can be considered in women with pelvic adhesion causing fallopian tube obstruction.
4. A male produces testosterone and spermatozoa for the duration of life, from puberty until old age. Data suggest, however, that spermatozoa count and motility may decline approximately two-fold with age. Men may also develop erectile dysfunction, libido and orgasm failures with age.
5. Endocrine disorders, genetic disorders, and varicocele are causes of infertility in men.

Chapter 15

Sexuality, Heterosexuality and Homosexuality

Human sexuality, human heterosexuality and possible causes of human homosexuality are addressed here. This chapter examines *Male and Female Sexuality and Testosterone* and its homosexual ramifications. *The Genetics of the X and Y Chromosomes* and possible causes of sexual abnormalities and homosexuality are investigated, as are *Psychological and Youth Issues*. An overall summary is presented, *Sexuality and Homosexuality*. It is suggested that you also read Chapter 13: Sex and the Brain, and Chapter 22: Fetal gender and gonadal development to receive a full story.

Male and Female Sexuality and Testosterone

Clearly, the Mullerian and Wolffian ducts, or female and male reproductive mechanisms, develop side-by-side in fetuses (see Chapter 22). If a fetus produces testosterone the Wolffian duct or male reproductive tubes (epidydimis, prostate and are vas deferens) are developed, and the female Mullerian tubes (uterus, fallopian tubes and vagina) are degraded. If testosterone is not produced, the Mullerian duct develops, and the Wolffian duct is degenerated. Testosterone seemingly controls the sexual accessory development of a fetus (Chapter 22).

Estrogen and progesterones are commonly conjugated to proteins and cannot cross the blood-brain barrier. Testosterone and androgens are not necessarily conjugated and so can cross into the brain. Research now shows that in both men and women testosterone and related androgens act on a sexual dimorphic nucleus in the preoptic area of the hypothalamus. This drives libido or sexual attractiveness, and sexual sensations. As such, it appears that testosterone drives sexual development or sexual accessory formation in the fetus, and sexuality or sexual sensation in the adult male and female [1-10].

Normal heterosexual males have much higher circulating testosterone concentrations than heterosexual females [1-11]. Normal concentrations are 4080 – 9560 pg/ml in 25-39-year-old men and 3190 – 8660 pg/ml in 25-30-year-old men [10,11]. In contrast, concentrations have a mean of 225 pg/ml in 34-37-year-old women, and 207 pg/ml in >41-year-old women [10,11].

Taken together, circulating testosterone concentrations in heterosexual women are about 1/20th of levels in men. As published, some homosexual men have normal or high testosterone concentrations. Most homosexual men, however, have unduly low blood testosterone concentrations [6-9]. Similarly, many gay women have unduly high male-like testosterone concentrations [6-9]. Unduly high and unduly low testosterone concentrations can clearly affect human sexuality at the level of the fetus and sexual differentiations and at adult ages in terms of sexual sensation or sexual feelings. Unduly high and unduly low testosterone levels may be the result of genetic abnormality (see next section), or it may also be the result of just normal bodily endocrine extremes. As such, high natural testosterone production and low natural testosterone production may be a significant cause of homosexuality [1-10].

Both males and females can lose appropriate testosterone production due to age, menopause, pituitary problems and other issues. Males and females upon losing testosterone can lose libido, sexual sensation and in men, erection capabilities. Testosterone replacement therapy in the form of a pill or dermal gel can extensively fix these medical problems [1-10].

Genetics of the X and Y Chromosomes

In particular, the Y chromosome, or male chromosome, and its contents can affect our sexuality, and how a person can be destined to be heterosexual or homosexual. Most notably, the sex-related region of the Y chromosome (SRY) region of the Y chromosome, which includes genes for the formation of the testis, for testosterone and the formation of a penis, can very much control the sexual outcome in life.

The sex of the fetus comes from the haploid sets in the fertilized embryo. All maternal oocytes have an X chromosome. If the ovum is fertilized by an X sperm then the fetus normally has a 46,XX diploid chromosome set, and so will be female. If the ovum is fertilized by a Y sperm then the fetus normally has a 46,XY diploid chromosome set, and so will be male. Complications occur in chromosome pairing and in chromosome replication. If there is an additional chromosome 13, 18 or 21 made, then there is a trisomy. This is most commonly caused by a break in DNA on a chromosome leading to needless replication or replacement. Trisomy 13, 18 and 21 are called Patau's syndrome, Edward's syndrome and Down's syndrome, which are associated with major neurological abnormalities. An extra chromosome or trisomy and a missing chromosome or monosomy can complicate the sex chromosomes.

Turner's Syndrome (45,X) is a monosomy leading a person to have one X chromosome. This occurs in 1 in 2,500 newborn female babies. The person is most commonly phenotypically identified as a female, although is infertile. Growth and height problems, short stature, swelling of hands and feet, no sexual development and cognitive defect are common complications of this phenotype. Patients can be treated with sexual steroid hormone replacement therapy and can develop normal sexuality or homosexuality [12,13].

Triple X syndrome is a relatively common trisomy in females (47,XXX). It occurs in 1 in 1,000 newborn females. The person is phenotypically identified as a female. This syndrome has minimal complications and does not commonly interfere with menstrual cycle or fertility. Triple X can, in rare cases, cause delayed development or even ovarian or other sexual abnormalities [14].

Klinefelter's syndrome (47,XXY) is also relatively common, occurring in 1 in 1,000 newborn males. The person phenotypically is a male. The most common complications are reduced male fertility, low sperm count and small testicles. Lastly, 47,XXY also occurs at a rate of approximately 1 in 1,000 newborn males. Phenotypically, the person is a male [15,16]. While the male may have normal fertility, fast growth is common and some mental retardation is common. Klinefelter's syndrome males are unduly commonly inclined toward homosexuality [15,16].

Lastly, 47,XYY also occurs at a rate of approximately 1 in 1,000 newborn males. Phenotypically, the person is a male. While the male may have normal fertility, fast growth is common and some mental retardation is common. XYY syndrome causes aggressiveness and impulsiveness in a person, and a higher risk towards crime. An XXY syndrome male may also be more inclined towards homosexuality.

SRY is a group of genes coding for the development of the testis, the penis and testosterone, and is located at the end of the short arm of the Y chromosome; this is considered the SRY zone. If during male meiosis this group of SRY genes can be translocated from a Y chromosome to an X chromosome. An XY fetus can be generated with no SRY genes (translocated to a male X chromosome) or no signal to generate testis; no testosterone, no penis and no male characteristics [17,18]. Phenotypically, this XY fetus could be recognized at birth – wrongly - as a female (46,XY-SRY). SRY translocation problems can affect all SRY genes or just one of them. Whichever way, it can lead to sexual confusion [17,18].

Alternatively, an XX fetus with SRY translocation can get the SRY genes and the signals to make testis, generate testosterone, make a penis and have a male phenotype (46,XX+SRY) [17,18]. Such a fetus may also be wrongly identified as being male. Unfortunately, both (46,XY-SRY) mistaken females and (46,XX+SRY) mistaken males are infertile. But none have any other non-sexual, genetic or neurological problems. Studies with aborted fetuses and animals suggest that the occurrence of SRY syndromes, 46,XY-SRY females and 46,XX+SRY males may be quite high (1 in 100 pregnancies?); however, the incidence is a matter of conjecture. It has to simply be considered as a cause for sexual confusion, homosexuality, and infertility [17,18].

In male fetuses, the mullerial inhibiting signal (MIS) is coded for by a gene in the SRY segment of the Y chromosome. As such, the MIS signal can be absent in 46,XY-SRY individuals, leading to development of the Müllerian duct. In 46,XX+SRY individuals, MIS destroys the Müllerian duct leading to there being no vagina, uterus or fallopian tube. MIS signals the degeneration of the Müllerian duct. Similarly, testosterone promotes the development of the Wolffian duct, the formation of the prostate, epididymis and vas deferens [17,18].

In the female fetus, if MIS is absent, the Müllerian duct develops. The Müllerian duct induces formation of the vaginal plate which initiates formation of the vagina, fallopian tubes and uterus. The absence of testosterone leads to the degeneration of the Wolffian duct.

Unquestionably, sexual genetic errors, whether Turner's syndrome, triple X syndrome or Klinefelter's syndrome, or SRY translocation, can defeat or destroy the reproductive system leading to issues such as homosexuality [12-18].

Are genetic defects and unduly low or high testosterone production the only biological causes of homosexuality? The work of Simon LeVay, Dean Hamer, and a small group of researchers concerned to distinguish biological and genetic influences on sexual behavior has discredited much of the loose rhetoric that has been used about homosexuality. In August 1991 LeVay, a neuroscientist who now directs the Institute of Gay and Lesbian Education in southern California, published in the magazine *Science* findings from autopsies of men and women of known sexual preference [19]. He found that a tiny region in the center of the brain - the interstitial nucleus of the anterior hypothalamus (INAH) - was, on average, substantially smaller in nineteen gay men who died from AIDS than among sixteen heterosexual men [19]. Is brain development a further biologic cause of homosexuality?

Psychological and Youth Issues

Unquestionably, psychological and youth issues and stress are a third major reason for homosexuality [20-23]. Males who have negative interactions or become scared of females may become homosexuals, as can females who have negative and stress interactions with males or become scared of males [20-23].

Sexuality and Homosexuality

All told, there appear to be three basic reasons for a male or female to become homosexual rather than heterosexual; unduly high or low testosterone production, genetic trisomy, monosomy and SRY defects, and psychological, youth and stress issues [1-23]. Other possible reasons (further research is needed) include brain INAH development. Whichever the reason males choose to become homosexual, whether it is one of these three reasons, or simply choice, homosexuals are homosexuals. In the USA and many other Western countries homosexuality is accepted. In some nations, most notably Moslem nations, it is not acceptable, regardless of whether a genetic nature is proven. Medical findings and their sexual complications need to be accepted.

References

[1] Swaab DF, Chung WC, Kruijver FP, Hofman MA, Ishunina TA. Sexual differentiation of the human hypothalamus. *Adv Exp Med Biology* 2002;511:75-100.

[2] Dohler KD. The pre- and postnatal influence of hormones and neurotransmitters on sexual differentiation of the mammalian hypothalamus. *Int Rev Cytology* 1991;131:1-57.

[3] Savic I, Garcia-Falgueras A, Swaab DF. Sexual differentiation of the human brain in relation to gender identity and sexual orientation. *Prog Brain Res* 2010;186:41-62.

[4] Kula K, Slowikowska-Hilczer J. Sexual differentiation of the human brain. *Przegl Lek* 2000;57:41-44.

[5] Wu MV, Manoli DS, Fraser EJ, Coats JK, Tollkuhn J, Honda S, Harada N, Shah NM., Estrogen masculinizes neural pathways and sex-specific behaviors. *Cell* 2009;139:61-72.

[6] Balthazart J, Jani O, Ball GF. Do sex differences in the brain explain sex differences in the hormonal induction of reproductive behavior? What 25 years of research on the Japanese quail tells us. *Horm Behav* 1996;30:627-661.

[7] Low Uterine Testosterone Levels Determine Homosexual Behavior in Males. http://news.softpedia.com/news/Low-In-Utero-Testosterone-Levels-Determine-Homosexual-Behavior-in-Males-52005.shtml

[8] Starká L, Šipová I, Hynie J. Plasma testosterone in male transsexuals and homosexuals. *J Sex Res* 1976;11:134-138.

[9] Pillard RC, Rose RM, Sherwood M. Plasma testosterone levels in homosexual men. *Arch Sexual Behav* 1974;3:453-458.

[10] Zitzmann M, Nieschlag E. Testosterone levels in healthy men and the relation to behavioural and physical characteristics: facts and constructs. *Euro J Endocrinol* 2001; 144:183-197.

[11] Sowers MF, Beebe JL, McConnell D, Randolph J, Jannausch M. Testosterone Concentrations in Women Aged 25–50 Years: Associations with Lifestyle, Body Composition, and Ovarian Status. *Am J Epidemiol* 2001: 153: 256-264.

[12] Turner's syndrome. http://learn.genetics.utah.edu/content/disorders/whataregd/turner.

[13] Morgan T. Turner Syndrome: Diagnosis and Management. *Am Fam Physician* 2007;76:405-417.

[14] Lanktree MB, Fantus IG, Hegele RA. Triple X syndrome in a patient with partial lipodystrophy discovered using a high-density oligonucleotide microarray: a case report. *Journal Med Case Rep* 2009;3:8867-9969.

[15] Living With XXY/Klinefelter Syndrome. http://www.angelfire.com/wy/XXY/XXYLegacy/ MyStory.html

[16] Diamond M, Watson LA. Androgen Insensitivity Syndrome and Klinefelter's Syndrome. *Child and Adol Psych Clin N Amer* 2004;13:623-640

[17] Genomic resource centre, Genetic Components of Sex and Gender, World health organization. http://www.who.int/genomics/gender/en/index1.html.

[18] Horton R. Is homosexuality inherited? Frontline. http://www.pbs.org/wgbh/ pages/frontline/shows/assault/genetics/nyreview.html

[19] LeVay S. A Difference in hypothalamic structure between heterosexual and homosexual men. *Science* 1991;2153:1034-1037.

[20] Dorner G, Schenk B, Schmiedel B, Ahrens L. Stressful events in prenatal life of bi- and homosexual men. *Exp Clin Endocrinol* 1983;81:83-87.

[21] Parental Stress feminizes and demasculizes the behavior of males. *Science,* 1972; 83-84.

[22] Bradley SJ, Oliver GD, Chernick AB, Zucker KJ. Experiment of nurture: ablation, penis at 2 months, sex reassignment at 7 months, and a psychosexual follow-up in young adulthood. *Pediat* 1998;102:e9-e16.

[23] Beaman W, Cannizzaro L, Goldman C. The Evolution of the Medical Definition of Homosexuality. https://confluence.cornell.edu/display/WWC/The+Evolution+of+the+Medical+Definition+of+Homosexuality.

Key Points

1. Sexual abnormalities and homosexuality may be due to genetic monosomy or trisomy, Turner's syndrome, triple X syndrome or Klinefelter's syndrome. They may be due to meiotic error or SRY syndromes, with translocation of key Y chromosome gene to the X chromosome. Abnormalities may be due to overproduction or underproduction of the critical hormone testosterone, either in the fetus or in the adult. Other possibilities include brain abnormalities involving the INAH and other critical regions. Sexual abnormalities may otherwise be psychological or involving stress and childhood interactions.

Chapter 16

Sperm Activation

Coitus leads to the release of semen into the vagina and uterus. The fact that the sperm enters the vagina and uterus does not mean that it will propel its way to the ovum or that the ovum will be fertilized. If mature spermatozoa are simply incubated with oocytes *in vitro* fertilization either does not occur at all, or takes many hours to complete. If spermatozoa are taken from a uterus or fallopian tubes two hours after coitus, they are, however, capable of immediate fertilization. These sperm that have visited the uterus or fallopian tube are clearly more active or are capacitated. What we understand occurs to sperm on entering an estrogen-primed uterus or fallopian tube is called sperm capacitation. The sperm also cannot penetrate the zona pellucida or shell of an ovum without going through the acrosome reaction, a second form of activation needed for penetrating an ovum. Here we describe these two activation protocols.

Spermatozoa Capacitation

Sperm enters the vagina and proceeds through the uterus to the fallopian tube. The sperm is propelled by the movement of the flagella or the spermatozoa tail. In order for sperm to reach the fallopian tube, it must be activated or capacitated. The capacitation process has two segments that activates the sperm, boosting its propulsion and preparing it for entering the oocyte vicinity (Figure 16.1).

Firstly, (Segment 1) a change occurs in sperm capacitation in the movement characteristics of the spermatozoa, to a hyperactive state. The wave-like patterns of the sperm tail or flagella are made stronger, leading to wider amplitude strokes or much more efficient movements, when sperm are swimming in the uterus and fallopian tubes. Classically, a pre-capacitation spermatozoon appears motionless under a microscope, while a post-capicatation spermatozoon appears wiggling (Figure 15.1).

Secondly, (Segment 2) a change occurs in the surface membrane making spermatozoa responsive to signals encountered in the vicinity of the oocyte. An acrosome reaction occurs, leading to increased calcium permeability, leading to a rise in intracellular calcium levels. Calmodulin-binding proteins are stripped from the spermatozoa surface, yet again promoting calcium permeability. As a result of elevated calcium, adenyl cyclase activity within the spermatozoa rises. This leads to cyclic AMP production and to increased phosphorylation of proteins. Spermatozoa motility is enhanced accordingly (Figure 16.1).

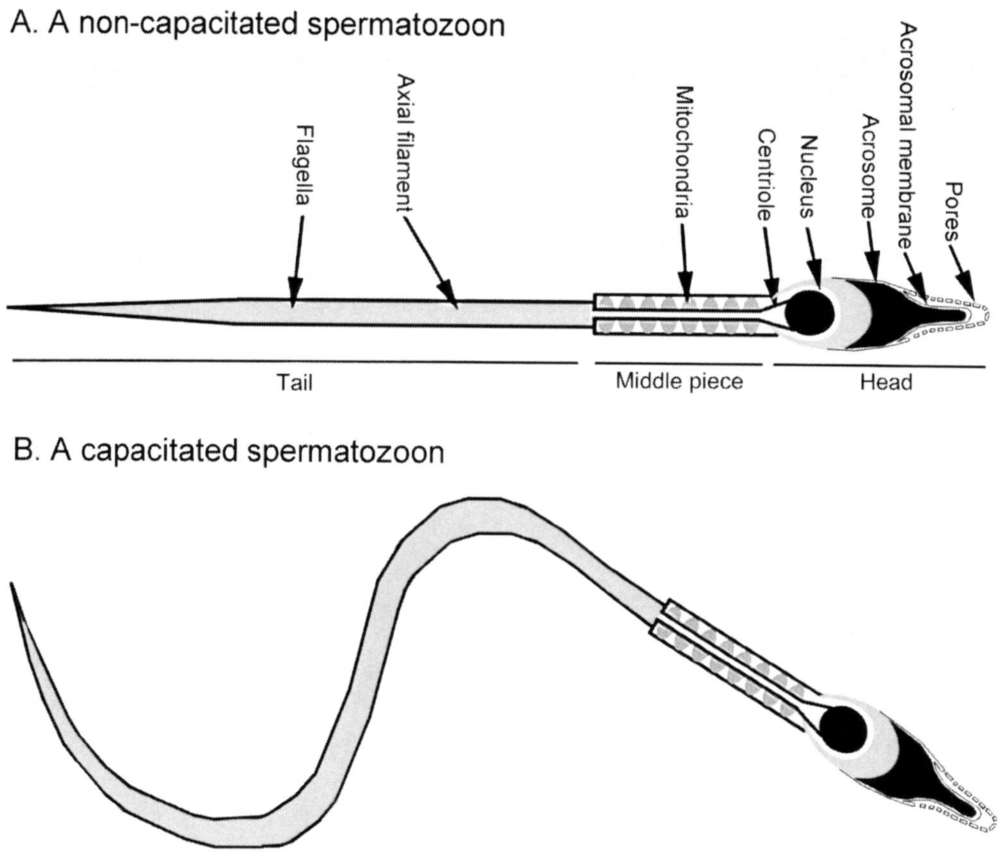

Figure 16.1. The spermatozoon and capacitation.

Spermatozoa Acrosome Reaction

As sperm comes into contact with the zona pellucida surrounding the ovum, the oocyte acrosome reaction occurs. This acrosome reaction gives the spermatozoa the needed changes to burn its way through the zona pellucida and to fertilize the oocyte. The porous membrane stuck to the head of spermatozoa swells in the acrosome reaction. The porous membrane is lost as it swells and fuses with the underlying acrosome membrane (Figure 16.2). This reaction, like spermatozoa capacitation, leads to a large increase in intracellular calcium. An agent secreted by the zona pellucida, called ZP3, activates this acrosome reaction. With the loss of the porous membrane comes the release of proteolytic enzymes such as hyaluronidase as acronsin, needed for penetration of the zona pellucida in the fertilization procedure.

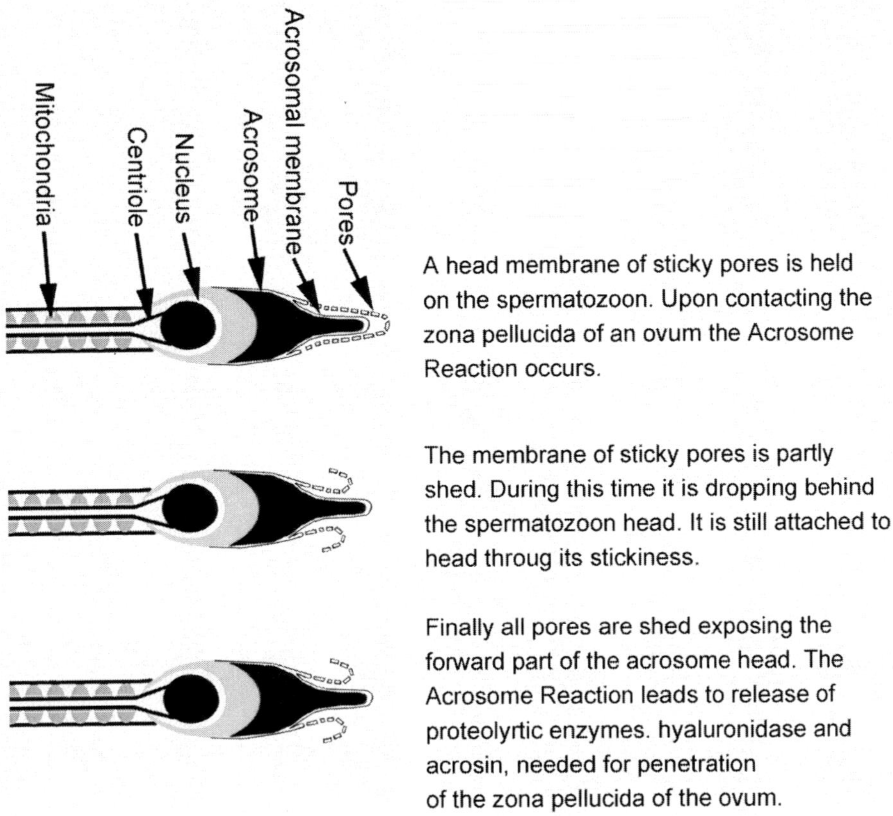

Figure 16.2. Acrosome Reaction.

References

[1] Taguma K, Nakamura C, Ozaki A, Suzuki C, Hachisu A, Kobayashi K, Mochida K, Ogura A, Kaneda H, Wakana S. A practical novel method for ensuring stable capacitation of spermatozoa from cryopreserved C57BL/6J sperm suspension. *Exp Anim* 2009;58:395-401.

[2] Parrish JJ, Susko-Parrish J, Winer MA, First NL. Capacitation of bovine sperm by heparin. *Biol Reprod* 1988;38:1171-1180.

[3] Salicioni AM, Platt MD, Wertheimer EV, Arcelay E, Allaire A, Sosnik J, Visconti PE. Signalling pathways involved in sperm capacitation. *Soc Reprod Fertil Suppl* 2007;65:245-259.

[4] Breitbart H. Intracellular calcium regulation in sperm capacitation and acrosomal reaction. *Mol Cell Endocrinol* 2002;187:139-144.

[5] Berger T, Turner KO, Meizel S, Hedrick JL. Zona pellucida-induced acrosome reaction in boar sperm. *Biol Reprod* 1989;40:525-530.

[6] Inoue N, Satouh Y, Ikawa M, Okabe M, Yanagimachi R. Acrosome-reacted mouse spermatozoa recovered from the perivitelline space can fertilize other eggs. *Proc Natl Acad Sci USA* 2011;108:20008-200011.

[7] Hoshi M, Nishigaki T, Ushiyama A, Okinaga T, Chiba K, Matsumoto M. Egg-jelly signal molecules for triggering the acrosome reaction in starfish spermatozoa. *Int J Dev Biol* 1994;38:167-174.

[8] Zeginiadou T, Papadimas J, Mantalenakis S. Acrosome reaction: methods for detection and clinical significance. *Andrologia.* 2000;32:335-343.

[9] Florman HM, Jungnickel MK, Sutton KA. Regulating the acrosome reaction. *Int J Dev Biol* 2008;52:503-510.

[10] Litscher ES, Wassarman PM. Characterization of mouse ZP3-derived glycopeptide, gp55, that exhibits sperm receptor and acrosome reaction-inducing activity in vitro. *Biochem* 1996;35:3980-3985.

Key Points

1. The fallopian tube mucosa nourishes the moving oocyte, zygote or conceptus. The smooth muscle of the fallopian tube wall constricts and contracts, leading to a vacuum-like effect in the fallopian tube, causing the propulsion of the embryo.
2. Capacitation of spermatozoa is essential for spermatozoa success in the uterus and fallopian tubes. Capacitation causes the tail to make wider and stronger movements in the uterus and fallopian tubes. It also changes the surface membrane, making spermatozoa responsive to signals received in the vicinity of the oocyte. Calcium permeability of the spermatozoa is greatly increased. This leads to cyclic AMP production and increased spermatozoa motility.
3. In order for a sperm to penetrate the zona pellucida it must go through the acrosome reaction. The acrosome membrane merges with the spermatozoa porous membrane, then becomes exteriorized. The acrosome reaction is activated by ZP3.

Chapter 17

Fertilization and Blastocyst Formation

Oocyte Propulsion through Fallopian Tube

The ovulated oocyte, surrounded by a zona pellucida and cumulus cells, is picked up after ovulation and placed in the fimbriae of the fallopian tube and transported through the fallopian tube to the uterus. The fallopian tube mucosa, or moist tissue, nourishes the moving oocyte or zygote (fertilized oocyte). Secretions from the peg cells in the fallopian tube provide nourishment to the oocyte or zygote. The smooth muscle wall of the fallopian tubes constricts and contracts providing a squeezing vaccum-like propulsion of the oocyte through the fallopian tube length. This constriction and contraction of the fallopian tube is promoted by prostaglandins and by estradiol; it effectively moves the oocyte or zygote from the ovary, through the fallopian tube to the uterus for fertilization (if not already fertilized) and implantation.

Fertilization

From the acrosome reaction the exteriorized spermatozoon membranes become proteolytic enzymes. These digest a path through the zona pellucida through which the spermatozoon passes. Penetration through the zona pellucida shell takes 5-20 minutes (Figure 17, panel 1). The head of the spermatozoon then fuses with the plasma membrane of the oocyte (Figure 17.1, panel 2). Only spermatozoon that have undergone the acrosome reaction are capable of permeating the zona pellucida and are capable of fusing with the oocyte plasma membrane. Calcium from the spermatozoon is required for the fusing process. Once fusing occurs, the spermatozoon freezes all movement. Within 1-3 minutes of fusing a dramatic increase occurs in free calcium in the oocyte. This lasts 2-3 minutes and then repeats itself in waves over and over again.

As soon as fusion occurs the oocyte becomes a zygote. The zygote must first prevent further spermatozoon from fertilizing it. Secondly, it must complete the second stage of meiosis. These remaining stages take approximately 20 hours to complete. In the follicle only the first stage of meiosis occurred, terminating in second meiotic metaphase-2. The elevated calcium waves cause the cortical granules, in the perivitelline space after a sperm penetrates the zona pellucida, to fuse (Figure 17.1 panels 1 and 2). Upon fusing the cortical granules release their contents into the perivitelline space. Among their contents are enzymes which link the glycoproteins within the zona pellucida together, cross-linking them, making the zona pellucida impenetrable to further spermatozoa.

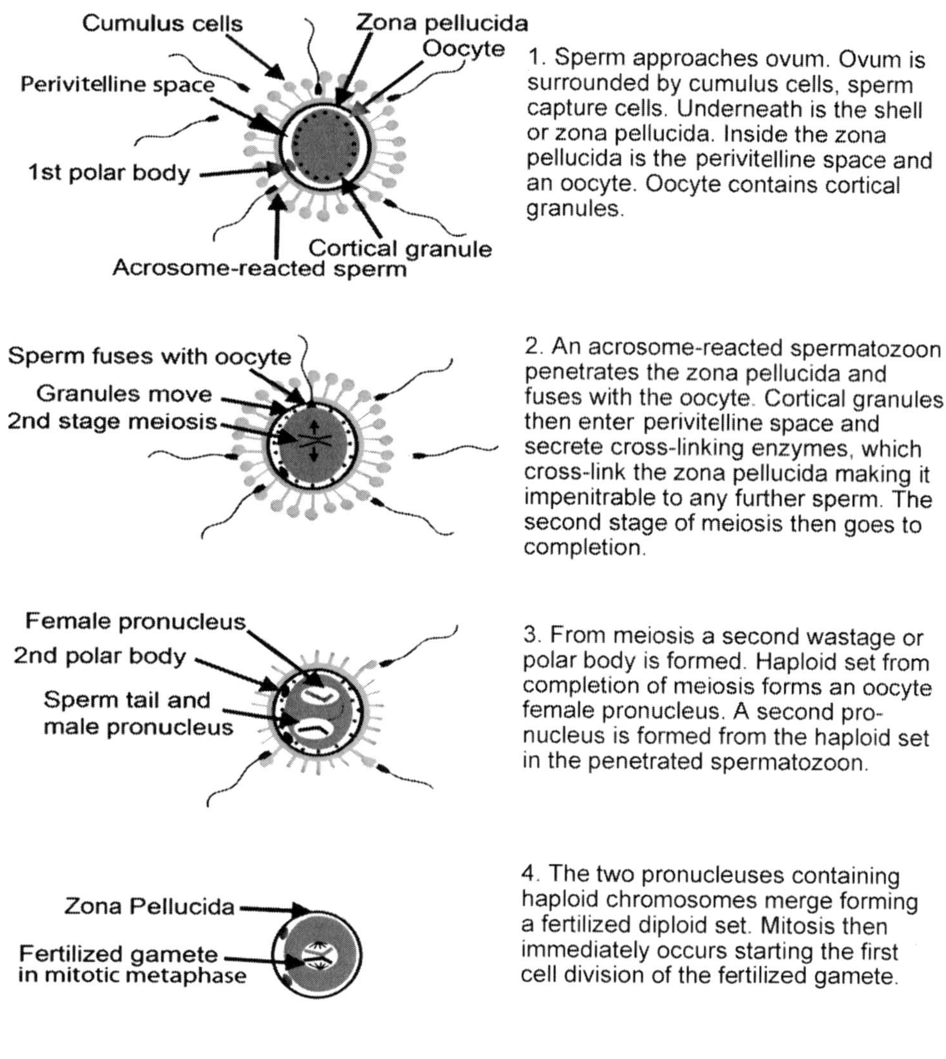

Figure 17.1. The steps of fertilization.

The arresting of meiosis in metaphase-2 in the follicle prior to ovulation is caused by failure of "maturation promoting factor (MPF)." In response to the intracellular calcium, MPF levels cause meiosis to go to completion following spermatozoon penetration. With completion of meiosis a second polar body is formed and extruded from the oocyte (Figure 17.1 panel 3). The haploid set from meiosis forms with the nuclear membrane the female pronucleus in the oocyte cell (Figure 17,1, panel 3). After the spermatozoon has entered the oocyte and the nuclear membrane has broken down, a new membrane forms around the chromatin, forming a male pronucleus in the oocyte (Figure 17.1, panel 3). At this time the male pronucleus contains the male haploid set from the spermatozoa and the female pronucleus contains the female haploid set from the oocyte. The pronuclear membranes then break down; the parental haploid sets mix in a single nucleus to make a fertilized diploid set. A mitotic metaphase spindle is formed (Figure 17.1, panel 4). Approximately 24 hours after the diploid set is formed mitosis occurs together with first cell division, making two identical cells.

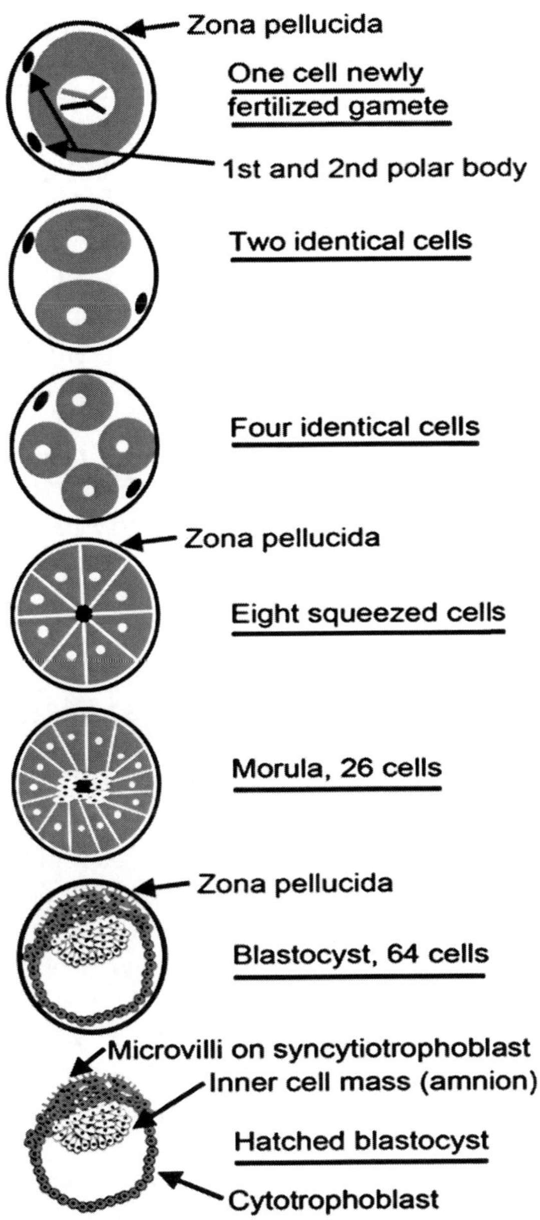

Figure 17.2. Growth of an embryo into a morula and blastocyst.

Morula and Blastocyst Formation

The zygote or conceptus then proceeds through cellular divisions. It takes approximately 1 day to go from one to two identical cells, 2 days to go from 2 cells to 4 cells, approximately 3 days to go to a 16-cell morula, and 5 days to go to a 32-cell blastocyst. During this time, the conceptus remains approximately the same size, limited by the extension of the zona pellucida. The end result is the cells becoming smaller and smaller to fit the same space (Figure 17.2). The conceptus cells produce multiple growth factors, insulin-like growth factor-1 and -2 (IGF-1 and IGF-2), transforming growth factors α, ß1 and ß2 (TGFα, TGFß1 and TGFß1), epidermal growth factor (EGF) and platelet-derived growth factor A (PDGF-A). All the growth factors are autocrine acting back on the conceptus to promote growth.

At around 8-16 cells the conceptus undergoes differentiation to form a morula (Figure 17.2). The cells divide into chorion cells (red cells shown in Figure 17.2) and amnion cells or "inner cell mass" (white cells shown in Figure 17.2). The chorion cells are destined to become the placenta trophoblast cells and the amnion cells are destined to become the fetus. Approximately two days later a blastocyst forms (Figure 17.2). The blastocyst comprises cytotrophoblast cells deriving from the morula chorion and an inner cells mass, destined to be the fetus. The trophoblast cells surround a blastocoelic cavity filled with blastocoelic fluid. The formation of blastocysts and expansion of the blastocoelic cavity is promoted by EGF and TGFa.

As the blastocyst approaches the endometrial lining, the blastocyst protective barrier, the zona pellucida is lost or hatched (Figure 17.2). There is evidence that signaling occurs between the hatched blastocyst and the endometrial wall, involving estradiol production and placental hCG released by the blastocyst. Syncytiotrophoblast cells are formed and the blastocyst grows microvilli. These microvilli are used for attachment of the blastocyst to the decidualized uterine epithelium.

Twins and Multiple Pregnancies

The zona pellucida also functions in pregnancies to prevent the conceptus from coming apart. If the conceptus does break apart forming two distinct groups of cells or multiple groups of cells, monozygotic (coming from one zygote) twins or multiple pregnancies results. These are genetically identical twins. Generally, monozygote twins come from cells that have split prior to 12 days after fertilization (Figure 17.3). After 12 days monozygotic twinning leads to conjoint pregnancies (Figure 17.3).

Di-, tri-, tetra-, penta-, hexa- and hepta-zygotic twins result from independent spermatozoa fertilizing independent oocytes. Normally in women, just one oocyte is ovulated each menstrual cycle. Occasionally two and rarely three separate oocytes are ovulated. Promotion of ovulation with human chorionic gonadotropin, and *in vitro* fertilized pregnancies in which multiple zygotes are placed in the uterus, increases the chances of a multiple zygotic pregnancy.

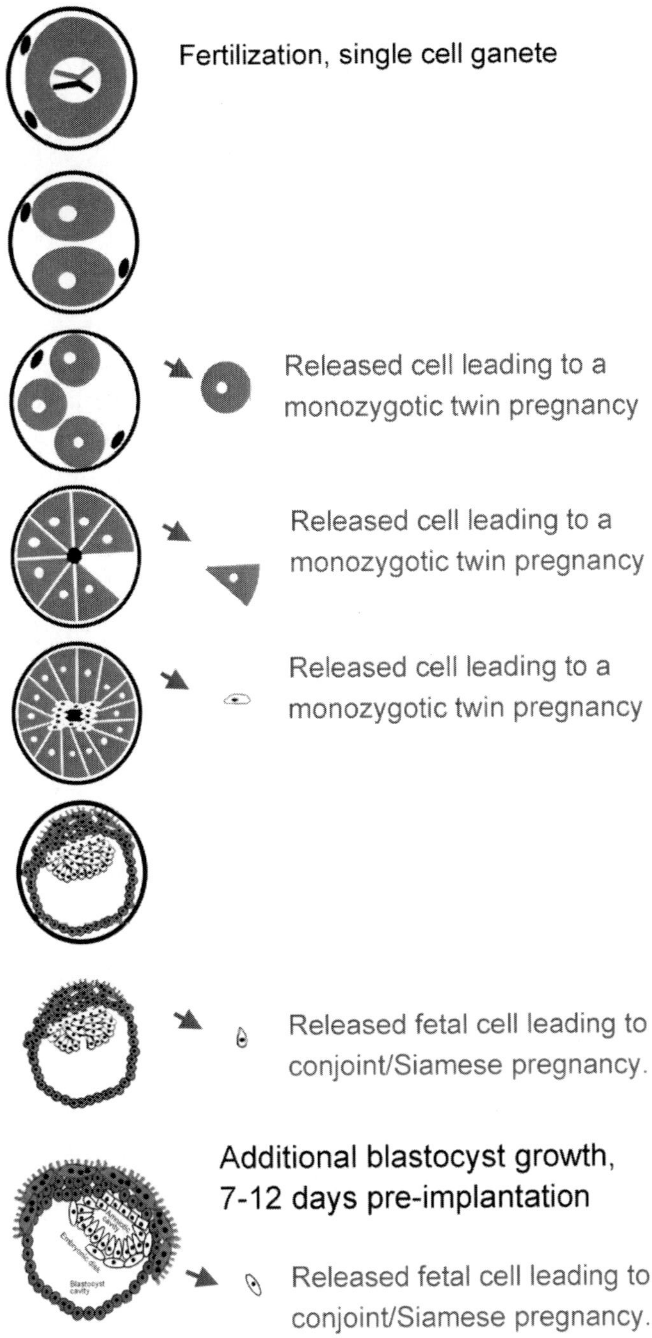

Figure 17.3. Monozygotic twins and conjoint twins.

The statistical odds of having a twin or multiple pregnancy are 1 in 90 pregnancies; 1 in 135 for multiple zygotic pregnancies, and 1 in 270 for monozygotic or identical pregnancies.

Conjoint twinning or multiple pregnancies occurs in approximately 1 in 50,000 pregnancies. A conjoint twinning occurs when cells break apart at 12-15 days after fertilization. All conjoint pregnancies are identical or monozygotic. These cells split after multiple differentiations occur, or cells lose an all-fetus function, leading to Siamese twins or pregnancies that share certain organs (Figure 17.3). A high proportion of conjoint pregnancies fail, not making it to term.

The Human Reproduction Model

Fertilization and blastocyst formation, and (to complete things) implantation of the blastocyst to cause a pregnancy (Chapter 19) totals the human reproductive picture with a positive result; a pregnancy. Presented here is a figure representing all aspects of human reproductive biology, outlining the growth of a follicle leading to a dominant follicle and ovum, and how the testis intricately makes sperm (Figure 17.4). Also shown is the way in which the sperm can be capacitated and can undergo the acrosome reaction leading to fertilization. Finally shown is the way in which the embryo can become a morula and blastocyst leading to implantation and human pregnancy. By putting it all together as outlines, one gets an overall or general picture of human reproduction as a process (Figure 17.4), including how it is all intricately controlled by hormones, and how it is all complexed into one simple network (Figure 17.4).

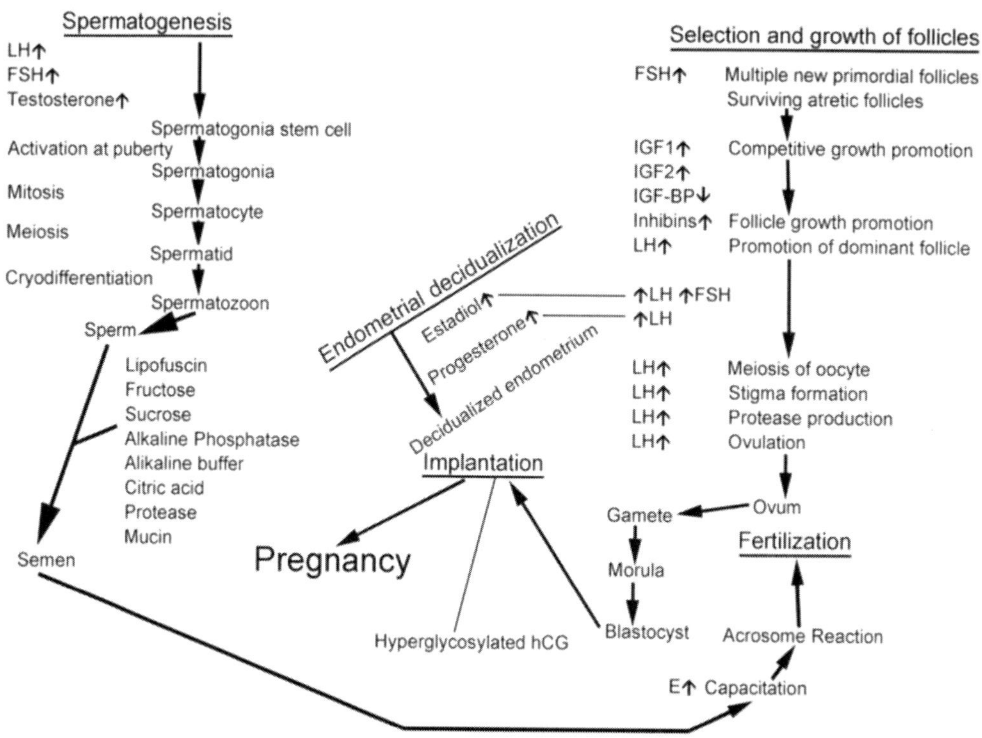

Figure 17.4. Outline of the pathways of human reproduction.

I have placed a poster copy of this figure on the wall of my office. If anyone wants a copy they should contact me: P.O. Box 950, Angel Fire NM 87710. Powerpoint slides of all figures and tables are also available at this address for lecturers using this book for teaching. I sometimes spend considerable periods staring or meditating at the figure's pathway intricacies. I am basically a researcher specializing in the hormone hCG. To my name I have the evolution of hCG, the discovery of hyperglycosylated hCG and its structure and biological functions, and multiple minor discoveries. Yes, I got to put hyperglycosylated hCG on the figure as the autocrine which controls human implantation [1-4]. That is not much; my mind wants to add further steps to this complex figure.

References

[1] de Paula WBM, Lucas CH, Agip AA, Vizcay-Barrena G, Allen JF. Energy, ageing, fidelity and sex: oocyte mitochondrial DNA as a protected genetic template. *Philos Trans Royal Soc Lond Biol Sci* 2013; 368(1622):20120263.

[2] Taunton J, Rowning BA, Coughlin ML, Wu M, Moon RT, Mitchison TJ, Larabell CA. Actin-Dependent Propulsion of Endosomes and Lysosomes by Recruitment of N-Wasp. *J Cell Biol* 2000;148:519–530.

[3] Hoodbhoy T, Talbot P. Mammalian cortical granules: contents, fate, and function. *Mol Reprod Dev* 1994;39:439-448.

[4] Kim NH, Funahashi H, Abeydeera LR, Moon SJ, Prather RS, Day BN. Effects of oviductal fluid on sperm penetration and cortical granule exocytosis during fertilization of pig oocytes in vitro. *J Reprod Fertil* 1996;107:79-86.

[5] Miller DJ, Gong X, Decker G, Shur BD. Egg cortical granule N-acetylglucosaminidase is required for the mouse zona block to polyspermy. *J Cell Biol* 1993;123:1431-1440.

[6] Romar R, Coy P, Gadea J, Rath D. Effect of oviductal and cumulus cells on zona pellucida and cortical granules of porcine oocytes fertilized in vitro with epididymal spermatozoa. *Anim Reprod Sci* 2005;85:287-300.

[7] Clift D, Schuh M. Restarting life: fertilization and the transition from meiosis to mitosis. *Nat Rev Mol Cell Biol* 2013;14:549-562.

[8] Egerszegi I, Alm H, Rátky J, Heleil B, Brüssow KP, Torner H. Meiotic progression, mitochondrial features and fertilisation characteristics of porcine oocytes with different G6PDH activities. *Reprod Fertil Dev* 2010;22:830-838.

[9] Nagy ZP, Liu J, Joris H, Devroey P, Van Steirteghem A. Time-course of oocyte activation, pronucleus formation and cleavage in human oocytes fertilized by intracytoplasmic sperm injection.*Hum Reprod* 1994;9:1743-1748.

[10] Misamore MJ, Stein KK, Lynn JW. Sperm incorporation and pronuclear development during fertilization in the freshwater bivalve Dreissena polymorpha. *Mol Reprod Dev* 2006; 73:1140-1148.

[11] Strelchenko N, Verlinsky O, Kukharenko V, Verlinsky Y. Morula-derived human embryonic stem cells. *Reprod Biomed Online* 2004;9:623-629.

[12] Johnson MH, Ziomek CA. The foundation of two distinct cell lineages within the mouse morula. *Cell.* 1981;24:71-80.

[13] Doetschman TC, Eistetter H, Katz M, Schmidt W, Kemler R. The in vitro development of blastocyst-derived embryonic stem cell lines: formation of visceral yolk sac, blood islands and myocardium. *J Embryol Exp Morphol* 1985;87:27-45.
[14] Rossant J. Stem cells from the Mammalian blastocyst. *Stem Cells.* 2001;19:477-482.
[15] Zwijnenburg PJ, Meijers-Heijboer H, Boomsma DI. Identical but not the same: the value of discordant monozygotic twins in genetic research. *Am J Med Genet Neuropsychiatr Genet* 2010;153B:1134-1149.
[16] Schachter M, Raziel A, Friedler S, Strassburger D, Bern O, Ron-El R. Monozygotic twinning after assisted reproductive techniques: a phenomenon independent of micromanipulation. *Hum Reprod* 2001;16:1264-1269.
[17] From monsters to modern medical miracle: Selected moments from the history of conjoined twins. http://www.nlm.nih.gov/hmd/conjoined/index.html
[18] Spitz L. Conjoined twins. *Prenat Diagn* 2005;25:814-819.
[19] Sasaki Y, Ladner DG, Cole LA Hyperglycosylated hCG the source of pregnancy failures. *Fertil Steril,* 2008; 89:1871-1786.
[20] Cole LA. Hyperglycosylated hCG and Pregnancy Failures. *J Reprod Immunol* 2012;93:119-122.
[21] Cole LA. Chapter 7: hCG and Hyperglycosylated hCG, Promoters of Villous Placenta and Hemochorial Placentation. *The Placenta: Development, Function and Diseases,* Nicholson R (ed). Nova Publishers, 2013.
[22] Cole LA, Hyperglycosylated hCG, A Review, *Placenta,* 2010; 8: 853-664.

Key Points

1. The spermatozoa crosses the zona pellucida using proteases to burn a hole. The spermatozoa then fuses with the oocyte plasma membrane.
2. Fusion of the spermatozoa with the plasma membrane makes the oocyte a zygote. The elevated calcium causes the cortical granules to fuse and release their contents. Among their contents is an enzyme that cross-links glycoproteins in the zona pellucida, sealing it and preventing further spermatozoa from penetrating it.
3. Upon fusion of the spermatozoa with the plasma membrane the second stage of meiosis commences and reaches completion.
4. A male pronucleus and female pronucleus form; each contain their haploid set.
5. When the contents of the male pronucleus and female pronucleus come together they immediately enter mitotic metaphase as part of cell division.
6. The 2 cells rapidly divide to make 4 cells, 8 cells and 16 cells. At the 8 cell of 16 cell stage differentiation occurs into chorion and amnion cells and a morula is formed. Cell growth is promoted by growth factors.
7. Growth factors promote the formation and growth of the blastocoelic cavity and a blastocyst is formed and grows. The blastocyst is constructed of trophoblast cells and the inner cell mass, or cells destined to become the fetus.

Chapter 18

Hydatidiform Mole

At the end of the last chapter a model was presented examining all male and female reproductive biology and how it all fits together (Figure 17.4). Hydatidiform mole is the medical example of a complete failure, or failure of the pathways that are meant to lead to normal pregnancy.

Hydatidiform Mole

Hydatidiform mole means a mole resembling a hydatid or cyst. A hydatid is a larval cyst of tapeworm that may be filled with fluid. A hydatidiform mole is a pregnancy comprising primarily placental tissue. Like a tapeworm cyst, it can be a complete reproductive disaster. A hydatidiform mole can be complete or partial. A complete hydatidiform mole comprises only cystic placenta tissue; a partial hydatidiform mole, in contrast, can contain cystic placenta and some fetal tissue. Both disorders have bizarre pathophysiologies that defy the concepts of human reproduction and human sexuality (Figure 18.4).

Hydatidiform moles occur in the United States and other western countries at an incidence of 1 in 900 pregnancies. Most hydatidiform moles are spontaneously aborted, raising the occurrence to approximately 1 in 400 pregnancies in the west [1,2]. The incidence of hydatidiform mole in Indonesia and the Philippines may be as high as 1 in 145 pregnancies [3], or 1 in 60 pregnancies when considering spontaneous abortions [1,2]. Hydatidiform moles are most common in young pregnancies in women not completing puberty, and in older pregnancies prior to menopause. Hydatidiform moles are a benign mass. Hydatidiform moles - most notably, complete hydatidiform moles - can, however, become invasive, malignant or cancer-like. Moles can also be readily transformed into choriocarcinoma or trophoblastic cancers.

Complete Hydatidiform Mole

If an ovum is produced without a haploid set of chromosomes due to failure in the first or second stage of meiosis, it will lead to an empty ovum. An empty ovum is a candidate for a complete hydatidiform mole pregnancy. A sperm penetrates the zona pellucida of the ovum then the spermatic haploid set searches for a maternal haploid set within the egg to join. When one is not found the sperm deposits its haploid set as the ovum's prime haploid set. One of two things can then happen. The deposited haploid set can duplicate, generating a diploid set or, if the cortical granules fail to block further sperm from penetrating the zona pellucida, a second sperm can penetrate the ovum, depositing its haploid set in a pronucleus and fertilizing the egg (Figure 18.1). Complete hydatidiform mole is the only condition in which you can have a dispermic diandrogenous all paternal XX or XY embryo.

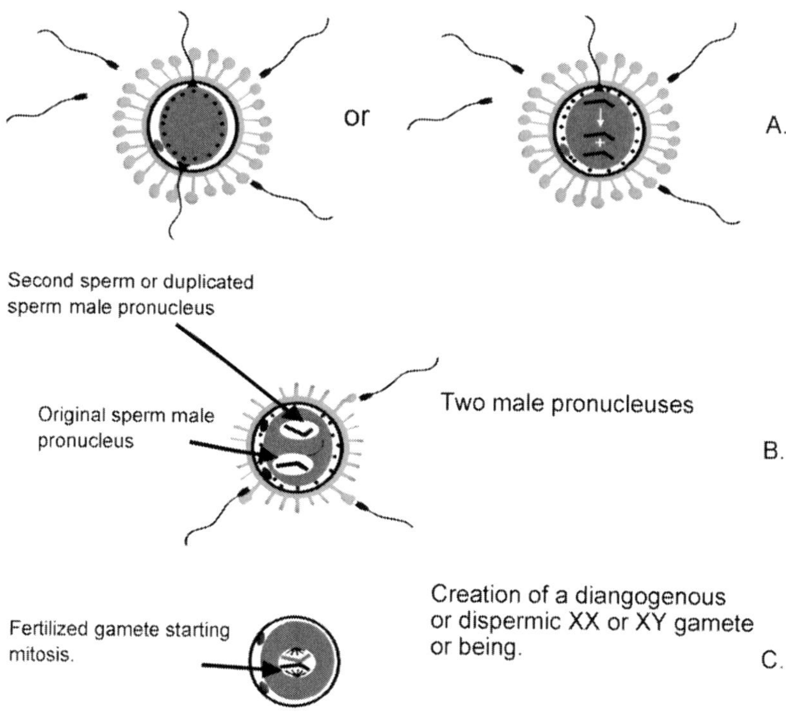

Figure 18.1. Complete hydatidiform mole.

A diploid XX or XY (not YY) embryo is formed. The zygote divides, forming 2 identical cells, 4 identical cells, 8 identical cells and 16 identical cells in the normal way. Then a morula is formed which normally divides into amnion (fetal tissue) and chorion (placental tissue). In the complete hydatidiform mole case, the morula will fail to divide the tissue into amnion and chorion and by default will become 100% chorion. The chorionic being divides further to form a chorion-only blastocyst with no fetal mass, and then implants. The being is only composed of chorion tissue, without an amnion to absorb the transferred nutrient. The chorion becomes strings of hygromatous cysts containing the nutrients normally transferred by the placenta to a fetus. As shown in Figure 18.2, a washed hysterectomy of a complete hydatidiform mole, the uterus is filled with hundreds of hygromatous cysts. When viewed after hysterectomy it appears like a bowl of red cherries (Figure 18.2).

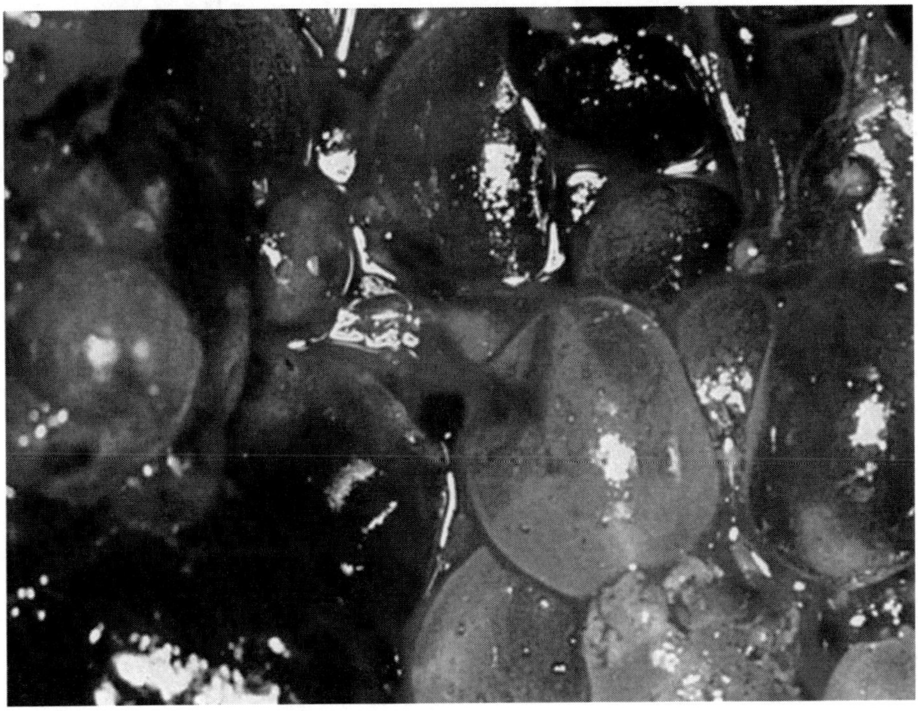

Figure 18.2. A complete hydatidiform mole at hysterectomy.

The complete hydatidiform mole pregnancy comprises only hygromatous cysts. Normally the woman will look unduly large for the gestation age of her pregnancy. The human chorionic gonadotropin (hCG) levels may be 2 to 10–fold higher than those seen in a pregnancy with the sheer mass of trophoblastic tissue. Look for a pregnancy case with placenta hCG greater than 100,000 miu/ml.

Normally, a complete mole is first discovered by ultrasound. It yields a snowflake-like pattern from cystic trophoblast tissue upon ultrasound and no fetus. A complete hydatidiform mole is removed by dilation and curettage, normally at 8 weeks to 16 weeks of gestation. The problem with complete hydatidiform moles is that some trophoblast tissue may remain following dilation and curettage. In one in four cases this tissue may start invading the uterus (invasive hydatidiform mole) using a process analogous to pregnancy implantation (see Chapter 19), hyperglycosylated hCG-driven invasion. The tissue may invade through the uterus to other organs. In complete hydatidiform mole cases the total hCG is normally high, approximately 250,0000 mIU/ml. In complete hydatidiform mole cases, if a plateau is observed in the decline of hCG following dilation and curettage an invasive mole is indicated, Alternatively, if hCG levels, after declining to less than 1 mIU/ml and becoming undetectable, start to rise, an invasive mole is diagnosed. In both cases chemotherapy is started. The chemotherapy recommended is methotrexate, and actinomycin D if resistance is found to methotrexate.

As commonly found, when circulating placental hCG concentrations dip below 300 mIU/ml, a plateau in reduction can occur. This is quiescent gestational trophoblastic disease. Either apoptosis or chemotherapy has destroyed the invasive cells, the root cytotrophoblast cells. All that remains is fused syncytiotrophoblast cells, which neither grow nor invade. In these cases chemotherapy will not work. The patient needs to be carefully followed for approximately six months until the residual syncytiotrophoblast tissue goes through apoptosis or disappears.

Approximately 1 in 40 cases of complete hydatidiform mole develop into choriocarcinoma, a highly invasive malignancy. Invasive hydatidiform mole tissue can be histologically characterized as invasive villous placenta tissue. Choriocarcinoma can be characterized as invasive cytotrophoblastic tissue with no placental villous elements. Invasive choriocarcinoma should be treated by an EMA-CO combination chemotherapy procedure. Week one is etoposide, methotrexate and actinomycin D, and week two, cyclophosphamide and onvocin (vincristine). Choriocarcinoma spreads quickly from the uterus to the lungs, and on to the brain.

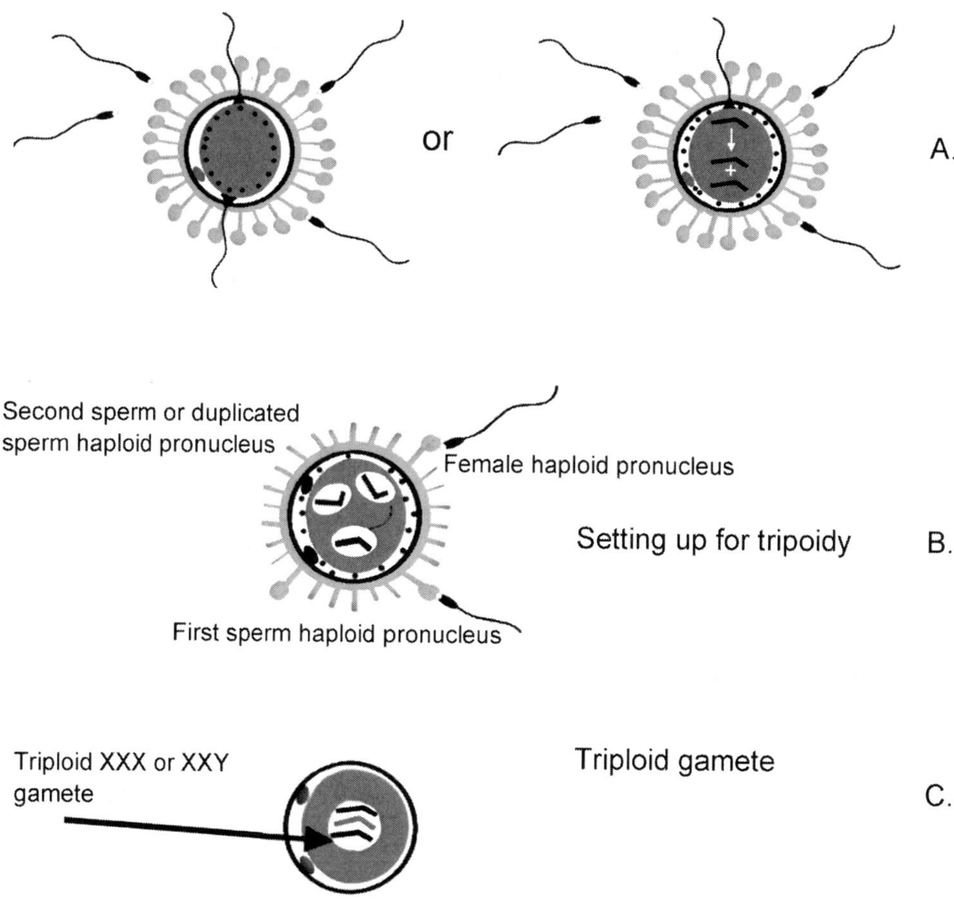

Figure 18.3. Partial hydatidiform mole.

Occasionally in the USA one observes a complete hydatidiform mole conjoint with a normal pregnancy, as a dizygotic twin. This twin can be monitored very carefully by ultrasound during pregnancy. The biggest danger is the one-in-four chance of the mole becoming invasive, and one-in-40 chance of it becoming choriocarcinoma. If it is not invasive, the pregnancy could make it, with careful management, to term. Otherwise, it all should be terminated as early as possible. If the mole shows signs of any invasion the pregnancy should be immediately terminated because it will invade the normal pregnancy and invade the mother.

Partial Hydatidiform Mole

A partial hydatidiform mole is a triploid pregnancy and another strange complication of the reproductive process (Figure 18.4). As described in the previous chapter (Chapter 17), fertilization is an intricate process. Part of this process is the cortical granules. As illustrated in Figure 18.1, upon sperm penetration the granules enter the perivitelline space and secrete enzymes that cross-link the zona pellucid, making it impenetrable to further sperm. This limits the ovum to penetration by one sperm. Partial hydatidiform mole is what happens when this corticle granule process fails, and an egg can be penetrated by multiple sperm (Figure 18.3).

If a sperm penetrates an ovum with an ovum haploid chromosome set, and is unable to pair its haploid set with the ovum's haploid set, a partial hydatidiform mole may result. This sperm haploid set can duplicate, or if the cortical granule process fails, the egg can be fertilized by another sperm. The three haploid sets, two deriving from sperm or a duplicated haploid set, and one being the ovum's haploid set, form three pronucleuses (Figure 18.3). The three pronucleuses merge, forming a triploid XXY or XXX embryo (Figure 18.3). This type of hydatidiform mole is partly differentiated at the morula stage, and partly differentiated there afterwards. The result is a mixture of placenta hygromatous cysts and some fetal elements (Figure 18.4).

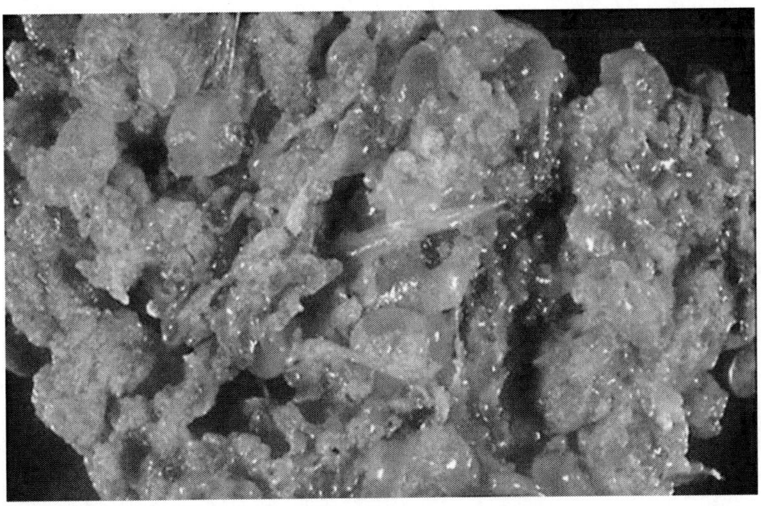

Figure 18.4. Partial hydatidiform mole after hysterectomy.

I have personally dissected a few partial hydatidiform mole masses (Figure 18.4). It can be quite unpleasant. One can dissect one's way through cystic and placenta tissues to suddenly come across an intact, fully-formed finger. It is haunting.

Partial hydatidiform moles rarely become invasive like complete partial moles. Very commonly, partial hydatidiform moles cause miscarriage of pregnancy. In some countries dilation and curettage is not performed when a partial hydatidiform mole is suggested by ultrasound. The mole is allowed to remain until the person has a miscarriage.

It is important to differentiate between a complete and partial hydatidiform mole correctly using cytogenetics on the dilation and curettage product. A complete mole is traditionally diploid, while a partial mole is triploid. A complete hydatidiform mole must be distinguished from a partial hydatidiform mole because of the invasive nature of the complete mole. In both cases, both complete and partial, weekly placental hCG measurements are suggested until the concentration reaches <1 mIU/ml. At that point, placental hCG should be measured three months further to ensure that recurrence or invasive mole is not a possibility.

References

[1] Takeuchi S. Immunology of spontaneous abortion and hydatidiform mole. *Am J Reprod Immunol* 1980;1:23-28.

[2] Yapar EG, Ayhan A, Ergeneli MH. Pregnancy outcome after hydatidiform mole, initial and recurrent. *J Reprod Med* 1994;39:297-299.

[3] Baxton CL. Management of patients with hydatidiform mole. *Ann NY Acad Sci* 1959;80: 121-124.

[4] Sebire NJ, Fisher RA, Foskett M, Rees H, Seckl MJ, Newlands ES. Risk of recurrent hydatidiform mole and subsequent pregnancy outcome following complete or partial hydatidiform molar pregnancy. *Br J Obset Gynecol* 2003;110:22-26.

[5] Sebire NJ, Foskett M, Paradinas FJ, Fisher RA, Francis RJ, Short D, Newlands ES, Seckl MJ. Outcome of twin pregnancies with complete hydatidiform mole and healthy co-twin. *Lancet* 2002 22;359:2165-2166.

[6] Cole LA, Muller Y. hCG in the Management of Quiescent and Chemorefractory Gestational Trophoblastic Diseases, *Gynecol Oncol* 2010;116:3-9.

[7] Vejerslev LO, Fisher RA, Surti U, Wake N. Hydatidiform mole: parental chromosome aberrations in partial and complete moles. *J Med Genet.* 1987; 24: 613–615.

[8] Barut A, Arikan I, Harma M, Harma MI, Barut F, Coskan A. Recurrent partial hydatidiform mole. *J Pak Med Assoc* 2011;61:1016-1017.

[9] Teng NN, Ballon SC. Partial hydatidiform mole with diploid karyotype: report of three cases. *Am J Obstet Gynecol* 1984;150:961-964.

[10] Szulman AE, Philippe E, Boué JG, Boué A. Human triploidy: association with partial hydatidiform moles and nonmolar conceptuses. *Hum Pathol* 1981;12:1016-1021.

[11] Devriend K. Hydatidiform mole and triploidy: the role of genomic imprinting in placental development. *Human Reprod Upd* 2005;11:137-142.

Key Points

1. Complete mole is a complication of pregnancy in which an empty ovum is produced without haploid set. This may be fertilized by a single sperm. Its haploid set may be duplicated, creating two pronucleuses and a diandrogenous XX or XY being. Alternatively, the ovum may be fertilized by two sperm leading to two pronucleuses.
2. Partial mole is a complication of pregnancy. In this syndrome, either a single sperm's haploid set is duplicated leading to three pronucleuses (one from sperm, one from the duplicated haploid set, and one is the ovum's haploid set); alternatively, if cortical granules are failing to seal the zona pellucid, then two sperm and the egg can generate the three pronucleuses. Either way, it is XXY or XXX triploid.
3. It is essential to distinguish the karyotypes of hydatidiform moles. Complete mole is diploid and partial mole is triploid. This will clearly differentiate the two disorders.

Pregnancy

Chapter 19

Implantation and Pregnancy Failure

Implantation

Deep invasion to one-third the thickness of the myometrium (implantation) and hemochorial placentation permits very efficient nutritional exchange in humans. The blastocyst implants in the decidua then continues to invade deeper. With time, the placental cells take on a villous structure and then start hemochorial placentation (efficient placentation, maternal blood surrounding villous structure)[1-5].

As the blastocyst approaches the endometrial lining, the blastocyst protective barrier, the zona pellucida, is lost or hatched (Figure 19.1, Panel A). There is evidence that signaling occurs between the hatched blastocyst and the endometrial wall prior to implantation and attachment, involving hCG, estradiol and EGF released by the blastocyst syncytiotrophoblast cells (Figure 19.1, Panel B). The syncytiotrophoblast microvilli attach to structures called the glycocalyx or pinopodes on the uterine epithelium. Literally, the blastocyst microvilli are held on to these structures (Figure 19.2, Panel C). Cytotrophoblast cells signaled by hyperglycosylated hCG invade the uterine epithelium and underlying stromal tissue, in finger-like manners (Figure 19.2, Panel C), digging a hole in the uterine surface and effectively implanting the entire blastocyst in the uterus. Science shows that autocrine hyperglycosylated hCG made by cytotrophoblast cells binds a TGFβ receptor leading to metalloproteinase and collagenase-led invasion [1].

As soon as implantation starts, the endometrial lining becomes the decidua of pregnancy. Once implanted, the blastocyst differentiates its cytotrophoblast cells by fusion to syncytiotrophoblast cells (Figure 19.2, panel D). This differentiation is driven by hCG. The blastocyst at 4.5 weeks of gestation is a mixture of invasive cytotrophoblast cells and hCG-producing syncytiotrophoblast cell. The hCG produced enters the maternal circulation, driving progesterone production by the ovarian corpus luteum and starting angiogenesis or growth of uterine spiral arteries. The hyperglycosylated hCG made by the cytotrophoblast cells drives invasion of the blastocyst deeper into the uterus. As shown in Figure 19.3, the cytotrophoblast cells form a column to drive invasion. Eventually, by approximately 5 weeks of gestation the blastocyst has invaded itself deep enough into the decidua for the uterine epithelium to seal itself closed (Figure 19.3). The sealing closed is something unique to humans [1-5].

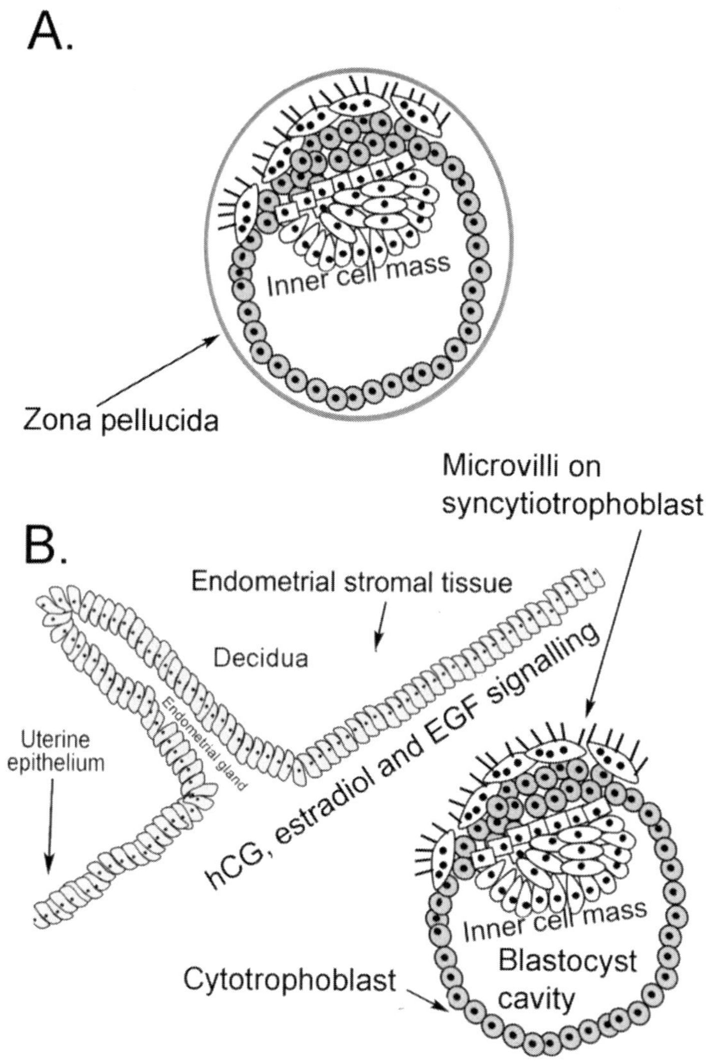

Figure 19.1. Blastocyst preparing for implantation at 3 weeks of menstrual cycle. Blastocyst is surrounded by shell or zona pellucida (Panel A). Blastocyst was hatched, losing zona pellucida, and is now communicating with decidua prior to implantation (Panel B).

Pregnancy Failure

Failure to implant properly is a major cause of biochemical pregnancies and spontaneous abortions in pregnancy [7-9]. As shown by Norwitz et al., Semprini and Simon, Wilcox et al. Walker et al. [10-12], and multiple other investigators, most (>70%) biochemical pregnancies or early failures are due to the failure of pregnancies to implant appropriately. Similarly, most first and second trimester spontaneous abortions or failures of pregnancy are due to failure of pregnancies to implant appropriately. The remainder of biochemical pregnancies and spontaneous abortions are due to hydatidiform mole or gross genetic abnormality [7-12].

Figure 19.4 shows data from 133 woman eager to achieve pregnancy. Women were followed with daily urines through multiple menstrual cycles until pregnancy was achieved. Concentrations of total hCG and hyperglycosylated hCG were measured in the day of implantation of pregnancy (first day of production of total hCG, >1 mIU/ml).

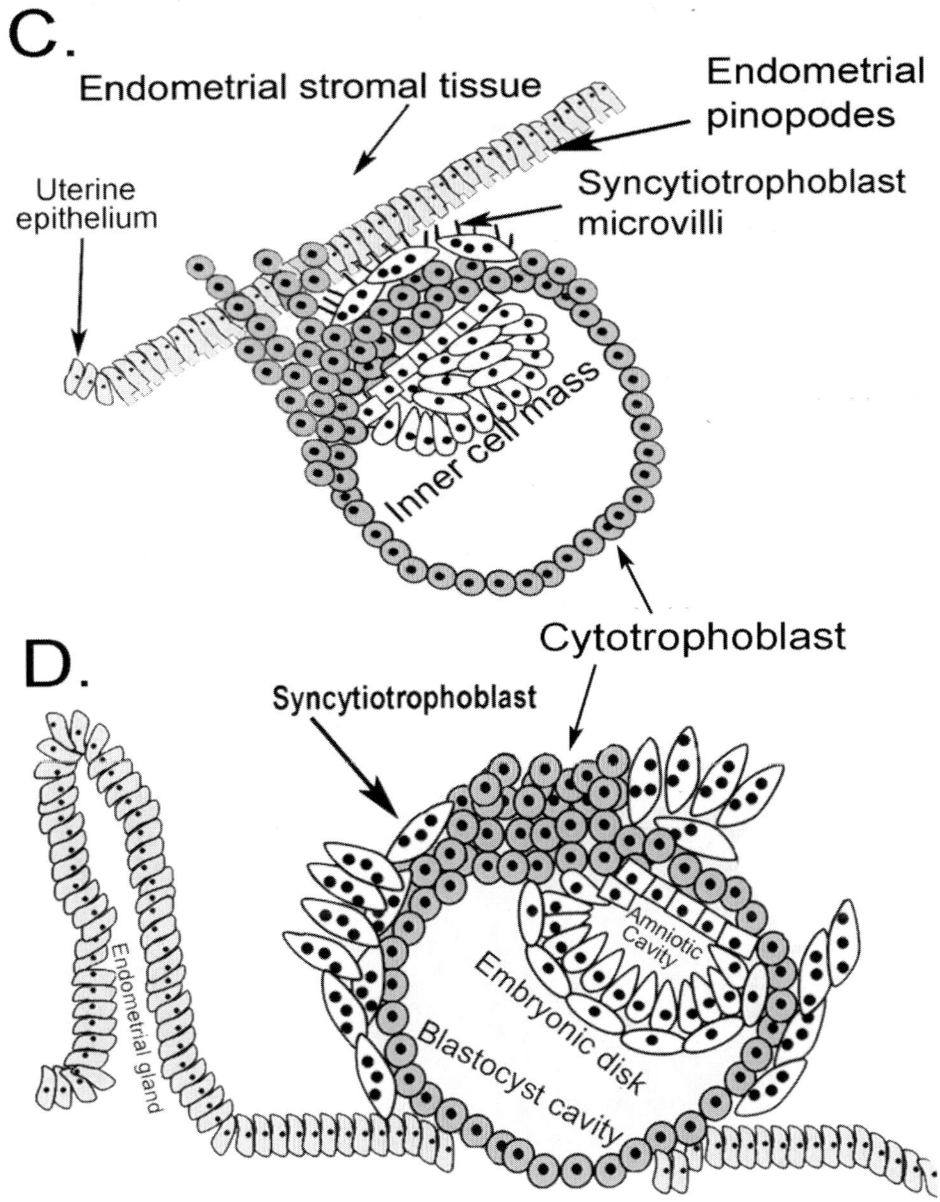

Figure 19.2. Blastocyst implanting in endometrial lining (decidua), starting implantation at 3-4 weeks of gestation. The blastocyst shows how syncytiotrophoblast microvilli attach to uterine epithelium pinopodes or to the glycocalyx. The blastocyst shows fingers of cytotrophoblast cells invading the uterus in implantation, penetrating the uterine epithelium and the underlying endometrial stroma tissue.

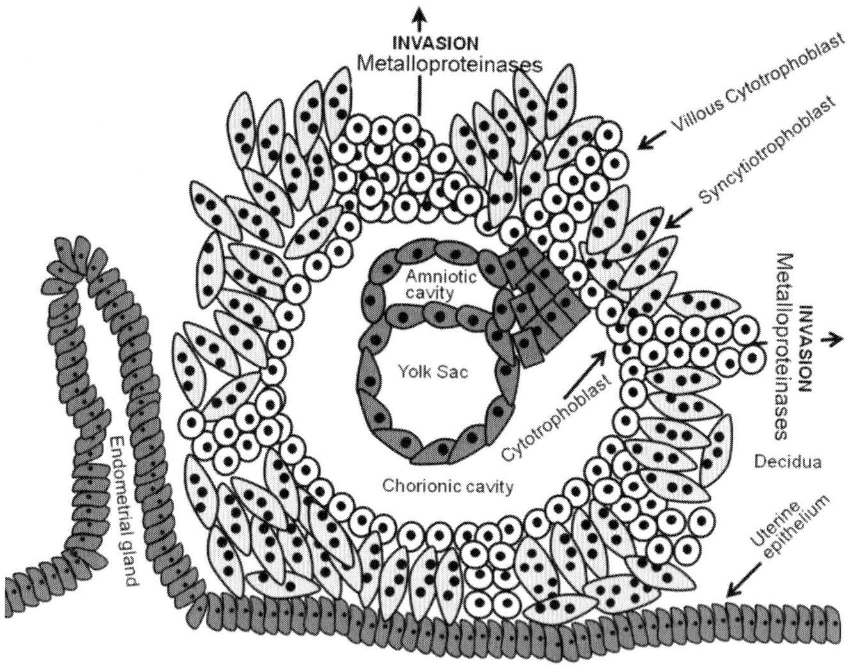

Figure 19.3. The cytotrophoblast cells form a column to drive invasion. Eventually, by approximately 5 weeks of gestation the blastocyst has invaded itself deep enough into the decidua for the uterine epithelium to seal itself closed. The sealing closed is something unique to humans.

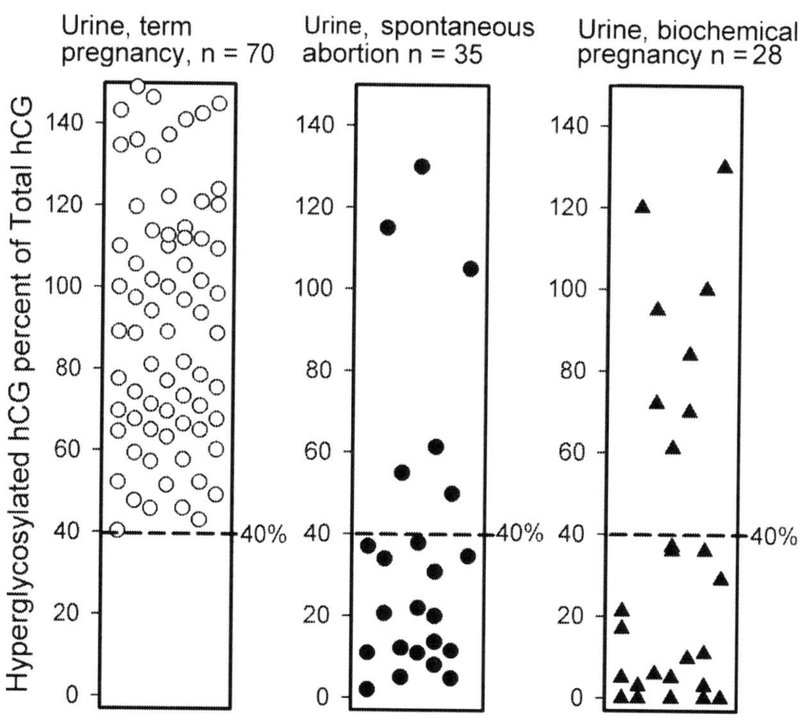

Figure 19.4. Concentration of hyperglycosylated hCG (hyperglycosylated hCG as a percentage of total hCG) on day of implantation in 133 women achieving pregnancy.

As shown in Figure 19.4, sufficient hyperglycosylated hCG to signal appropriate implantation was present in 70 of 70 term pregnancies and in 6 of 35 spontaneous abortion outcome pregnancies and 8 of 28 biochemical outcome pregnancies. As inferred, hyperglycosylated hCG drives pregnancy implantation and that spontaneous abortion and biochemical pregnancy are due to insufficient hyperglycosylated hCG production [13].

References

[1] Berndt S, Blacher S, Munaut C, Detilleux J, Evain-Brion D, Noel A, Fournier T, Foidart JM (2013) Hyperglycosylated human chorionic gonadotropin stimulates angiogenesis through TGF-ß receptor activation. *J FASEB* 27:1309-1321

[2] Wilcox AJ, Baird DD, Weinberg CR. Time of implantation of the conceptus and loss of pregnancy. *N Engl J Med 1999*;340:1796-1799.

[3] Bazer FW, Wu G, Spencer TE, Johnson GA, Burghardt RC, Bayless K. Novel pathways for implantation and establishment and maintenance of pregnancy in mammals. *Mol Hum Reprod* 2010;16:135-152.

[4] Stewart DR, Overstreet JW, Nakajima ST, Lasley BL. Enhanced ovarian steroid secretion before implantation in early human pregnancy. *J Clin Endocrinol Metab* 1993; 76:1470-1476.

[5] Nepomnaschy PA, Weinberg CR, Wilcox AJ, Baird DD. Urinary hCG patterns during the week following implantation. *Hum Reprod* 2008;23:271-277.

[6] Kleinhaus K, Perrin M, Friedlander Y, Paltiel O, Malaspina D, Harlap S. Paternal age and spontaneous abortion. *Obstet Gynecol* 2006;108:369-377.

[7] Thom DH, Nelson LM, Vaughan TL. Spontaneous abortion and subsequent adverse birth outcomes. *Am J Obstet Gynecol* 1992;166:111-116.

[8] Gray RH, Simpson JL, Kambic RT, Queenan JT, Mena P, Perez A, Barbato M. Timing of conception and the risk of spontaneous abortion among pregnancies occurring during the use of natural family planning. *Am J Obstet Gynecol* 1995;172:1567-1772.

[9] Wilcox AJ, Baird DD, Weinberg CR. Time of implantation of the conceptus and loss of pregnancy. *N Engl J Med* 1999;340:1796-1799.

[10] Norwitz ER, Schust DJ, Fisher SJ, (2001). Implantation and the survival of early pregnancy, *New Engl J Med* 2001;345, 1400-1408.

[11] Semprini AE, Simon G. Not so efficient reproduction. *Lancet* 2000;356, 257-258.

[12] Walker EM, Lewis M, Cooper W, Marnie M, Howie PW. Occult biochemical pregnancy: fact or fiction? *Br J Obstet Gynaecol* 1988;95:659-663.

[13] Wilcox AJ, Weinberg, CR, Baird DD: Risk factors for early pregnancy loss. *Epidemiol* 1990; 1:382–385.

[14] Hyperglycosylated hCG and Pregnancy Failures. *J Reprod Immunol* 2012;93:119-122.

Key Points

1. It is important to understand the principal of implantation, how the blastocyst is hatched, and that invasion is led by cytotrophoblast cells, as well as how the blastocyst and the uterine epithelium attach through microvilli and the glycocalyx structure.
2. Cytotrophoblast cells produce hyperglycosylated hCG, which binds a TGFβ receptor. This promotes invasion and growth of cytotrophoblast cells.
3. Biochemical pregnancy and spontaneous abortion are primarily due to inappropriate implantation. This is due to inefficient production of hyperglycosylated hCG.

Chapter 20

Placental Function: Hemochorial Placentation

Hemochorial placentation is a term for advanced placental function involving blood and the placenta and the transfer of nutrients to the fetus. Hemochorial placentation is the principal function of a placenta.

The implanting blastocyst at 5 - 5.5 weeks of pregnancy is 60% syncytiotrophoblast cells (fused cells with 3-6 nucleii) and 40% cytotrophoblast cells (roots cells mononuclear). The 5-5.5 week structure has developed multiple columns of cytotrophoblast cells stretching from the fetal core to the blastocyst surface (Figure 20.1). What happens from this point is directed at generating villous tissue for efficient hemochorial placentation and a fetus. First the blastocyst cavity grows and expands, and becomes the amniotic cavity. Secondly, the cytotrophoblast cells driven by hyperglycosylated hCG invade the uterus deeper and deeper, invading through the decidua and into the myometrium, reaching approximately one-third the thickness of the uterine muscular wall (myometrium)[4-12].

As shown in Figure 20.1, the columns of cytotrophoblast cells grow outwards and deeper into the myometrium. The growth of cytotrophoblast cells in column structures is driven by hyperglycosylated hCG. Hyperglycosylated hCG is a cytotrophoblast autocrine, antagonizing a TGFβ receptor and promoting cell growth and invasion [1,2]. hCG promotes differentiation of the growing cytotrophoblast cells into syncytiotrophoblast cells. The combined effect of hyperglycosylated hCG and hCG is villous placenta tissue outgrowth (Figure 20.2)[1-3]. Figure 20.2 shows the start of outgrowth; villous placenta tissue at 6 weeks' gestation [4-15].

Villous structures have an anchor villous. At the end of the anchor villous is a disc of extravillous cytotrophoblast cells (Figure 20.3), which produces hyperglycosylated hCG. They also having floating villi; two, three or four sidearms or floating villi in each villous structure (Figure 20.3). All are made of cytotrophoblast cells surrounded by syncytiotrophoblast cells and terminally differentiated syncytiotrophoblast cells with 10 to 40 nuclei (Figure 20.2 and 20.3). The floating villi are the active villi that transport nutrients, glucose, oxygen and other essentials from the surrounding tank of maternal blood, into their fetal circulation (Figure 20.4). Under the influence of hCG, a maternal spiral artery grows to meet the developing placenta structure, and an umbilical circulation grows to link the growing villous placenta and the fetus (Figures 20.2, 20.3 and 20.4)[4-15].

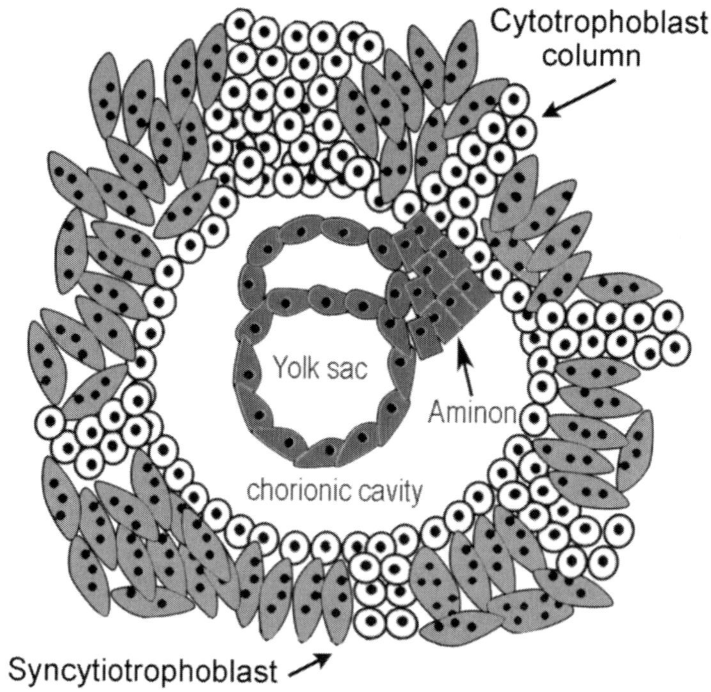

Figure 20.1. Blastocyst implanted into uterus at 5 – 5.5 weeks' gestation. Picture shows formation of cytotrophoblast columns.

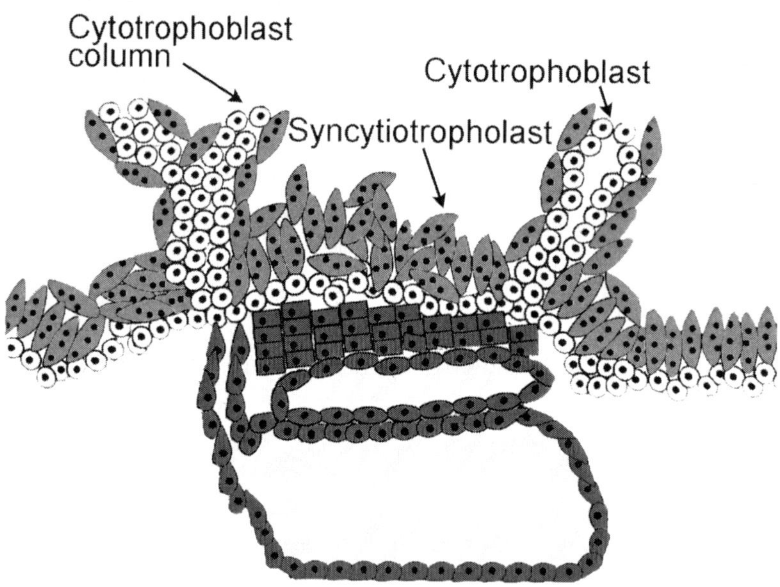

Figure 20.2. Villous trophoblast formation at 6 weeks of gestation, formation of cytotrophoblastic columns.

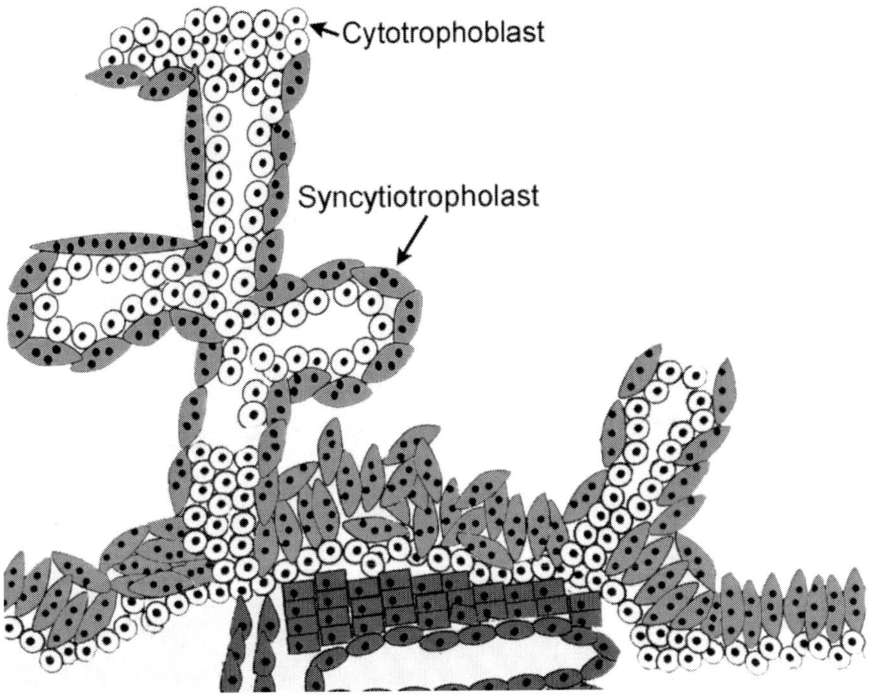

Figure 20.3. Villous trophoblast at 7-8 weeks' gestation.

The developed villous placenta at around 8-10 weeks of gestation fits in a tank of maternal blood and efficiently provides fetal nutrition (Figure 20.4). The maternal blood fills the placental tanks. There are approximately 4-6 tanks inside each placenta. The blood is then filtered across singly syncytiotrophoblast cells into a floating villous. The nutrients are immediately taken up by the umbilical circulation and travel to the fetus.

Over the course of the first trimester of pregnancy the active hemochorial placentation system is built, and implanted into the myometrium. Figure 20.4 shows a mature placenta at 10 weeks of gestation with hemochorial placentation. This shows a fetus in the uterus linked to the placenta by the umbilical cord. The only barrier between maternal blood and the fetal circulation is syncytiotrophoblast cells and possibly underlining cytotrophoblasts cells. The remaining maternal blood after entering the tanks is removed through the maternal draining venous lakes. The umbilical veins transfer the blood to the fetus. At parturition the entire placental structure with 4-6 blood-filled tanks is delivered [4-15].

Recent research shows that hyperglycosylated hCG stimulation of placental growth and invasion is critical in both the first and second trimesters of pregnancy [3,10]. If hyperglycosylated hCG is deficient in the second trimester of pregnancy, hemochorial placentation may lose efficiency. The maternal body develops hypertensions to force the tank-villous placenta filtration model (Figure 20.4), and preeclampsia may result [10].

Hemochorial placentation first evolved with the first appearance of CG and hyperglycosylated CG in lower simian primates. With the appearance of CG and hyperglycosylated CG the appearance of hemochorial placentation was automatic. Hyperglycosylated hCG drive the growth of villous placenta, and the invasion deep into the myometrium [11]. hCG drives the continuous fusing of growing cytotrophoblast cells to form syncytiotrophoblast cells [3]. hCG also drives the growth of the maternal uterine spiral artery and the umbilical circulations [3,12-15]. All told, development of hemochorial placentation appears to be the principal job of the hCG and its variants.

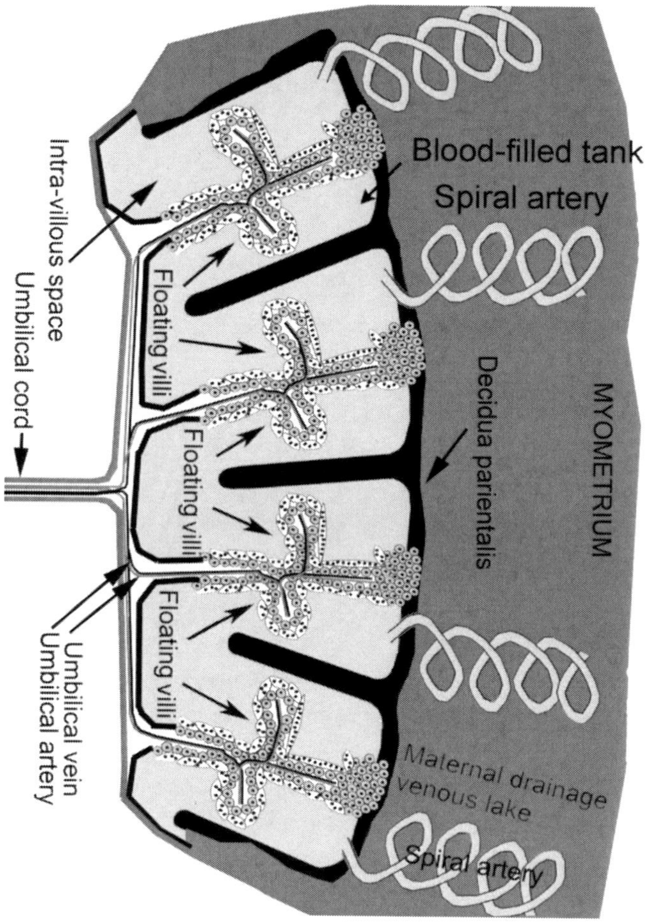

Figure 20.4. Functioning hemochorial placentation at 10 weeks' gestation.

References

[1] Berndt S, Blacher S, Munuat C, Detilleux J, Evain-Brion D, Noel A, Fournier T, Foidart JM (2013) Hyperglycosylated human chorionic gonadotropin stimulates angiogenesis through TGF-ß receptor activation. *J FASEB* 27:1309-1321

[2] Butler SA, Ikram MS, Mathieu S, Iles RK (2000) The increase in bladder carcinoma cell population induced by the free beta subunit of hCG is a result of an anti-apoptosis effect and not cell proliferation. *Brit J Cancer* 82:1553-1556.

[3] Shi QJ, Lei ZM, Rao CV, Lin J (1993) Novel role of human chorionic gonadotropin in differentiation of human cytotrophoblasts. *Endocrinol* 132;387-395.

[4] Chakraborty D, Rumi MA, Konno T, Soares MJ. Natural killer cells direct hemochorial placentation by regulating hypoxia-inducible factor dependent trophoblast lineage decisions. *Proc Natl Acad Sci USA* 2011;108:16295-16300.

[5] Enders AC, Welsh AO. Structural interactions of trophoblast and uterus during hemochorial placenta formation. *J Exp Zool* 1993 Sep 1;266(6):578-87.

[6] Wulff C, Wilson H, Dickson SE, Wiegand SJ, Fraser HM. Hemochorial placentation in the primate: expression of vascular endothelial growth factor, angiopoietins, and their receptors throughout pregnancy. *Biol Reprod* 2002;66:802-812.

[7] Enders AC, Carter AM. Placenta. Review: The evolving placenta: different developmental paths to a hemochorial relationship. *J Placenta* 2012;33:S92-S98.

[8] Rasweiler JJ. Development of the discoidal hemochorial placenta in the black mastiff bat, Molossus ater: evidence for a role of maternal endothelial cells in the control of trophoblastic growth. *Am J Anat* 199;191:185-207.

[9] Moll W, Künzel W, Herberger J. Hemodynamic implications of hemochorial placentation. *Eur J Obstet Gynecol Reprod Biol* 1975;5:67-74.

[10] Bahado-Singh RO, Oz AU, Kingston JM, Shahabi S, Hsu CD, Cole LA. The role of hyperglycosylated hCG in trophoblast invasion and the prediction of subsequent pre-eclampsia. *Prenat Dagn* 22:478-481, 2002.

[11] Cole LA. hCG and Hyperglycosylated hCG, Promoters of Villous Placenta and Hemochorial Placentation. *Placenta: Functions, Development and Disease,* Nova Publishers, 2013, in press.

[12] Toth P, Li X, Rao CV, Lincoln SR, Sanfillipino JS, Spinnato JA, Yussman MA. Expression of functional human chorionic gonadotropin/human luteinizing hormone receptor gene in human uterine arteries. *J Clin Endocrinol Metab* 1994;79:307-315

[13] Zygmunt M, Herr F, Keller-Schoenwetter S, Kunzi-Rapp K, Munstedt K, Rao CV, Lang U, Preissner KT. Characterization of human chorionic gonadotropin as a novel angiogenic factor. *J Clin Endocrinol Metab* 2002;87:290-5296.

[14] Rao CV, Li X, Toth P, Lei ZM. Expression of epidermal growth factor, transforming growth factor-alpha and their common receptor genes in human umbilical cords. *J Clin Endocrinol Metab* 1995;80:1012-1020.

[15] 1Rao CV, Li X, Toth P, Lei ZM, Cook VD. Novel expression of functional human chorionic gonadotropin/luteinizing hormone receptor in human umbilical cords. *J Clin Endocrinol Metab* 1993;77:1706-1714.

Key Points

1. It is important to understand the principle of hemochorial placentation, and the anatomy of the placenta.
2. It is important to understand the principle of implantation; how the blastocyst is hatched, and that invasion is led by cytotrophoblast cells, as well as how the blastocyst and the uterine epithelium attach through microvilli and the glycocalyx structure.
3. It is also important to understand how villous structures are produced which lead to hemochorial placentation.

Chapter 21

The Hormones of Pregnancy

Chapter 19 covers hyperglycosylated hCG and implantation of pregnancy. Chapter 20 covers hyperglycosylated hCG and placental hCG and hemochorial placentation. This cChapter 21 covers the principle functions of placental hCG and hyperglycosylated hCG. Chapter 22 covers sex steroids and fetal gender, and Chapter 23 covers oxytocin and other hormones and parturition. Here we examine the functions of placental hCG and hyperglycosylated hCG in pregnancy, and other critical hormones produced during pregnancy. Human placental lactogen (hPL) and human placental growth hormone (hPGH) are important in pregnancy, as are the sex steroids. The sex steroids, estrone, estradiol and estriol, and progesterone are made at much higher serum concentrations in pregnancy than are observed during the menstrual cycle.

Placental hCG, Other Actions

Placental hCG has multiple critical functions outside of implantation and hemochorial placentation in pregnancy. Firstly, from 3.5 weeks to 7 weeks of gestation placental hCG maintains progesterone production by the corpus luteum of the ovary as the GnRH-LH source of the menstrual cycle dies off (Chapter 4 and Chapter 6). Placenta hCG keeps corpus luteal progesterone levels rising. At around 7 weeks of gestation, villous placental syncytiotrophoblast cells take over progesterone production (Figure 21.1) [1-4]. In many respects, detection of progesterone in a mother is a pregnancy test.

Other functions of placental hCG include suppression of immuno-rejection of the fetal placenta unit by the mother. hCG suppresses macrophage phagocytosis of the foreign beings by promoting a macrophage migration inhibiting factor [5-8]. hCG also has a role in preventing uterine myometrial contractions during the course of pregnancy [9-11]. It is thought that the diminution of hCG as pregnancy reaches parturition allows contractions [9-11]. Research now shows that the fetal kidney and liver form a variant of hCG during pregnancy, which directly promotes fetal organ growth. Receptors have been demonstrated on multiple fetal organs, which disappear at parturition [12-15]. Other functions of placental hCG raise many questions. Placenta hCG receptors have been found in the human brain stem of pregnant women [16,17]. What role do these have during pregnancy? This needs a lot of investigation. It is thought that hCG action on these receptors may cause the classical hyperemesis or morning sickness associated with pregnancy [16,17].

Hyperglycosylated hCG

Hyperglycosylated hCG is an essential autocrine produced during pregnancy made by cytotrophoblast cells. As discussed in Chapter 19, hyperglycosylated hCG first role is in implantation of pregnancy, maintenance of deep invasion by the placenta deep into the uterus. Hyperglycosylated hCG also has a major function in forcing the placenta to grow during pregnancy, growth in line to increasing fetal weight. Hyperglycosylated hCG promotes cytotrophoblast cell growth. Under the influence of hCG cytotrophoblast cells fuse to make syncytiotrophoblast cells. Thus placental mass ,cytotrophoblasts and syncytiotrophoblast cells or mass of villous placental tissue propogates throught the length of pregnancy

Human Placental Lactogen and Human Placental Growth Hormone

The pituitary gland produces human growth hormone (hGH). Little or no GH is produced, however, during pregnancy. The placental trophoblast cells make 2 hGH-related molecules during the course of pregnancy, human placental lactogen (hPL) and human placenta growth hormone (hPGH). Pituitary GH is a 191 amino acid protein hormone. hPL is a 190 amino acid protein hormone; it is extremely similar to hGH, with 85% common amino acid sequence. hPGH is a 191 amino acid protein hormone; it has 93% amino acid sequence homology with hGH. All 3 variants of growth hormone have a molecular weight of approximately 22,000. The genes coding hGH, hPL and hPGH are all close to each other on chromosome 17, suggesting duplication and common ancestry. The name human placental lactogen was chosen many years ago with the discovery of this placental hormone. Initial experiments showed that this molecule had lactogen-like bioactivity in animal models, hence the name. Modern research shows that hPL acts biologically in humans like hGH, controlling glucose levels and promoting growth. The lactogenic activity has not been confirmed in humans so the hormone's name is rather confusing.

hPL and hPGH primarily function to ensure a steady supply of glucose and amino acids for the fetus in mothers. Both hPL and hPGH have anti-insulin properties in mothers, decreasing maternal insulin sensitivity and thus raising maternal glucose levels, to supply glucose to the fetus. When fetal demands generate hypoglycemia in mothers, increased levels of hPL and hPGH produced by the syncytiotrophoblast cells convert increasing amounts of maternal fat to glucose (β-oxidation and gluconeogenesis). This meets fetal demands. Early in gestation, progesterone promotes an increased appetite in mothers. Excess glucose in pregnant mothers is then converted to fats (glycolysis and lipid synthesis) and stored. Later in pregnancy, hPL and hPGH mobilize this stored fat as glucose (lipolysis and gluconeogenesis) for the fetus. These fat deposits are the root of an important pathway in pregnancy, since late in pregnancy maternal tissues become progressively less sensitive to insulin, leading to higher maternal glucose levels. hPL and hPGH can also enter the fetal circulation and promote fetal growth. Studies show that hPGH concentrations in fetal circulation can be directly correlated with fetal growth in humans in the third trimester of human pregnancy. hPGH can promote glycogenesis in the fetuses, permitting storage of excess sugars for use by the fetus at times of nutritional deficiency.

The concentration of hPL rises from 10 ng/ml to 5000 ng/ml in serum during the course of pregnancy. hPL concentrations follow placenta size. hPGH concentrations in serum increase from <1 to 14 ng/ml as pregnancy advances, following a similar placenta size course. Neither hPL nor hPGH hormones have a specific receptor of their own in the mother and fetus and they bind the common hGH receptor in the mother and fetus to invoke metabolic functions, promoting lipolysis and gluconeogenesis to raise serum glucose levels and to promote fetal growth. Unduly low hPL levels in the fetus (amniotic fluid) are a predictor of intrauterine growth restriction (IUGR).

Estrogens

All three estrogens, E1 estrone, E2 estradiol and E3 estriol, are produced during pregnancy. Their synthesis and aromatization are somewhat different in pregnancy than during the menstrual cycle (see Chapter 4). In the synthesis of estrone (E1) and estradiol (E2), the fetal adrenal gland and the maternal adrenal gland produce a dehydroepiandrosterone-sulfate (DHEA-sulfate). This is the substrate. The placenta converts this molecule to androstenedione and on into testosterone. Then a placental aromatase converts androstenedione and testosterone to estrone (E1) and estradiol (E2) (Figure 4.8). High concentrations of estrogens are produced during pregnancy. The principal form of estrogen made in pregnancy is estriol (E3). Estriol (E3) is an estrogen with little use in the menstrual cycle [2,4,5,6,7]. The fetal adrenal makes DHEA-sulfate which is hydroxylated to 16α-hydroxy-DHEA-sulfate in the fetal liver. The fetal liver converts this to 16α-hydroxyandrostenedione which is passed to the placenta where aromatase converts this to estriol (Figure 4.8).

As shown in Figure 21.1, estradiol predominates during most of the course of pregnancy, but estriol uniquely, little used in the menstrual cycle, reaches higher concentrations, <100 ng/ml, in the third trimester of pregnancy. In the case of all three estrogens, levels in pregnancy exceed concentrations made during the menstrual cycle. Estrogens are lipids and are generally not water soluble molecules. A high proportion of estrogens are conjugated, existing as estrogen-sulfate or estrogen-glucurinide to enhance solubility. Some estrogens remain unconjugated; these may adhere to an albumin or another protein to permit transport in serum. Looking at pregnancy serum, for instance, approximately 33% of estrone is conjugated, 87% of estradiol is conjugated, and 94% of estriol is conjugated. Figure 21.1 shows the total concentrations of E1, E2 and E3 during pregnancy, conjugated plus unconjugated steroids.

Estrogens have multiple functions during pregnancy. Estrogens have a key function during building tissue. Estrogens accomplish this by either increasing the size or the number of tissues, vessels, and blood cells. Estrogens are a major factor in the increased size of the uterus and thickening of the uterine wall. During pregnancy, the uterus increases in size to contain the developing pregnancy. Uterine growth and thickening of the uterine wall are promoted by estrogens. Uterine size and fetal size are coordinated by placental hCG. The uterus grows from 60 grams in weight to 1200 grams during the course of pregnancy.

Estrogens are responsible for an increased lymphatic and nerve supply to the uterus during pregnancy. Estrogens also promote the growth of uterine veins to accommodate blood flow. Uterine veins may dilate up to 60 times larger than prepregnant states, in order to produce adequate drainage for the large uteroplacental venous output. Estrogens contribute to the increase in the maternal breast size. The numbers and size of ducts increase, vascularity increases, and the nipples and areolae become larger. This is dealt with in greater detail in Chapter 25.

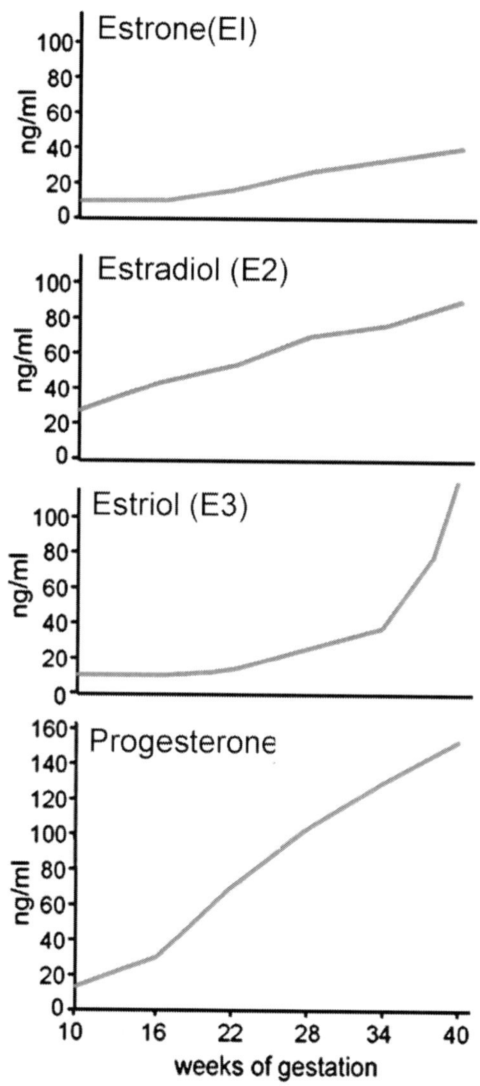

Figure 21.1. Concentration of sex steroids in maternal serum during pregnancy.

Estrogens change the composition of maternal blood. Estrogens cause an increase in serum-binding proteins, the proteins that bind and carry unconjugated sex steroids during pregnancy. There is a significant increase in the number of white blood cells in the blood due to estrogen action, leukocytosis of pregnancy. There is also an increase in the fibrinogen content of blood. As a result, blood clots or coagulates occur more readily. This decreases the risk of hemorrhage in pregnancy, but also increases the risk of blood clots or thrombosis.

There are numerous publications relating estrogen production in cell proliferation to fetal growth and well-being. Estrogen promotes anabolism or growth in the fetus in general, in fetal organs and fetal body and musculature. Estrogens soften connective tissue and collagen tissues during pregnancy. Estrogens, along with the hormone relaxin, relax pelvic joints and ligaments, and increase mobility of nipple tissue. In late pregnancy, fibers of the uterine cervix become swollen. This is preparing the cervix for dilation at parturition. A list of proven functions of estrogens in pregnancy is listed in Table 21.1.

Table 21.1. Functions of estrogens during pregnancy

1.	Increase uterine mass, thickening uterine wall;
2.	Increase uterine lymphatics and nerve response;
3.	Expand uterine venous output;
4.	Maternal blood, serum binding proteins increase, white blood cells increase, fibrinogen content increase;
5.	Increase maternal breast size, number of ducts, enlarge nipple and areolae;
6.	Fetal anabolism or growth promoter;
7.	Soften connective tissue/collagen, preparation of cervix for birth.

Progesterone

Progesterone has multiple roles relating to pregnancy and the development of the fetus. Prior to implantation, progesterone converts the endometrium to its secretory stage, expanding the epithelial lining to prepare the uterus for implantation. If pregnancy does not occur, progesterone levels decrease leading to menstruation. During implantation progesterone decreases the maternal immune response to allow for the acceptance of the pregnancy.

Progesterone stimulates the growth of breast tissue during pregnancy, most notably an increase in breast lobes. Milk glands and ducts develop in preparation for lactation. During this developmental stage, the presence of progesterone inhibits lactation. Progesterone inhibits prolactin, so that it is only at parturition when progesterone levels fall that lactation can occur. This subject is dealt with in detail in Chapter 25.

During pregnancy the cervix is closed with a thick, mucus plug. This mucus plug protects the pregnancy from bacteria. Decrease in progesterone levels causes the loss of the mucus plug at parturition. Progesterone is important for the fetal adrenal gland. Progesterone acts as a substrate for the adrenal glands to make glucocorticoids and mineralocorticoids. Rising fetal cortisol produced from progesterone in the fetal adrenal gland signifies the onset of labor/parturition in humans. Figure 21.1 shows maternal blood progesterone levels during pregnancy. Table 21.2 lists proven functions for progesterone during pregnancy.

Table 21.2. Functions of progesterone during pregnancy

1. Prepares endometrium and endometrial lining for implanting pregnancy;
2. Decreases maternal immune response to foreign invading tissue;
3. Promotes breast growth, blocking lactation during pregnancy;
4. Releases cervical plug at parturition;
5. Provides a substrate for fetal adrenal gland synthesis of glucocorticoids.

References

[1] Aschheim S, Zondek B. Das Hormon des hypophysenvorderlappens. testobjekt zum Nachweis des hormons. *Klin Wochenschr* 1927;6:248-252.

[2] Schmitt EJ, Barros CM, Fields PA, Fields MJ, Diaz T, Kluge JM, Thatcher WW. A cellular and endocrine characterization of the original and induced corpus luteum after administration of a gonadotropin-releasing hormone agonist or human chorionic gonadotropin on day five of the estrous cycle. *J Anim Sci* 1996;74:1915-1929

[3] Strott CA, Yoshimi T, Ross GT, Lipsett MB. Ovarian physiology: relationship between plasma LH and steroidogenesis by the follicle and corpus luteum; effect of hCG. *J Clin Endocrinol Metab* 1969;29:1157-1167.

[4] Mochtar MH, Hogerzeil HV, Mol BW. Progesterone alone versus progesterone combined with HCG as luteal support in GnRHa/HMG induced IVF cycles: a randomized clinical trial. *Hum Reprod* 1996;11:1602-1605.

[5] Akoum A, Metz CN, Morin M. Marked increase in macrophage migration inhibitory factor synthesis and secretion in human endometrial cells in response to human chorionic gonadotropin hormone. *J Clin Endocrinol Metab* 2005;90:2904-2910

[6] Matsuura T, Sugimura M, Iwaki T, Ohashi R, Kanayama N, Nishihira J. Anti-macrophage inhibitory factor antibody inhibits PMSG-hCG-induced follicular growth and ovulation in mice. *J Assist Reprod Genet* 2002;19:591-595.

[7] Wan H, Marjan A. Cheung VW, Leenen PJM, Khan NA, Benner R, Kiekens RCM. Chorionic gonadotropin can enhance innate immunity by stimulating macrophage function. *J Leukocyte Biol* 2007;82:926-933.

[8] Noonan FP, Halliday WJ, Morton H, Clunie GJA: Early pregnancy factor is immunosuppressive. *Nature* 1879;278:649-651.

[9] Reshef E, Lei ZM, Rao CV, Pridham DD, Chegini N, Luborsky JL. The presence of gonadotropin receptors in nonpregnant human uterus, human placenta, fetal membranes, and decidua. *J Clin Endocrinol Metab 1990*;70:421-430.

[10] Eta E, Ambrus G, Rao V. Direct regulation of human myometrial contractions by human chorionic gonadotropin. *J Clin Endocrinol Metab* 1994;79:1582-1586.

[11] Edelstam G, Karlsson C, Westgren M, Löwbeer C, Swahn ML. Human chorionic gonadatropin (hCG) during third trimester pregnancy. *Scand J Clin Lab Invest* 2007;67: 519-525.

[12] Goldsmith PC, McGregor WG, Raymoure WJ, Kuhn RW, Jaffe RB. Cellular localization of chorionic gonadotropin in human fetal kidney and liver. *J Clin Endocrinol Metab* 1983;57:54-61.

[13] Abdallah MA, Lei ZM, Li X, Greenwold N, Nakajima ST, Jauniaux E, Rao CV. Human Fetal nongonadal tissues contain human chorionic gonadotropin/ luteinizing hormone receptors. *J Clin Endocrinol Metab* 2004;89:952-956.

[14] Rao CV. Chapter 11: Paradigm shift on the targets of hCG actions. In: H*uman chorionic gonadotropin* (hCG). Ed. Cole LA, Elsevier, Oxford UK, 2010, pp 131-135.

[15] McGregor WG, Raymoure WJ, Kuhn RW, Jaffe RB. Fetal tissues can synthesize a placental hormone. Evidence for chorionic gonadotropin β-subunit synthesis by human fetal kidney. *J Clin Invest* 1981;68:306-309.

[16] Lei ZM, Rao CV, Kornyei J, Licht P, Hiatt ES. Novel expression of human chorionic gonadotropin/luteinizing hormone receptor gene in brain. E*ndocrinol* 1993;132:262-270.

[17] Rao CV: Immunocytochemical localization of gonadotropin and gonadal steroid receptors in human pineal glands. *J Clin Endocrinol Metab* 1997;82:2756-2757.

[18] Pedersen JF, Sørensen S, Ruge S. Human placental lactogen and pregnancy-associated plasma protein A in first trimester and subsequent fetal growth. *Acta Obstet Gynecol Scand* 1995;74:505-508.

[19] Giampietro O, Ferdeghini M, Scatena P. Human placental lactogen (hPL) deficiency in a normal pregnancy. *Postgrad Med J* 1984; 60: 689–690.

[20] *Human placental Lactogen, New York Times health Guide.* http://health.nytimes.com/health/guides/test/human-placental-lactogen/overview.html.

[21] Pedersen NG, Juul A, Christiansen M, Wøjdemann KR, Tabor A. Maternal serum placental growth hormone, but not human placental lactogen or insulin growth factor-1, is positively associated with fetal growth in the first half of pregnancy. *Ultrasound Obstet Gynecol* 2010;36:534-541.

[22] Albrecht ED, Pepe GJ. Estrogen regulation of placental angiogenesis and fetal ovarian development during primate pregnancy. *Int J Dev Biol* 2010;54:397-408.

[23] Panagiotopoulou K, Katsouyanni K, Petridou E, Garas Y, Tzonou A, Trichopoulos D. Maternal age, parity, and pregnancy estrogens. *Cancer Causes Control* 1990;1:119-124.

[24] Telleria CM, Zhong L, Deb S, Srivastava RK, Park KS, Sugino N, Park-Sarge OK, Gibori G. Differential expression of the estrogen receptors alpha and beta in the rat corpus luteum of pregnancy: regulation by prolactin and placental lactogens. *Endocrinol* 1998;139:2432-2442.

[25] Ortiz ME, Ortiz RE, Garfield R, Zepeda AJ, Croxatto HB. Progesterone, but not luteal estrogen, is required for the establishment of pregnancy in the new world monkey Cebus apella. *Am J Primatol* 2007;69:1131-1140.

[26] Verhaegen J, Gallos ID, van Mello NM, Abdel-Aziz M, Takwoingi Y, Harb H, Deeks JJ, Mol BW, Coomarasamy A. Accuracy of single progesterone test to predict early pregnancy outcome in women with pain or bleeding: meta-analysis of cohort studies. *Brit Med J* 2012;345:e6077.

[27] Norwitz ER, Phaneuf LE. Progesterone Supplementation and the Prevention of Preterm Birth. *Rev Obstet Gynecol* 2011; 4: 60–72.

[28] Haluska GJ, Cook MJ, Novy MJ. Inhibition and augmentation of progesterone production during pregnancy: effects on parturition in rhesus monkeys. *Am J Obstet Gynecol* 1997;176:682-691.

[29] Siiteri PK, Febres F, Clemens LE, Chang RJ, Gondos B, Stites D. Progesterone and maintenance of pregnancy: is progesterone nature's immunosuppressant? *Ann N Y Acad Sci* 1977;286:384-397.

Key Points

1. Placental hCG has multiple other functions during pregnancy, promoting corpus luteal progesterone production from 3.5 weeks to 7 weeks, preventing gestational trophoblastic disease. Placental hCG has also been shown to have a function in preventing immunosuppression and macrophage suppression of the foreign feto-placenta unit. The functions include suppression of contractions during the course of pregnancy and permitting them at term. A fetal hCG has been identified, produced by the fetal liver and kidney; this seemingly promotes the growth of fetal organs.
2. While it is important to know that estrogens and progesterone are essential for mammary development, it is not essential to fully understand the other functions of these steroids in pregnancy.
3. The use of hPL to modulate maternal glucose concentration for the fetus is important to understand, as is the storage of lipids in the mother for glucose reserve.
4. It needs to be understood that estriol is the major estrogen produced in the third trimester of pregnancy.
5. It is important to understand the interrelationship between hLG and hPGH and growth hormone, and that these molecules are simply growth hormone variants.

Chapter 22

Fetal Gender and Gonadal Development

Fetal Growth and Metabolism

Fetal growth is quite slow to around 20 weeks' gestation (Figure 22.1). At 8 weeks of gestation the fetus weighs just 0.0025 pounds; by 12 weeks of gestation 0.03 pounds, by 16 weeks of gestation 0.22 pounds, and by 20 weeks of pregnancy 0.66 pounds. Weight increase very much increases in a logarithmic-like manner as pregnancy advances, reaching means of 1.32, 2.22, 3.75, 5.78 and 7.63 pounds at 24, 28, 32,36 and 40 weeks of gestation [1].

Maternal health and nutrition are important for fetal growth and fetal health. Fetal health and nutrition are hindered by smoking and drug use. Maternal nutrition in pregnancy can have enduring effects on the health of the offspring, influencing mental and emotional health, susceptibility to cardiovascular disease and onset of non-insulin dependent diabetes mellitus.

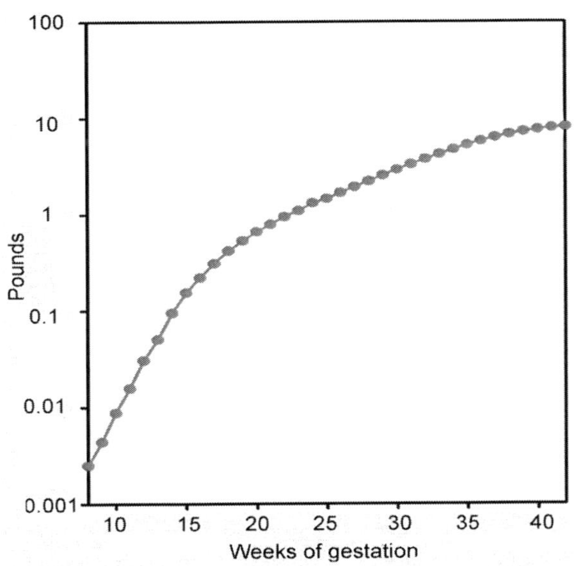

Figure 22.1. Weight gain of fetus during pregnancy, average weight at birth 7.16 pounds.

Carbohydrate or glucose is the principal nutrient of fetuses. Approximately 50% of the calories taken by fetuses should be glucose. Oxygen intake is also important. Maternal pulmonary ventilation increases 40% during pregnancy. The fetus has limited capability of gluconeogenesis or glucose generation. The fetus totally relies on the mother for obtaining needed glucose. As dealt with in the preceding chapters, the mother utilizes human placental lactogen (hPL) and human placental growth hormone (hPGH) to generate glucose needed by the fetus from her diet and from her fat storage [1].

Fetal Sexuality

The sex of the fetus comes from the haploid sets in the fertilized embryo. The genetic determinant of sex is the presence of the Y chromosome. The haploid set in a fertilized maternal ovum all have an X chromosome. If the ovum is fertilized by an X sperm (chromosome 23), then the fetus normally has a 46,XX diploid chromosome set, so will be female. If the ovum is fertilized by a Y sperm (chromosome 23), then the fetus normally has a 46,XY diploid chromosome set, so will be male [2,3].

Multiple complications occur in haploid chromosome meiosis and in chromosome replication. If there is an additional chromosome number 13, 18 or 21 generated then there is a trisomy. This is most commonly caused by a break in DNA on a chromosome leading to needless replication or replacement. Trisomy 13, 18 and 21 are called Patau's syndrome, Edward's syndrome and Down's syndrome, respectively. All are associated with gross neurological abnormalities. An extra chromosome or trisomy and a missing chromosome or monosomy can complicate the sex chromosome or chromosome pair 23.

Syndromes include Turner's Syndrome (45,X), a monosomy leading to a person with one X chromosome. This occurs in 1 in 2,500 newborn female babies. The person is phenotypically identified as a female, although infertile. Short stature and cognitive defect are common complications of this phenotype. Triple X syndrome is a common trisomy in females (47,XXX). It occurs in 1 in 1,000 newborn females. The person is phenotypically identified as a female. This syndrome has minimal complications and does not commonly interfere with menstrual cycle or fertility. Klinefelter's syndrome (47,XXY) is quite common, occurring in 1 in 1,000 newborn males. The person phenotypically is a male. The most common complications are reduced male fertility, low sperm count and small testicles. Lastly, 47,XYY also occurs at a rate of approximately 1 in 1,000 newborn males. Phenotypically, the person is a male. While the male may have normal fertility, fast growth is common and some mental retardation is also common [2,3].

SRY stands for <u>S</u>ex-related <u>R</u>egion of <u>Y</u> chromosome. A group of genes coding for the development of the testis is located at the end of the short arm of the Y chromosome; this is considered the SRY zone. If, during male meiosis, this group of genes is translocated to the X chromosome, and XY fetus (no SRY) can be generated with no signal to generate testis, no testosterone, and no male characteristics, it is phenotypically recognized as a female (46,XY^{-SRY}). Alternatively, an XX fetus (with SRY) can have the signals to make testis, generate testosterone and have a male phenotype (46,XX^{SRY}). Unfortunately, both (46,XY^{-SRY}) females and (46,XX^{SRY}) males are infertile, but have no other genetic or neurological problems. Studies with aborted fetuses and animals suggest that the occurrence of SRY syndromes (46,XY^{-SRY} females and 46,XX^{SRY} males) may be quite high; however, the incidence is a matter of conjecture. It has to simply be considered as a cause of infertility [2,3].

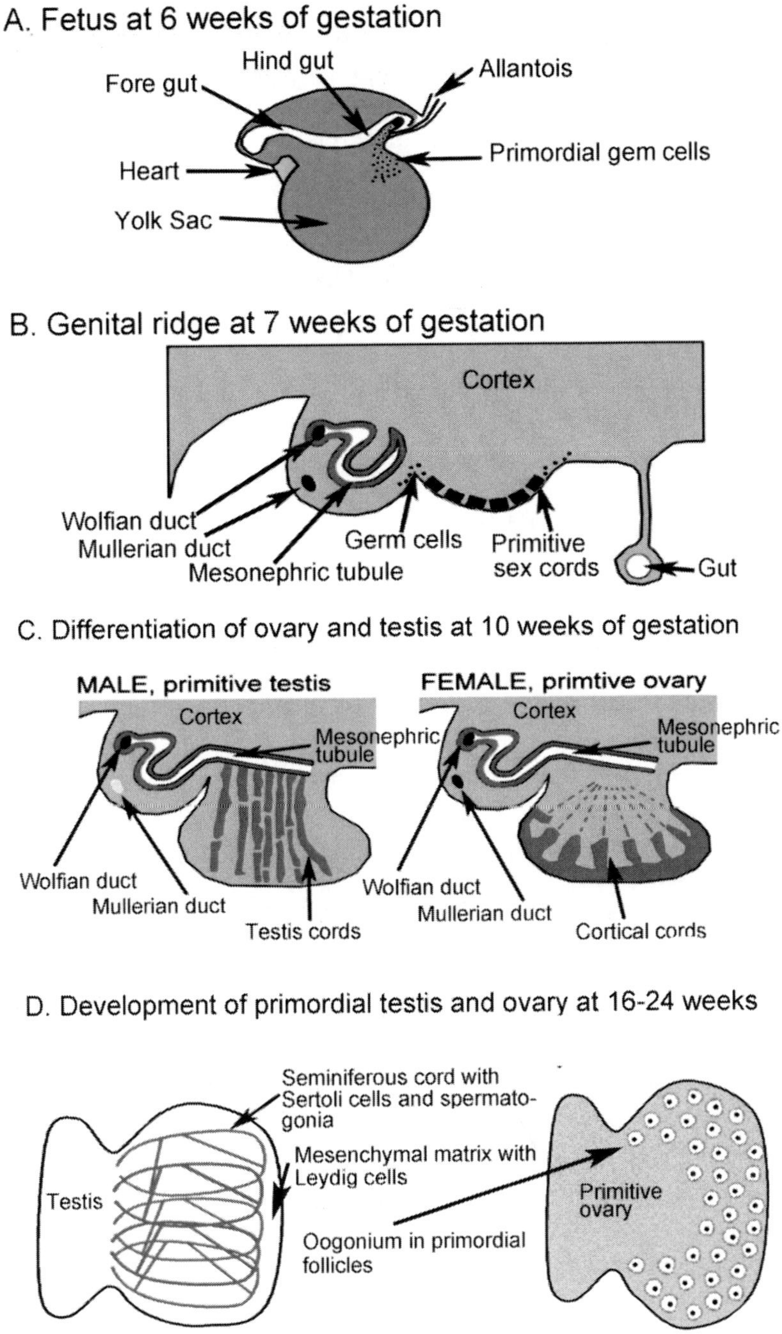

Figure 22.2. The development of gonads with fetal maturity.

Fetal Gonad Differentiation

Fetal gonad development starts around 6 weeks of gestation. At this time no sexual differentiation occurs (Figure 22.2 section A). The primordium (primordial structure) is undifferentiated primordial germ cells, formed in the yolk sac near the developing allantois (Figure 22.2 section A). These cells first migrate to the genital ridge (Figure 22.2 section B). The genital ridge cells differentiate, forming the germinal epithelium at around 8 weeks' gestation. The migration to the genital ridge is driven by amoeboid movement. The genital ridge produces a chemotactic substance to enhance primordial germ cell attraction. Over the following weeks the primordial germ cells form the primitive undifferentiated sex cords on the germinal epithelium (Figure 22.2 section B). An incomplete signal at this point can result in hermaphroditism. The differentiation and formation of the primitive testis and primitive ovary occurs at the genital ridge (Figure 22.2 section B)[4-10].

In the male karyotype, that having a Y chromosome and SRY set of genes, the undifferentiated sex cords enlarge at around 10 weeks' gestation and form the primitive testis (Figure 22.2 section C). The primordial germ cells within the sex cords, the testis cords, differentiate into immature sperm cells or spermatogonia with the formation of the primitive testis on the genital ridge at around 16-20 weeks of gestation (Figure 22.2 section C).

Ovarian gonad differentiation follows testicular differentiation with a 2-4 weeks' delay. Initially, the sex cords formed by the primordial germ cells proliferate (Figure 22.2 section B) in the germinal epithelium forming primordial oocytes or oogonia. The sex cords then form on the genetic ridge, developing to the primitive ovary (Figure 22.2 section C). Oogonia then form from the germ cells. Basically, small clusters then form around these oogonia. This initiates the formation of primary follicles characteristic of the ovary. In these follicles, mesenchymal cells secrete an outer basement membrane. The mesenchymal cells then give rise to the granulosa cells of the follicle. The granulosa cells and oogonia together form oocytes and primordial follicles which fill the primary ovary (Figure 22.2 section D). This describes the early development of the ovary and testis [4-10].

Fetal Reproductive Accessory Organ Differentiation

Sexual differentiation of reproductive accessory organs is dependent totally on secretory products produced by the primordial testis, formed as described above. These are Müllerian-inhibiting substance (MIS) made by cells destined to be Sertoli cells, and testosterone produced by the cells destined to be Leydig cells. If these secretory products are present, the fetus develops as a male. If these secretory products are absent, then the fetus will always develop as a female. No equivalent absolute signal is made by the primordial ovary. In fact, a castrated female fetus (primitive ovary removed) still develops female accessory organs [11-18].

While the fetal gonads develop from one primordium, the primordial germ cells, the reproductive accessory organs develop from two parallel sets of sex-specific organ-generating canals, the Wolffian duct and Müllerian duct (Figure 22.3 panel A). Both are present in all early fetuses. If primitive testes are present and MIS and testosterone are secreted, the Wolffian duct will develop into an epididymis, vas deferens and prostate gland, and the Müllerian duct will be degenerated (Figure 22.3 panel B Male). If MIS and testosterone are absent, then the Müllerian duct will develop into fimbria, a fallopian tube, a uterus and a vagina, and the Wolffian duct will be degenerated (Figure 22.3 panel B Female). Figure 22.3 panel B shows partial differentiation in the male and female at 17 weeks of gestation. The primitive Wolffian and Müllerian ducts develop parallel to the male and female urinary tracts. As the kidney and urinary tract develops, so does the Wolffian and Müllerian ducts (Figure 22.3]. When either sex system develops the other duct system degenerates [11-18].

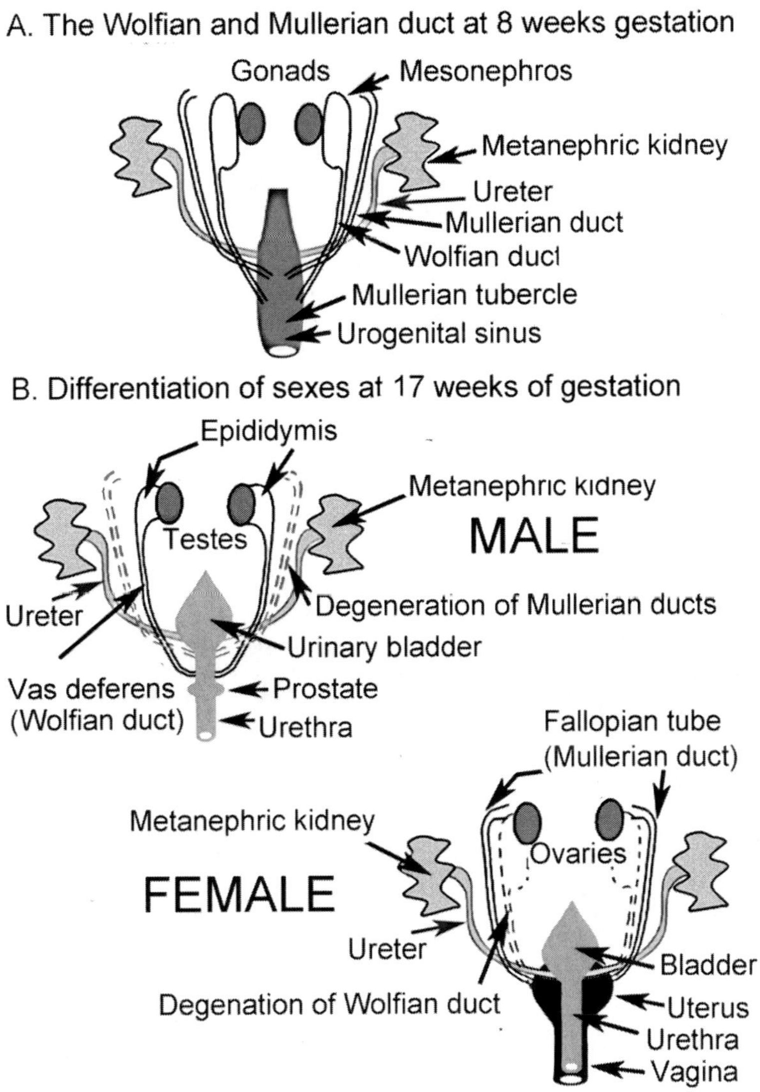

Figure 22.3. Fetal reproductive accessory organ differentiation.

In male fetuses, MIS is coded for by a gene in the SRY segment of the Y chromosome. As such, the MIS signal is absent in 46,XY^{-SRY} individuals, leading to the development of the Müllerian duct. In 46,XX^{SRY} individuals, MIS destroys the Müllerian duct, leading to there being no vagina, uterus or fallopian tube. MIS signals the degeneration of the Müllerian duct. Similarly, testosterone promotes the development of the Wolffian duct, the formation of the epididymis and vas deferens. In males the prostate forms at the base of the disappearing Müllerian tubercle in the position of the urogenital sinus (Figure 22.3, panel A)[11-18].

In the female fetus, if MIS is absent, the Müllerian duct develops. The Müllerian duct induces formation of the vaginal plate which initiates formation of the vagina and uterus (Figure 21.2, panel B). The Müllerian duct also differentiates into the fallopian tube (Figure 22.3, panel B). The absence of testosterone leads to the degeneration of the Wolffian duct [11-18].

References

[1] Mongelli M, Gardosi J. Fetal growth. *Curr Opin Obstet Gynecol* 2000;12:111-115.

[2] Efrat Z, Perri T, Ramati E, Tugendreich D, Meizner I. Fetal gender assignment by first-trimester ultrasound. *Ultrasound Obstet Gynecol* 2006;27:619-621.

[3] Devaney SA, Palomaki GE, Scott JA, Bianchi DW. Noninvasive fetal sex determination using cell-free fetal DNA: a systematic review and meta-analysis. *J Am Med Assoc* 2011 ;306:627-636.

[4] Bartha JL, Finning K, Soothill PW. Fetal sex determination from maternal blood at 6 weeks of gestation when at risk for 21-hydroxylase deficiency. *Obstet Gynecol* 2003; 101:1135-1136.

[5] Dominguez MM, Liptrap RM, Basrur PK. Steroidogenesis in fetal bovine gonads. *Can J Vet Res* 1988;52:401-406.

[6] McLaren A, Buehr M. Development of mouse germ cells in cultures of fetal gonads. *Cell Differ Dev* 1990;31:185-195.

[7] Modi DN, Sane S, Bhartiya D. Accelerated germ cell apoptosis in sex chromosome aneuploid fetal human gonads. *Mol Hum Reprod* 2003;9:219-225.

[8] Francavilla S, Cordeschi G, Properzi G, Concordia N, Cappa F, Pozzi V. Ultrastructure of fetal human gonad before sexual differentiation and during early testicular and ovarian development. *J Submicrosc Cytol Pathol* 1990;22:389-400.

[9] Taketo T, Saeed J, Roberge S, Matsuo N, Koide SS. Regulation of testicular differentiation and testosterone production in the fetal mouse gonad in vitro. *J Steroid Biochem Mol Biol* 1991;38:523-531.

[10] Rabinovici J, Jaffe RB. Development and regulation of growth and differentiated function in human and subhuman primate fetal gonads. *Endocr Rev* 1990;11:532-557.

[11] Gray LE, Ostby J, Furr J, Wolf CJ, Lambright C, Parks L, Veeramachaneni DN, Wilson V, Price M, Hotchkiss A, Orlando E, Guillette L. Effects of environmental antiandrogens on reproductive development in experimental animals. *Hum Reprod Update*. 2001;7:248-264.

[12] Zhang FP, Poutanen M, Wilbertz J, Huhtaniemi I. Normal prenatal but arrested postnatal sexual development of luteinizing hormone receptor knockout (LuRKO) mice. *Mol Endocrinol* 2001;15:172-183.

[13] Barsoum I, Yao HH. The road to maleness: from testis to Wolffian duct. *Trends Endocrinol Metab* 2006;17:223-228.
[14] Bok G, Drews U. The role of the Wolffian ducts in the formation of the sinus vagina: an organ culture study. *J Embryol Exp Morphol.* 1983 Feb;73:275-95.
[15] Mege JL, Sabatier-Laval E, Mure PY, Vargas B, Dubois R, Takvorian P, Dodat H. Malformations of Wolffian duct derived male genital organs (epididymis, vas deferens, seminal vesicules, ejaculatory ducts). *Prog Urol* 1997;7:262-269.
[16] Mauch RB, Thiedemann KU, Drews U. Anat Embryol (Berl). The vagina is formed by downgrowth of Wolffian and Müllerian ducts. *Graphical reconstructions from normal and Tfm mouse embryos.* 1985;172:75-87.
[17] Grynnerup AG, Lindhard A, Sørensen S. The role of anti-Müllerian hormone in female fertility and infertility - an overview. *Acta Obstet Gynecol Scand* 2012;91:1252-1260.
[18] Odi TO, Abdur-Rahman LO, Nasir AA. Persistent Mullerian duct syndrome: a case report and review of the literature. *Afr J Paediatr Surg* 2010;7:191-193.

Key Points

1. Fetal growth is quite slow to around 20 weeks of gestation, then becomes more and more rapid.
2. Most calories used by the developing fetus are from glucose.
3. Three sexual monosomies and trisomies are quite common, together accounting for 1 in 800 total pregnancies (1 in 2500 females, 1 in 1000 females and 1 in 1000 males). These are Turner's syndrome (45,X), Triple X (47,XXX) and Klinefelter's syndrome 47,XXY.
4. SRY (Sex Region of Y chromosome) is a key region of the Y chromosome including the critical gene for Müllerian-inhibiting substance. With meiosis SRY can be lost from the Y chromosome and gained on an X chromosome. As such, infertile 46,XX^{SRY} males and 46,XY^{-SRY} females can occur.
5. Development of the gonads starts at around 6 weeks of gestation with migration of primordial root germ cells, made in the yolk sac, to the genital ridge, where undifferentiated sex cords are formed and differentiation occurs.
6. In males (those with Y chromosome and SRY genes), the undifferentiated primitive sex cords differentiate to form the testis cords and then the primitive testis is formed at around 16-20 weeks' gestation.
7. Female fetuses (those lacking the Y chromosome and SRY genes) have the undifferentiated primitive sex cords. They form the ovarian cords and then the primitive ovary is formed approximately 2-4 weeks after male differentiation, or around 18-24 weeks' gestation.
8. All fetuses have by 8 weeks' gestation a parallel pair of Müllerian ducts and Wolffian ducts. The Wolffian duct develops in males forming an epididymis and a vas deferens. The Müllerian duct is degenerated in males. The Müllerian duct differentiates in females forming the fimbria, a fallopian tube, a uterus and upper vagina. The Wolffian duct is degenerated in females.

9. Müllerian-inhibiting substance (MIS) and testosterone are made by the primitive testis. These dictate the sex of the fetus. MIS causes the degeneration of the Müllerian duct. Testosterone promotes the differentiation of the Wolffian duct to form an epididymis and vas deferens. This is the solitary sexual differentiation signal; the primitive ovary forms no signal in the female.

Chapter 23

Parturition

Fetal Endocrinology and Preparation for Birth

The fetus needs to be delivered to survive. The fetus needs to develop mechanisms to prepare it for delivery. The rising levels of glucocorticoids as pregnancy approaches term have a key role in maturing the respiratory system to prepare for life dependent on self-breathed oxygen compared with life dependent on the free supply of maternal oxygen. Other critical anatomical changes and functional changes prepare the fetus for birth.

It has already been emphasized that human chorionic gonadotropin (hCG), human placental growth hormone (hPGH) and human estrogens (Chapters 14 and 21) have important roles in maternal physiology and fetal development (Table 23.1). Most fetal endocrinology glands have become functional by the end of the first trimester of pregnancy. Most of the fetal hormones have special functions just in fetal development. This is discussed here [1-4].

In the third trimester of pregnancy the fetal lungs go through a rehearsal. For several hours each day rapid movements of the diaphragm and lungs are made. These move amniotic fluids into and out of the lung. These movements are assumed to be practice for birth. Among the changes that occur at birth, the cardiovascular system must switch between a fetal circulatory system involving the placenta supplying oxygen/carbon dioxide gaseous exchange and a birth system in which the lungs provide gaseous exchange [1-4].

Thyroid Hormones

The secretion of thyroxine from the fetal thyroid gland becomes most apparent after 20 weeks' gestation. Thyroxine in the fetus is promoted by the pituitary thyroid stimulating hormone. Thyroxine is essential for normal development of the fetus. Fetal hypothyroidism is associated with poor fetal bone development and deficiency in fetal body hair. Most importantly, hypothyroidism is associated with retarded fetal behavior. This is because thyroxine is essential for normal differentiation of the brain (Table 23.1).

Table 23.1. Promotion of growth and differentiation of fetal organs by fetal endocrines

Hormone	Function in fetus
Human placental growth hormone	Function indicated in promotion of fetal growth
Human chorionic gonadotropin	Receptors found on lung, liver, kidney, spleen, intestines Function suggested in promoting fetal growth and development
Adrenocorticotropic hormone	Promoted formation of islets of Langerhans in pancreas
Adrenocorticotropic hormone	Control fetal glucocorticoid production
Thyroxine	Promotes differentiation of fetal brain
Thyroxine	Promotes bone development and fetal hair growth
Testosterone	Promotes sexual differentiation of the brain
Glucocorticoids	Promotes enzyme needed for surfactant synthesis
Glucocorticoids	Promotes fluid resorption in lung
Glucocorticoids	Regulates maturation of fetal islets of Langerhans in pancreas
Thyroid stimulating hormone	Controls fetal thyroxine production

Pancreatic Hormones

The islet of Langerhans cells of the pancreas are activated early in gestation. Development of these cells is apparently initiated by pituitary adrenocorticotrophic hormone (ACTH), and the action of adrenal glucocorticoids. The rate at which glucose is utilized by the fetus is largely controlled by fetal insulin, which becomes active at around 10 weeks of gestation [1-4].

Adrenal Hormones

Adrenal glucocorticoids have important functions in the fetus. Glucocorticoid production by the fetal adrenal (cortisol) is controlled by pituitary ACTH signaling. Cortisol is present in fetal blood at around 10 weeks of gestation, and blood levels increase as gestation progresses. After birth the adrenal gland undergoes structural changes [1-4].

The pressure required to expand the fetal lung changes as gestation advances. This is due to the synthesis of a surfactant, a phospholipid. The surfactant reduced the surface tension of pulmonary fluids in the lung, easing expansion. The surfactant synthesis starts in the middle trimester of pregnancy but is especially active in the two months before birth. Glucocorticoids have a major function in activating the enzyme needed for surfactant synthesis. Glucocorticoids are also responsible for converting noradrenalin to adrenalin to promote respiratory function and for synthesis of catecholamine receptors in the lung. Glucocorticoids aid fluid resorption in the lung at the time of birth (Table 23.1) [1-4].

Anterior Pituitary Hormones

The anterior lobe of the pituitary functions through most of fetal life. Growth hormone is produced, but research suggests that it has no clear function in fetal growth. Prolactin is produced, but has no clear function. TSH promotes thyroid hormone production and ACTH promotes adrenal function throughout gestation [1-4].

Testis

Male testes produce testosterone which can have sex-specific effects on the brain. Testosterone influences neural developments. Testosterone is a neuromodulator (Table 23.1).

Myometrium, Cervix, Oxytocin and Prostaglandin Action at Parturition

Prior to birth the fetus resides within its fetal membrane in the uterus (Figure 23.1). It is held in place by a firm cervix. Delivery requires contraction of the uterine myometrial muscle assisted by contractions of the muscles of the abdominal wall to expel the fetus, and ripening or softening of the cervix. These processes and the hormones and prostaglandins that promote these events are discussed here [5-10].

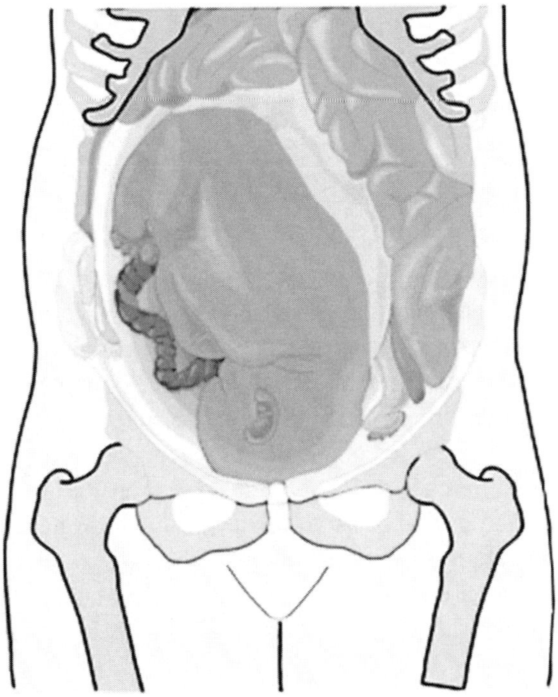

Figure 23.1. The fetus prior to parturition.

Myometrium Function during Parturition

The myometrium is mostly comprised of muscle, uterine spiral arteries and nerves. During the course of pregnancy estrogens increase the bulk of muscles. Contractions of the myometrium at parturition are dependent upon a rise of intracellular calcium. The calcium binds regulator sites on the proteins actin and myosin, leading to the expression of an ATPase and a contraction. Contractions are activated by prostaglandins and by oxytocin. Prostaglandins promote contractions by enhancing the supply of calcium from intracellular calcium stores. Data suggest that hCG may restrict contractions in pregnancy [11]. Evidence suggests that a decline in hCG at parturition may be necessary to permit myometrial contractions [11].

Cervix Function during Parturition

The cervix is important in retaining the fetus during pregnancy. The cervix is mostly composed of collagen fiber connective tissue to hold the cervix firmly and resist stretch with fetal growth. In order for the fetus to pass the cervix and into the birth canal for delivery the composition of the cervix must change by ripening or softening. At the time of parturition a reduction occurs in the collagen fiber content of the cervix, with marked increases in glycosaminoglycans which decrease the aggregation of the remaining collagen fibers. Metalloproteinases or digestive enzymes start to abound in the cervix as parturition approaches. These chew up the cervical proteins leading to a softening of the tissue [5-10].

Prostaglandins, in addition to promoting myometrial contractions, enhance cervical ripening. PGE_2 and $PGF_{2\alpha}$ both have roles in cervical ripening. Prostaglandins can be used clinically to facilitate cervical ripening during normal delivery.

Oxytocin Reflex Action

Oxytocin acts in a reflex-like way, with nerves in the cervix and myometrium, signaling the nervous release of the molecule. Oxytocin is a nonapeptide synthesized by hypothalamic neurons. It is transported axonally to the posterior lobe of the pituitary where it is released. The release of oxytocin occurs in response to a cervical or myometrial touch or stretch tactile signal. The nervous signal is transmitted through the spine to the brain stem and on to the hypothalamus leading to oxytocin release and oxytocin promotion of contractions. The entire cycle, tactile signal-brain stem-hypothalamus-oxytocin release-contraction is like a neuroendocrine reflex. The number of oxytocin receptors on the myometrium increases as parturition approaches. The abundance of oxytocin receptors on the myometrium increases significantly as parturition approaches. When oxytocin binds its receptor it directly leads to a contraction by lowering the muscular threshold at which a contraction occurs [5-10].

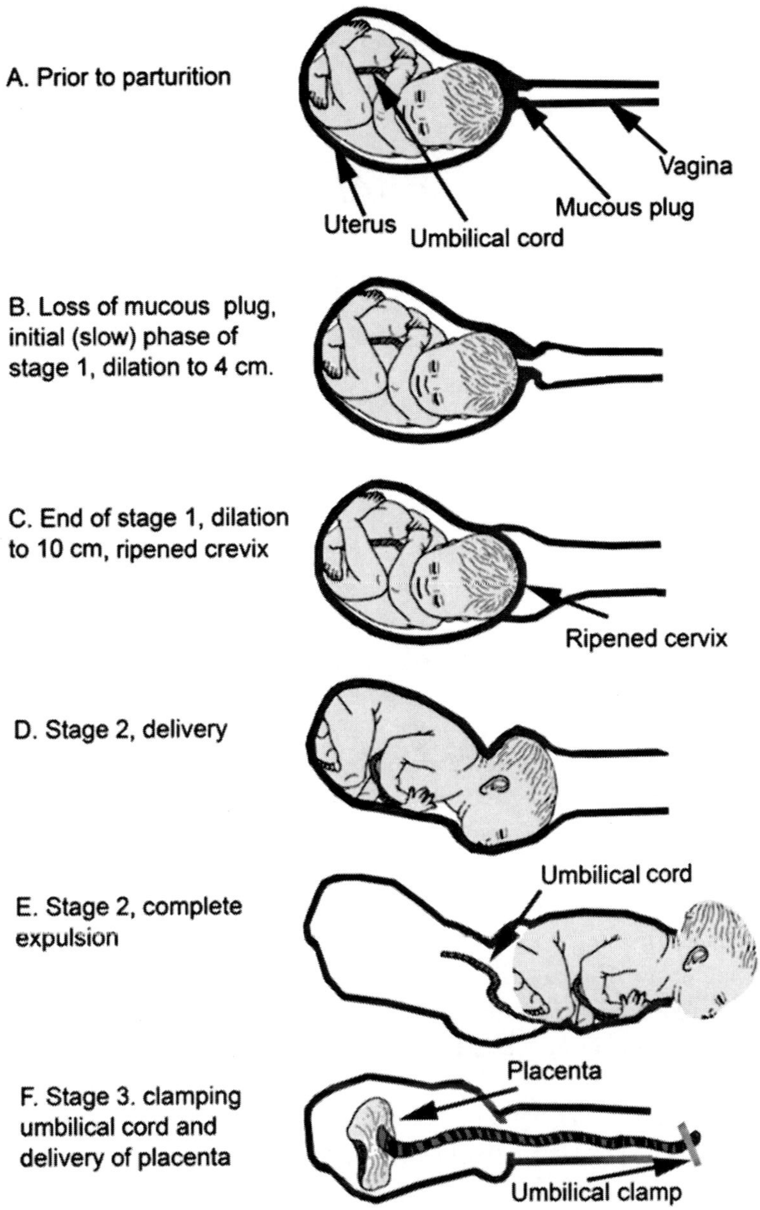

Figure 23.2. The stages of labor and delivery.

Prostaglandins and Initiation of Parturition

In most mammalian species the timing of parturition is due to glucocorticoids. These promote aromatase activity leading to estrogen synthesis. The estrogen produced promotes $PGF_{2\alpha}$ production by the uterus. This activates the events of parturition, promoting contractions and cervical ripening. In addition, oxytocin produced through the reflex-like action enhances contractions and promotes $PGF_{2\alpha}$. In humans, however, administration of adrenocorticotropic hormone to the fetus, which promotes fetal adrenal cortisol production, does not initiate parturition. In humans the pathways of initiation of parturition are very uncertain [5-10].

Labor and Delivery

In the preceding section the procedures that control onset of labor, or the processes by which the mother delivers a baby, were described. Premature labor is defined as delivery after viability (24 weeks gestation) or up to 37 weeks gestation. Term delivery is defined at 37-42 weeks gestation.

Labor is divided into 3 clear stages (Figure 23.2). The first stage comprises contractions of the myometrium (and abdominal muscles) and ripening of the cervix to permit delivery. Dilation of the cervix may be slow until 4 cm, and more rapid thereafter. The first stage is complete when the cervix has dilated to 10 cm. The second stage of labor starts with the cervix dilated to 10 cm and ends with expulsion of the fetus, or birth. The third stage begins with fetal delivery and ends after clamping of the umbilical cord with release and expulsion of the placenta (Figure 23.2)[12-15].

In the first stage of labor large contractions of the myometrium start occurring. Contractions start slowly and become more and more rapid as the first stage proceeds (Figure 23.2). The function of the early large contractions is to retract the lower uterine segment and cervix upwards to allow the vagina and uterus to align as a continuum or birth canal (Figure 23.2), through which the fetus is expelled. The occurrence of brachystasis reflects the properties of myometrial cells, whereby shortening of each muscle contraction occurs. Muscles contract, and rest, followed by a failure of the muscles to contract at such length. With each subsequent contraction further shortening of the muscle occurs. During this time in the first stage of labor ripening of the cervix is completed [12-15].

In the second stage of labor, the fully dilated cervix is brought up to the pelvic inlet. Subsequent uterine contractions and the resulting decrease in uterine volume push the fetus downward and through the birth canal (Figure 23.2). In the third stage, after the delivery of the fetus and clamping of the umbilical cord, the placenta, with further contractions, becomes detached from the uterine wall. Within a short time the placenta is expelled by uterine contractions. The first stage of labor commonly takes 8 hours (multiparous pregnancies) to 14 hours (nulliparous pregnancies). In the second stage of labor, expulsion of the fetus is quite rapid, taking less than an hour. The third stage of labor is also relatively rapid, approximately 30 minutes.

Parturition is a time when the fetus is very vulnerable, with the massive adjustments from placental respiratory respiration to lung respiratory respiration, and with the extreme pressure of delivery. The traditional approach is to monitor the fetal heart rate with a Pinard obstetric stethoscope or fetoscope. Modern methods include the electronic fetal monitor and telemetry. If fetal stress is detected during labor a Caesarian section can be indicated [12-15].

References

[1] McPherson RA, Khadka N, Moore JM, Sharma M. Are birth-preparedness programmes effective? Results from a field trial in Siraha district, Nepal. *J Health Popul Nutr* 2006; 24:479-488.

[2] Lothian JA. Safe, Healthy Birth: What Every Pregnant Woman Needs to Know. *J Perinat Educ* 2009;18:48–54.

[3] Chaim W, Mazor M. The relationship between hormones and human parturition. *Arch Gynecol Obstet.* 1998;262:43-51.

[4] Germain G, Ferre F. Hormones and parturition in primates. Ann *Endocrinol* 1987;48:311-321.

[5] Thomson AJ, Telfer JF, Young A, Campbell S, Stewart CJ, Cameron IT, Greer IA, Norman JE. Leukocytes infiltrate the myometrium during human parturition: further evidence that labour is an inflammatory process. *Hum Reprod.* 1999;14:229-236.

[6] Mesiano S. Myometrial progesterone responsiveness and the control of human parturition. *J Soc Gynecol Investig* 2004;11:193-202.

[7] Mitchell BF, Fang X, Wong S. Oxytocin: a paracrine hormone in the regulation of parturition? *Rev Reprod.* 1998 May;3:113-122.

[8] Blanks AM, Thornton S. The role of oxytocin in parturition. *Brit J Obstet Gynecol 2003*; 20:46-51.

[9] Karim SM. The role of prostaglandins in human parturition. *Proc R Soc Med 1971*;64:10–12.

[10] Challis JR, Lye SJ, Gibb W. Prostaglandins and parturition. *Ann N Y Acad Sci* 1997; 828:254-267.

[11] Eta E, Ambrus G, Rao V: Direct regulation of human myometrial contractions by human chorionic gonadotropin. *J Clin Endocrinol Metab* 1994;79:1582-1586.

[12] Al-Kuran O, Al-Mehaisen L, Bawadi H, Beitawi S, Amarin Z. The effect of late pregnancy consumption of date fruit on labour and delivery. *J Obstet Gynaecol.* 2011;31:29-31.

[13] O'Brien WF. The role of prostaglandins in labor and delivery. *Clin Perinatol* 1995; 22:973-984.

[14] Ehrenthal DB, Jiang X, Strobino DM. Labor induction and the risk of a cesarean delivery among nulliparous women at term. *Obstet Gynecol.* 2010;116:35-42.

[15] Delivery presentations. http://www.nlm.nih.gov/medlineplus/ency/article/002060.htm

Key Points

1. Thyroid hormone production is critical to a fetus in that it partially controls the differentiation and development of the brain.
2. Insulin is also critical for a fetus in controlling glucose usage.
3. Glucocorticoids such as cortisol are critical, promoting the formation of the surfactant needed for the birth lungs, promoting fluid resorption by the lung and promoting the formation of the islets of Langerhans early in pregnancy.

4. The myometrial muscle is the principal muscle of pregnancy contractions, and is essential for natural birth. Oxytocin and prostaglandins $PGF_{2\alpha}$ and PGE_2 promote contractions.
5. The cervix has to be ripened to permit expulsion of the fetus. Prostaglandins $PGF_{2\alpha}$ and PGE_2 promote ripening.
6. Labor and delivery occurs in 3 clear and separate stages. The first stage comprises contraction of the myometrium and ripening of the cervix, and dilation of the cervix to 10 cm. The second stage comprises expulsion and delivery of the fetus. The third stage comprises further myometrial contractions, detachment of the placenta and expulsion of the placenta.

Chapter 24

Perinatal Complications of Pregnancy

Hypertension in Pregnancy

Hypertension in pregnancy is a major complication of pregnancy, affecting as many as 15% of pregnancies. If blood pressure is greater than 140/90, pregnancy induced hypertension (PIH) is indicated (5-15% of pregnancies). If a patient also has proteinuria (urine protein greater than 0.3g / 24 h), then preeclampsia is indicated (5-10% of pregnancies). Severe PIH or preeclampsia is indicated by a blood pressure greater than 160/110 or by a significant proteinuria. PIH and preeclampsia often worsen as pregnancy advances, leading to HELLP syndrome (Hemolysis, Elevated Liver enzymes, Low Platelet syndrome) and eclampsia. These are marked by seizures and cerebro-vascular accidents in the mother. Hypertension in pregnancy is the greatest death threat during pregnancy.

All symptoms of PIH, preeclampsia, eclampsia and HELLP syndrome occur after 20 weeks' gestation, most commonly in the third trimester of pregnancy. Symptoms of PIH include hypertension as indicated by headaches, blurry vision and fatigue. Preeclampsia is indicated by proteinuria, decreased urine output and swelling of the face and hands, as well as swelling of the feet.

Much research in the last 20 years has focused on the causes of PIH and preeclampsia. Numerous publications now show that poor fetal nutrition, due to ineffective hemochorial placentation (see Chapter 20), poor placental invasion or insufficient blood flow to the uterus are causes of PIH/preeclampsia. The maternal cardiovascular system seemingly copes with these issues by raising the blood pressure. Poor villous invasion by cytotrophoblast cells in the first trimester of pregnancy can lead to ineffective hemochorial placentation, leading to potential fetal anoxia and PIH/preeclampsia (Chapter 20). This is why babies resulting from PIH and preeclampsia pregnancies are commonly unduly small at birth (less than 10th percentile).

Chapter 19 shows that hyperglycosylated hCG is at the root of placental invasion. As published, individuals who develop PIH and preeclampsia have unduly low hyperglycosylated hCG, or invasion signals, during the first trimester of pregnancy [5,6]. It appears that unduly low hyperglycosylated hCG at the time of implantation leads to failing pregnancies (Chapter 19), and that if a pregnancy produces sufficient hyperglycosylated hCG for implantation of pregnancy, but produces low hyperglycosylated hCG during the first or second trimester of pregnancy, it leads to PIH/preeclampsia after 20 weeks of gestation [5,6].

If a pregnancy is close to term, the best treatment for PIH/preeclampsia is to deliver the pregnancy. Otherwise, a combination of rest, consuming less salts, drinking 8 glasses of water a day, a high protein diet, calcium supplementation and baby aspirin is recommended. If blood pressure is severe, >160/110, blood pressure medications may be prescribed to avoid vascular accident in the mother.

Intrauterine Growth Restriction (IUGR)

IUGR is considered whenever the fetal weight is below the 10th percentile. The most common causes of IUGR are maternal behavior factors (see Table 24.1). Approximately 7% of pregnancies are considered IUGR. Alcohol use by a mother in the first trimester of pregnancy may lead to Fetal Alcohol Syndrome (FAS). However, alcohol use (as little as 2 drinks a day) in the second and third trimesters of pregnancy may cause IUGR.

Table 24.1. Causes of IUGR

1. Maternal behavior factors
Cigarette smoking
Alcohol use
Cocaine or other illicit drug use
Benzodiazepine or other prescribed drug use
Malnutrition or poor nutrition
2. Fetal factors
Chromosomal aberrations
Congenital factors, trisomy 13, 18, 21, Turner's syndrome
Multiple pregnancies, twins, triplets etc.
3. Infections
Syphilis
Cytomegalovirus
Rubella
Hepatitis B
HIV
Toxoplasmosis
Herpes simplex virus
4. Medical complications
PIH or preeclampsia
Maternal chronic heart disease
Uterine abnormalities

IUGR is categorized as symmetric or asymmetric. Symmetric refers to fetuses with poor growth velocity of the head, abdomen and long bones. Asymmetric refers to fetuses with poor growth of the abdomen and internal organs. IUGR is diagnosed by ultrasound by either fundal height (size of the uterus; from the top of the uterus to the top of the mother's pubic bone), or estimated fetal weight. If this is less than the 10th percentile for the gestational age, IUGR is considered. To determine if the baby is just small and growing normally or has IUGR, the baby's head circumference is compared to the baby's abdomen circumference. These are repeated with time. IUGR is indicated if a reduction in the abdomen circumference is noted compared to the head circumference. Decreased amniotic fluid volume is also an indicator of IUGR versus normal growth.

If IUGR is suspected, close fetal surveillance is recommended using ultrasound. Considerable fetal morbidity and mortality are associated with IUGR. This is caused by inadequate maternal-fetal circulation or fetal nutrition. Most fetuses with IUGR die after the 36th week of gestation. As such, the physician will need to carefully balance the risk of premature delivery (Caesarian section) in IUGR cases, with the risk of fetal death.

It is not possible to reverse, repair or undo IUGR. The best treatment may be bed rest, to increase blood flow to the uterus. Depending on the case, improved maternal diet may be recommended, along with dietary supplementation. While most infants from IUGR pregnancies live a healthy life, some have consequential cognitive and medical problems. Pregnancies with IUGR should be monitored for fetal heart rate and changes in fetal movement, amniotic fluid volume and umbilical artery. Doppler ultrasounds are recommended.

Preterm Labor (PTL)

PTL is any birth occurring, or starting to occur (preterm contractions) prior to the 37th week of gestation. Preterm births are a cause of infant deaths and lingering infant illnesses. PTL affects 12% of pregnancies in the USA. PTL occurs in women with a history of PTL, women with multiple fetus pregnancies, and women with certain uterine or cervical abnormalities. Multiple maternal behavioral factors can cause PTL; smoking, alcohol use in pregnancy, illicit drug use in pregnancy, domestic violence, stress, long working hours during pregnancy. Medical issues such as vaginal infection, sexually transmitted disease, PIH or preeclampsia and obesity can cause PTL.

Tests to predict PTL are currently limited. Commonly, the sign of PTL is regular uterine contractions or abdominal cramps. At this point, several medications can be used to extend imminent parturition. Magnesium sulfate is a tacolytic medication that can extend imminent parturition. Injection of progesterone can also extend imminent parturition. Generally speaking, parturition at 34 to 37 weeks of gestation leads to healthy infants without lung surfactant or other problems. Parturition prior to 34 weeks is a different issue. If a mother has PTL prior to 34 weeks she can be given glucocorticoids to speed the development of the lungs and the production of surfactant in the lungs.

References

[1] Sibai B, Dekker G, Kupferminc M. Pre-eclampsia. *Lancet* 2005;365:785-799.

[2] Bujold E, Roberge S, Lacasse Y, Bureau M, Audibert F, Marcoux S, Forest JC, Giguère Y. Prevention of preeclampsia and intrauterine growth restriction with aspirin started in early pregnancy: a meta-analysis. *Obstet Gynecol* 2010;116:402-414.

[3] Sibai BM. Diagnosis and management of gestational hypertension and preeclampsia. *Obstet Gynecol* 2003;102:181-192.

[4] Duley L. The global impact of pre-eclampsia and eclampsia. *Semin Perinatol.* 2009;33:130-137.

[5] Bahado-Singh RO, Oz AU, Kingston JM, Shahabi S, Hsu CD, Cole LA. The role of hyperglycosylated hCG in trophoblast invasion and the prediction of subsequent pre-eclampsia. *Prenat Dagn* 22:478-481, 2002.

[6] Brennan MC, Wolfe MD, Murray-Krezan CM, Cole LA, Rayburn WF. First Trimester Hyperglycosylated Human Chorionic Gonadotropin and Development of Hypertension/ Prenat Diagn 2013, in press.

[7] Unterscheider J, Daly S, Geary MP, Kennelly MM, McAuliffe FM, O'Donoghue K, Hunter A, Morrison JJ, Burke G, Dicker P, Tully EC, Malone FD. Optimizing the definition of intrauterine growth restriction: the multicenter prospective PORTO Study. *Am J Obstet Gynecol* 2013;208:e1-6.

[8] Mandruzzato G, Antsaklis A, Botet F, Chervenak FA, Figueras F, Grunebaum A, Puerto B, Skupski D, Stanojevic M. Intrauterine restriction (IUGR). *J Perinat Med* 2008;36:277-281.

[9] Wollmann HA. Intrauterine growth restriction: definition and etiology. *Horm Res.* 1998;49:1-6.

[10] Gilbert WM, Danielsen B. Pregnancy outcomes associated with intrauterine growth restriction. *Am J Obstet Gynecol 2003*;188:1596-1601.

Key Points

1. PIH affects as many as 15% of pregnancies; preeclampsia affects 5-10% of pregnancies. PIH is marked by a blood pressure of over 140/90 and preeclampsia by raised blood pressure combined with proteinuria. Eclampsia and HELLP syndrome are forms of advance preeclampsia with a blood pressure of greater than 160/110.
2. PIH and preeclampsia occur due to poor placental invasion or insufficient blood flow to the placenta. This may causes fetal anoxia.
3. The symptoms of PIH and preeclampsia include headaches, blurry vision, fatigue, decreased urine output, and swelling of the face, hands and feet.
4. IUGR is considered whenever fetal weight is below the 10th percentile. The most common causes of IUGR are maternal behavioral factors, such as smoking, alcohol use, drug use, medicine use and malnutrition. IUGR can also be caused by trisomy and monosomy fetuses and by multiple pregnancies. Reproductive tract infections, PIH/preeclampsia and maternal heart disease are also causes of IUGR.
5. If IUGR is suspected, close fetal surveillance with ultrasound is recommended.

6. PTL is any birth occurring prior to the 37th week of gestation. PTL occurs in women with a history of PTL, women with multiple pregnancies, and women with certain uterine and cervical abnormalities. Multiple maternal behavioral factors, such as smoking and alcohol use, can cause PTL.

Chapter 25

Mammary Gland and Breastfeeding

Mammary Development

The mammary glands of the breast are composed of approximately 20 lobular masses. In between the lobules and in front of the lobules is fat or adipose tissues. Each lobule is made up of clusters of alveoli, blood vessels and lactiferous ducts. The basic pregnancy breast structure is depicted in Figure 25.1. The alveolar cells in the lobules are responsible for milk synthesis post-partum.

At the start of puberty a breast comprises mostly lactiferous ducts (Figure 25.1). During puberty, estrogens promote the lactiferous ducts to branch. As menstrual cycles are established, estrogen and progesterone promote the formation and growth of lobules containing alveoli and adipose tissue, and breast size increases [1-5].

During early pregnancy, under the influence of rising estrogen and progesterone levels, the previously developed lactiferous ducts and the lobular alveolar system undergo major growth and hypertrophy. Under these progesterone and estrogen influences prominent lobules form, as shown in Figure 25.1; the alveoli become dilated (Figure 25.2). During the second trimester of pregnancy, under rising estrogen and progesterone levels, differentiation of the alveolar epithelial cells occurs into cells filled with endoplasmic reticulum and golgi, or into milk factory cells (Figure 25.3). At this time the cells start to accumulate a secretory material. Milk fat is synthesized in the endoplasmic reticulum of the alveolar epithelial cells. Fat globules slowly pass out through cell plasma membranes (Figure 25.3). Milk protein is synthesized in epithelial cells, from DNA transcription in the nucleus and translation in the endoplasmic reticulum. Milk sugar, or lactose production, occurs in the golgi apparatus. The enzyme galactosyltransferase links together glucose and galactose to make the lactose disaccharide. The hormone prolactin controls milk fat, milk protein and milk lactose synthesis. As shown in Figure 25.4, mammary gland milk production post-partum is totally controlled by the hormone prolactin [1-5].

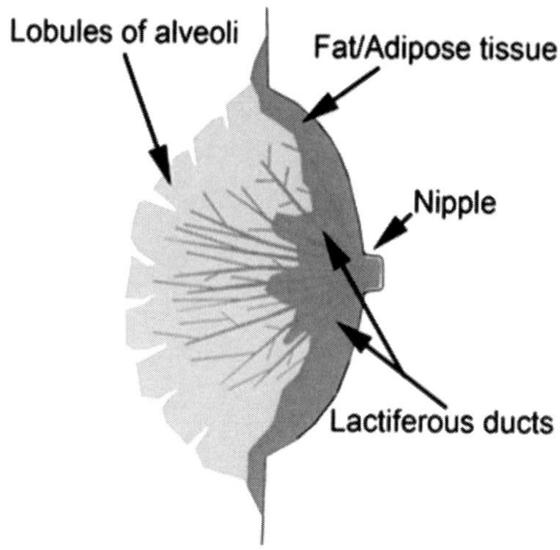

Figure 25.1. Breast of pregnant woman with developed lobules. Lobules consist of clusters of alveoli, which open into milk-collecting ducts.

At parturition, estrogen and progesterone levels drop down to barely detectable levels (Figure 25.4). In reality, human mammary glands are sufficiently developed by the second trimester to start breast milk production. The only reason milk production is not started at this time is because of the high levels of circulating estrogen and progesterone at this time. These steroid hormones inhibit milk production, which starts following their diminution at parturition [1-5].

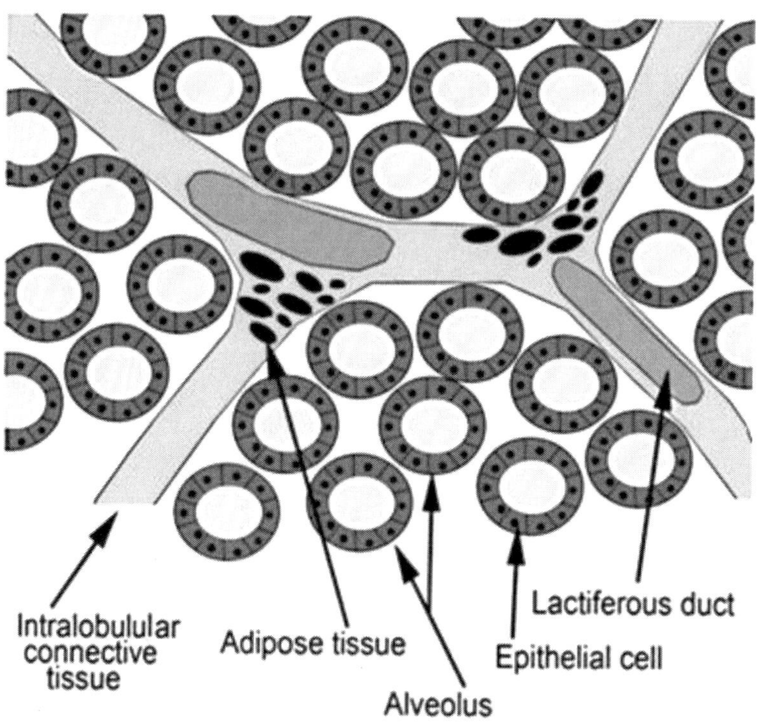

Figure 25.2 Microscopic structure of mammary lobules of alveoli during pregnancy.

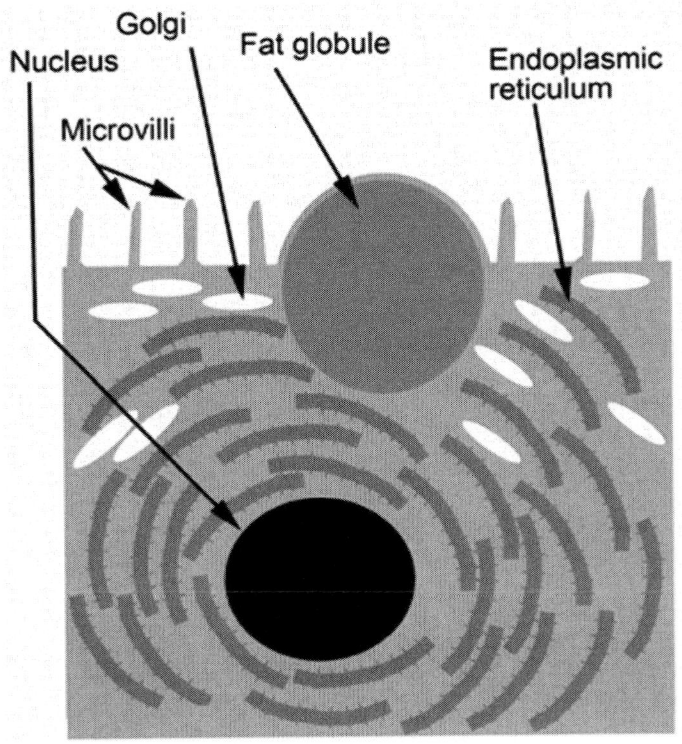

Figure 25.3. Drawing of ultrastructure of second trimester pregnancy alveolar epithelial cell. Drawing shows fat globule ready to exit cell.

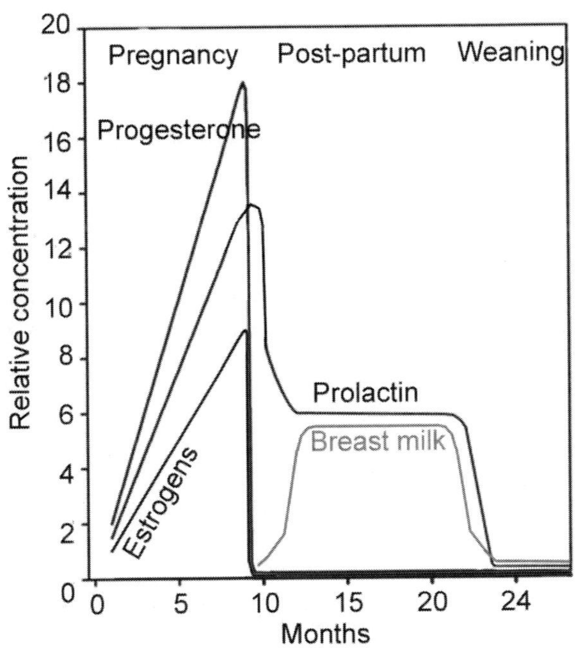

Figure 25.4. Relative concentrations of progesterone, estrogens, prolactin and breast milk production during pregnancy, post-partum and during weaning from breast milk.

After parturition, prolactin levels also decline, but they decline much slower than estrogen and progesterone levels (Figure 25.4). In the absence of suckling, the prolactin levels would decline to undetectable concentrations, and the newly initiated milk secretion would last only one month. However, nipple stimulation or suckling ensures prolactin production and prolonged milk synthesis. Upon suckling or breast stimulation two hypothalamic neurosecretory mechanisms are engaged. Firstly, there is a drop in hypothalamic dopamine secretion into the hypothalamic-hypophyseal tract, the portal system linking the hypothalamus and pituitary gland. Dopamine is an inhibitor of prolactin production by the pituitary. Secondly, there is an increase in hypothalamic production of prolactin releasing factor. This enters the hypothalamic-hypophyseal portal system and signals the lactotroph cells of the pituitary to produce more prolactin. The end result of suckling and these two neurosecretory mechanisms is greater production of prolactin, the milk stimulator. The greater the concentration of prolactin produced by the pituitary, the greater the concentration of breast milk produced [1-5].

Breastfeeding

Breast milk is optimal nutrition for a newborn baby. It comprises most water, containing lacose, fat, milk protein, free amino acids, major vitamin and minerals, it calorific value is 650 kcal/100ml. Milk suckling involves transport of milk from the alveolar luminina to the nipple. The milk ejection rate involves, as described, a suckling neurological response reaching the hypothalamus, a prolactin releasing factor signal to the lactrotroph cells from the hypothalamus, production of prolactin by the pituitary gland, and prolactin promoting milk sugar, protein and fat synthesis in the mammary gland [6-9].

Suckling is the most potent stimulus of milk ejection. The suckling reflex through the hypothalamus also activates oxytocin neurons in the hypothalamus, leading to release of oxytocin by the posterior pituitary gland. The oxytocin causes contractions in the myoepithelial cells surrounding the alveolar epithelial cells which make milk. The milk is effectively then squeezed or expelled into the lactiferous ducts facilitating breastfeeding. This squeezing or expulsion may cause milk to gush from the nipple.

Furthermore, milk expulsion can be conditioned to occur in response to other stimuli, such as baby's hunger or the baby crying. This suggests other nervous stimuli feeding through the brain into the hypothalamus, to promote the oxytocin neurons, and to promote milk ejection. Lactation can continue for months or years. During this period menstrual cycles may restart. They are usually restarted by 3-6 months following parturition, with invariable ovulation. This is the period of post-partum lactational amenorrhea or anovulation. The prolactin produced while breastfeeding may inhibit or suppress gonadotropin release by the gonadotrope cells, leading to anovulation and causing a weak contraception. It is called a weak contraception in that many sexually active mothers still achieve pregnancy during the first year of breast feeding [6-9].

When suckling is stopped, milk remains in the alveolar epithelial cells (Figure 25.3). This may cause distension. The alveolar wall may rupture due to the stored milk products. This effectively suppresses further milk secretion. As alveolar cells and other debris become phagocytosed by macrophages, the lobular structure of the breast becomes smaller and the ductal system in the breast starts to predominate. This whole closedown mechanism in the breast takes approximately 3 months [6-9].

References

[1] Russo J, Tay LK, Russo IH. Differentiation of the mammary gland and susceptibility to carcinogenesis. *Breast Cancer Res Treat* 1982;2:5-73.

[2] Soaje M, Deis RP. Opioidergic regulation of prolactin secretion during pregnancy: role of ovarian hormones. *J Endocrinol* 1997;155:99-106.

[3] Voogt JL, Lee Y, Yang S, Arbogast L. Regulation of prolactin secretion during pregnancy and lactation. *Prog Brain Res* 2001;133:173-185.

[4] Zinser GM, Welsh J. Accelerated mammary gland development during pregnancy and delayed postlactational involution in vitamin D3 receptor null mice. *Mol Endocrinol* 2004; 18:2208-2223.

[5] Booth BW, Boulanger CA, Smith GH. Alveolar progenitor cells develop in mouse mammary glands independent of pregnancy and lactation. *J Cell Physiol* 2007;212:729-736.

[6] Kramer MS, Aboud F, Mironova E, Vanilovich I, Platt RW, Matush L, Igumnov S, Fombonne E, Bogdanovich N, Ducruet T, Collet JP, Chalmers B, Hodnett E, Davidovsky S, Skugarevsky O, Trofimovich O, Kozlova L, Shapiro S. Breastfeeding and child cognitive development: new evidence from a large randomized trial. *Arch Gen Psychiatry* 2008;65:578-584.

[7] Ip S, Chung M, Raman G, Chew P, Magula N, DeVine D, Trikalinos T, Lau J. Breastfeeding and maternal and infant health outcomes in developed countries. Evid *Rep Technol Assess* 2007;153:1-186.

[8] Wolf JH. Low Breastfeeding Rates and Public Health in the United States. *Am J Public Health 2003*;93:2000–2010.

[9] Stuebe A. The Risks of Not Breastfeeding for Mothers and Infants *Rev Obstet Gynecol* 2009;2:222–231.

Key Points

1. Milk is very nutritious for a baby, comprising of lactose, fat, milk protein, free amino acids, major vitamins and minerals.
2. Milk production is totally controlled by prolactin through a suckling feedback cycle. Suckling leads to neurons in the hypothalamus producing prolactin releasing factor; this goes to the pituitary where lactotroph cells produce prolactin. Prolactin then promotes milk synthesis.
3. Prolactin promotes milk protein synthesis, fat synthesis and lactose synthesis in alveolar epithelial cells.
4. Estrogen and progesterone promote the growth and hypertrophy of lobules of alveoli during pregnancy. The alveoli differentiate during the second trimester of pregnancy into cells with numerous endoplasmic reticulum and golgi.

5. It is the drop in progesterone and estrone production of pregnancy at parturition that permits milk production to commence.
6. Suckling also stimulates oxytocin neurons in the hypothalamus. Oxytocin is produced by the posterior lobe of the pituitary. Oxytocin acts on myoepithelial cells, causing contractions which squeeze the milk into lactiferous ducts, facilitating milk ejection.

Chapter 26

Monosomies, Trisomies, Triploidies and other Genetic Abnormalities

Trisomies, Monosomies and Triploidies

A trisomy or monosomy occurs if the chromosome diploid pairs fail to separate properly during meiosis. The resulting ovum or spermatozoon may end up with a second copy (trisomy) or a missing copy (monosomy) of one entire chromosome. If a gamete results in fertilization and an embryo, the resulting embryo may also have an entire extra copy or missing copy of the chromosome.

Triploid conditions involve 69, 3 sets of 23, compared to 46 or two sets of 23 chromosomes. These occur due to failure of the cortical granules in the ovum, permitting fertilization by two sperm, or fertilization by one sperm and duplication of the sperm's haploid set [1-5].

Trisomy 16

Trisomy 16 is the most common trisomy in human pregnancies, occurring in approximately 1 in 75 pregnancies. This condition, however, always results in spontaneous abortion in the first trimester. No known case of trisomy has made it to term. Some babies are born with mosaic trisomy 16, with a mixture of normal cells and trisomy cells. These babies can survive to birth, and while in general they are small for their gestational age, the only established problem is ventricular septal defect (hole in the heart) [1-5].

Trisomy 21, Down Syndrome

Trisomy 21 or Down Syndrome is the most common trisomy leading to birth, affecting 1 in 691 pregnancies. Trisomy 21 leads to delays in physical growth, abnormal facial characteristics, and severe intellectual disability. The trisomy 21 child normally has an IQ of

50. Many grow up and live happily, possibly with employment. The risk for Down Syndrome pregnancy very much rises with age [1-5].

Trisomy 18, Edward's Syndrome

Trisomy 18 or Edward's Syndrome is a trisomy with an incidence of 1 in 6,000 pregnancies. Most pregnancies affected by trisomy 18 spontaneously abort and do not make it to term. Like trisomy 21, the risk for trisomy 18 pregnancy rises with age. The median life-span of a trisomy 18 newborn is 5-15 days. Most do not survive beyond a week or two weeks. A newborn has gross kidney malformations, facial defects and ventricular septal defects, with mental retardation.

Trisomy 13, Patau Syndrome

Trisomy 13 or Patau Syndrome has a 1 in 10,000 pregnancies incidence. Approximately one-half of trisomy 13 cases spontaneously abort during pregnancy. Approximately 80% of trisomy 13 births die within the first year of life. Newborns are mentally retarded with eye defects, abnormal genitalia, polydactyly (multiple fingers) and ventricular septal defects.

Monosomy X, Turner's Syndrome

Turner's Syndrome (45,X) is a monosomy leading a person to have one X chromosome. This occurs in 1 in 2,500 newborn female babies. The person is most commonly phenotypically identified as a female, although is infertile. Growth and height problems, short stature, swelling of hands and feet, no sexual development and cognitive defect are common complications of this phenotype. Patients can be treated with sexual steroid hormone replacement therapy and can develop normal sexuality or homosexuality.

Trisomy X Syndrome

Triple X syndrome is a relatively common trisomy in females (47,XXX). It occurs in 1 in 1,000 newborn females. The person is phenotypically identified as a female. This syndrome has minimal complications and does not commonly interfere with the menstrual cycle or fertility. Triple X can in rare cases cause delayed development or even ovarian or other sexual abnormalities [1-5].

Trisomy XXY, Klinefelter's Syndrome

Klinefelter's syndrome (47,XXY) is also relatively common, occurring in 1 in 1,000 newborn males. The person phenotypically is a male. The most common complications are reduced male fertility, low sperm count and small testicles. Lastly, 47,XXY also occurs at a rate of approximately 1 in 1,000 newborn males. Phenotypically the person is a male. While the male may have normal fertility, fast growth is common and some mental retardation is common. Klinefelter's syndrome males are unduly commonly inclined toward homosexuality [15,16].

Trisomy XYY, XYY Syndrome

Lastly, 47,XYY, XYY Syndrome also occurs at a rate of approximately 1 in 1,000 newborn males. Phenotypically the person is a male. While the male may have normal fertility, fast growth is common and some mental retardation is common. XYY syndrome causes aggressiveness and impulsiveness in a person, and a higher risk towards crime. An XXY syndrome male may be more inclined towards homosexuality [1-5].

Trisomy 22

Trisomy 22 affects 1 in 6,000 pregnancies. This condition, however, always results in spontaneous abortion in the first trimester. No known case of trisomy has made it to term. Some babies are born with mosaic trisomy 22, with a mixture of normal cells and trisomy cells. These babies can survive to birth, and while in general they are small for their gestational age, the problems range from cognitive deficiencies, unequal development of the two sides of the body (hemidystrophy), webbing of the neck, abnormal deviation of the elbows when extended (cubitus valgus), multiple pigmented moles or birthmarks, distinctive malformations of the head and face, and other physical abnormalities [1-5].

Trisomy 8, Warkany 2 Syndrome

Trisomy 8, Warkany 2 Syndrome affects 1 in 25,000 pregnancies. This condition, however, most commonly results in spontaneous abortion in the first trimester. Most babies making it through to parturition have mosaic trisomy 8, with a mixture of normal cells and trisomy cells. These babies can survive to birth, and while in general they are small for their gestational age, the problems range from psychomotor development problems to mental retardation or musculoskeletal abnormalities.

Triploid Syndrome

While triploidy may affect many pregnancies leading to first trimester spontaneous abortion, very few may make it to term. Those making it to term die within two weeks of birth. Most are born with growth retardation, and have facial defects, hypertelorism, colobomata, anomalous heart defects, renal hyperplasia and neural tube defects [1-5].

Partial Hydatidiform Mole, Triploid

Partial hydatidiform mole pregnancies are triploid. They do not generate an intact fetus, and mostly spontaneously abort. A mass develops that is mostly placental tissue and cystic placental tissue, and scattered fetal parts.

Table 26.1. Other Genetic Disorders

Genetic Syndrome	Approximate incidence	Chromosomes involved
Angelman syndrome	1 in 15,000	15
Apert syndrome	1 in 160,000	10
Canavan disease	1 in 6,400	17
Cri du chat	1 in 50,000	5
Cystic fibrosis	1 in 2,000	7
DiGeorge syndrome	1 in 4,000	22
Duchenne muscular dystrophy	1 in 7,000	X
Familial hypercholesterolemia	1 in 500	19
Galactosemia	1 in 57,000	
Glycogen storage diseases	1 in 50,000	
Hemophilia	1 in 10,000	X
Hereditary spherocytosis	1 in 5,000	8
Huntington's disease	1 in 15,000	4
Lysosomal acid lipase deficiency	1 in 40,000	
Marfan syndrome	1 in 4,000	15
Mucopolysaccharidoses	1 in 25,000	
Neurofibromatosis type I	1 in 2,500	17, 22
Neurofibromatosis type II	1 in 50,000	
Phenylketonuria	1 in 12,000	12
Polycystic kidney disease	1 in 1,250	16, 4
Prader–Willi syndrome	1 in 10,000	15
Sickle cell anemia	1 in 625	11
Tay-Sachs disease	1 in 3,000	15

Other Genetic Abnormalities

Table 26.1 lists 23 common genetic defects, out of a total catalog of approximately 200 known genetic defects. All involve damage to a chromosome or damaged genes or genes absent on a chromosome. Most commonly, genetic abnormalities involve intellectual disability, and commonly heart, nervous or muscular defect [1-5].

Detection

Today most pregnancy Trisomies, triploidies, monosomies and other abnormalties can be detedct by he combination of quadruple sreening and nuchal translucency mehods. New testsa are close on the horizon and should be available withone or two years, geta cell DNA methods seen promising for deteting genetically abnormal pregnancies, other teckniques such as urine mass spectrometry seeme very promising for the future.

References

[1] Molloy CA, Murray DS, Kinsman A, Castillo H, Mitchell T, Hickey FJ, Patterson B. Differences in the clinical presentation of Trisomy 21 with and without autism. *J Intellect Disabil Res* 2009;53:143-151.

[2] Avgidou K, Papageorghiou A, Bindra R, Spencer K, Nicolaides KH. Prospective first-trimester screening for trisomy 21 in 30,564 pregnancies. *Am J Obstet Gynecol* 2005; 192(:1761-1767.

[3] Trisomy 13. http://www.nlm.nih.gov/medlineplus/ency/article/001660.htm

[4] Down syndrome. http://www.nlm.nih.gov/medlineplus/downsyndrome.html

[5] Phelan MC, Curtis Rogers R, Michaelis RC, Moore CL, Blackburn W. Prenatal diagnosis of mosaicism for triploidy and trisomy 13. *Prenat Diagn* 2001;21:457-460.

Key Points

1. Most genetic abnormalitics, monosomies and trisomies result from an error in sperm or ovum meiosis. Triploidy most commonly results from fertilization of an ovum by multiple sperm or sperm haploid set duplication.
2. Most trisomies, monosomies and triploidies lead to intellectual retardation, facial disfiguration and heart ventricular septal defect.
3. Most trisomies, monosomies and triploidies are destroyed by spontaneous abortion of the pregnancy in the first trimester.

Puberty

Chapter 27

Adrenarche and Menarche in Girls

Adrenarche

Adrenarche is a forewarning of ensuing menarche that occurs in girls. Adrenarche occurs at 6-8 years of age. It arises from adrenal gland production of dehydroepiandrosterone (DHEA) and DHEA-sulfate. DHEA-sulfate can be aromatized by the adrenal gland to make limited amounts of estrogens. The limited estrogens promote initial breast development, and the DHEA, DHEA-sulfate and estradiol lead to initial pubic hair growth and initial axillary hair growth (Figure 27.1). The DHEA and DHAE-sulfate affect the brain, acting on the Sexually Dimorphic Nucleus of the hypothalamus, and the Amygdala of the temporal lobe promoting libido and aggressive behavior (Figure 27.1). Anabolic actions of DHEA and DHEA-sulfate lead to muscle growth. It is like the start of menarche except there is absolutely no ovarian processes or menstrual bleeding (Figure 27.1). Often parents become scared by adrenarche, thinking that something is wrong, and wondering why their child is going through puberty at such a young age [1-4].

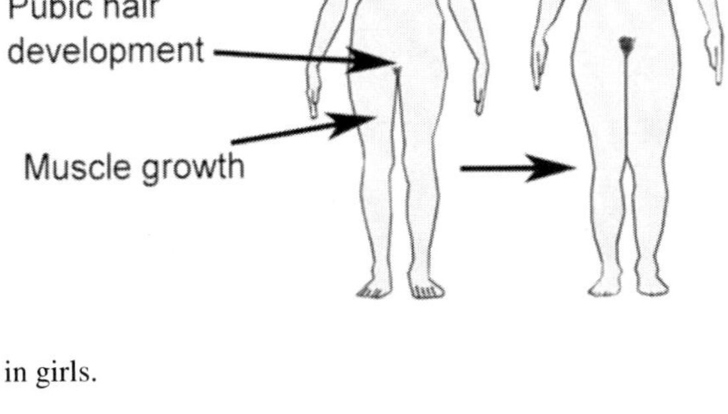

Figure 27.1. Adrenarche in girls.

Menarche

Menarche usually starts when girls are just 10-11 years old. It starts with a growth spurt usually between 10-11 years of age with an increase in both height and in fat depositions. Around 10-11 years of age initial breast buds develop, the pelvis widens and pubic hair growth continues. A year later, at 11-12 years of age, the ovaries start to mature, and the fallopian tubes, uterus, vagina, and breast areola all become pigmented. This may be the first sign of menarche. Over the next two years, 12-14 years age, the breasts fill out, axillary hair and pubic hair appear coarse, curly and abundant and menstrual bleeding can commence. In the next two years, by 14-15 years of age, the first ovulation may occur, making the person fertile; breast maturation completes, pubic hair becomes like an adult's, and sweat and subaceous glands develop, with voice deepening (See Table 27.1).

Table 27.1. Age range and signs of menarche

Age	**Activities**
10-11	Growth spurt begins, lasting 4 years, height increases, fat deposition occurs. Initial breast budding, pelvis widens, pubic hair starts.
11-12	Maturation of ovaries, and fallopian tubes, uterus, vagina, breast areola becomes pigmented, first sign of menses.
12-14	Filling of breast, axillary hair and pubic hair become coarse, curly and abundant, menses start.
14-15	First ovulation occurs, breast maturation is complete, pubic hair is like an adult's, final height is reached, sweat and subaceous glands develop, voice slightly deepens.

Table 27.2. Tanner staging of menarche

1. Breast development in menarche, Tanner staging (Illustrated in Figure 26.2):	
Stage 1.	Breast development, prior to age 10, there is virtually no breast, just a child's nipple.
Stage 2.	Areola and papilla are elevated, age 10-11.
Stage 3.	Breast is enlarged, areola larger and pigmented, no clear contours, age 11-12 (Figure 26.2).
Stage 4.	Breasts fill out, areola plus papilla form separate curves or mounds to the breast, they do not blend into a smooth curve of breast, age 12-14 (Figure 26.2).
Stage 5.	Adult or mature breast, areola part of general breast contour, papilla projects, Age 15+.
Pubic hair growth in menarche, Tanner staging (Illustrated in Figure 26.2):	
Stage 1.	Prepubertal, there is minimal hair.
Stage 2.	There is sparse, lightly pigmented hair, straight, around labia.
Stage 3.	There is darker hair, beginning to curl, increased amount of hair.
Stage 4.	There is coarse, curly abundant hair, but less than an adult.
Stage 5.	Adult; there is a feminine triangle spread to thighs, less coarse and curly.

Timing of menstruation has been advancing with years: in 1835 a girl of normal weight started puberty at age 15; in 1895 at age 13; in 1947 at age 12; in 1990 at age 11; and in 2010 at age 10. Menarche can occur up to two years earlier in an overweight girl. It appears that throughout the ages children are being better fed, becoming fatter, and are increasingly becoming ready to enter puberty earlier. Although a girl first ovulates at age 14-15, ovulation may be infrequent, with ovulation occurring in approximately 50% of menstrual cycles at age 16. It can rise in incidence to 70-80% of menstrual cycles by age 18. It could be correctly said that puberty is not over until a girl is 18 [5-8].

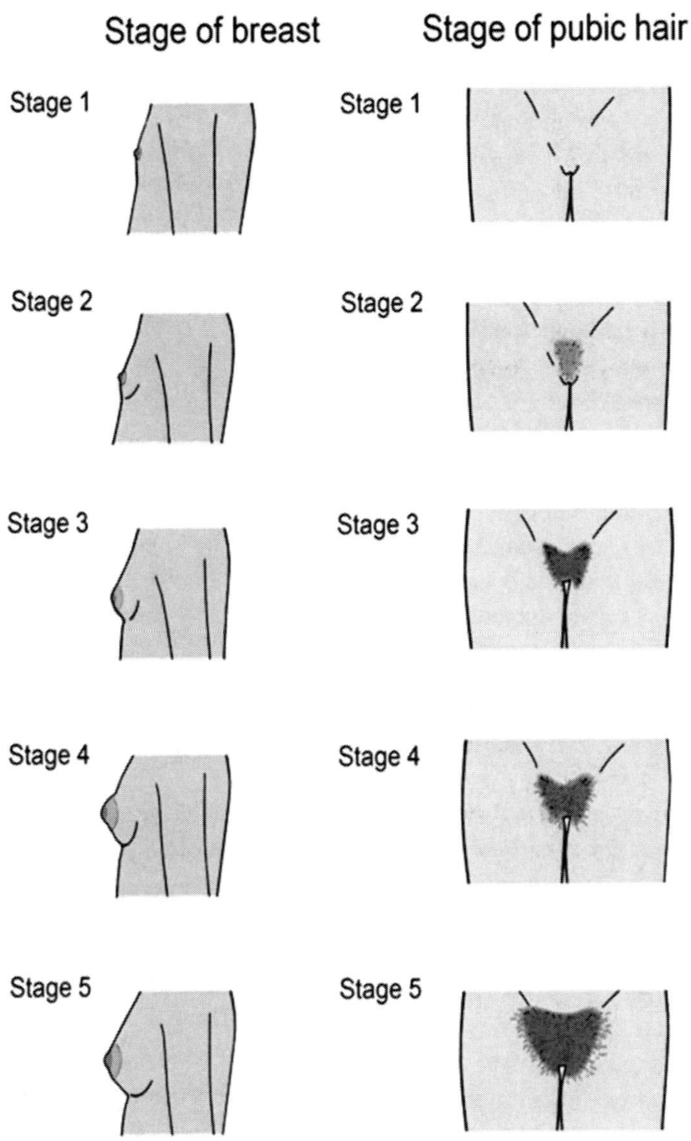

Figure 27.2. Tanner staging of breast development and pubic hair growth in girls.

Tanner Staging

The advancement of female menarche can be rated using Tanner staging (Table 27.2 and Figure 27.2). Following breast growth and the appearance of papilla marks comes Stage 1. The areola and papilla become expanded in Stage 2. In Stage 3 the breast becomes enlarged and pigmented with no clear contours. In Stage 4 the breast fills out but the areola has separate curves to the breast. Finally, in adult Stage 5 the areola becomes part of the breast contours.

Examining pubic hairs as an indicator of puberty development, Stage 1 is no pubic hair, and Stage 2 is minimal or initial pubic hair. In Stage 3 there is an increasing amount of hair; the hair is darker and beginning to curl. In Stage 4 there is more abundant coarse, curly hair. Finally, in adult Stage 5, there is the feminine triangle of abundant hair, which is spread to the thighs and is less coarse and less curly [5-8].

The Physiology of Starting the Menstrual Cycle

How does the menstrual cycle get started? What turns on the gonadotropin releasing hormone (GnRH), which in turn promotes the luteinizing hormone (LH) and follicle stimulating hormone (FSH) production, which drives androstenedione, estrogen and progesterone production during the menstrual cycle? LH and FSH promote growth and development of follicles, leading to ovulation. What starts these processes, leading to the first menses at age 12-14 and the first ovulation at age 14-15 [5-8]?

There are two theories being considered by numerous scientists today. In the KISS theory, the protein kisspeptin, a 53 amino acid protein, produced by the KISS-1 gene, binds the GPR54 receptor in the Sexually Dimorphic Nucleus within the hypothalamus; this directly initiates GnRH production, starting the menstrual cycle. Once GnRH starts LH and FSH production in the pituitary, estrogen and progesterone feed back controlling GnRH pulses [5-8].

There is also much science supporting a leptin theory. As the body builds up fat, leptin is produced. Leptin activates neuropeptide Y, a neuroinhibitor of GnRH that keeps GnRH turned off until the leptin signal is received at menarche. It is well known that overweight children, especially girls, tend to mature earlier than lean children. This has led to the hypothesis that the degree of body fatness may trigger the neuroendocrine events that lead to the onset of puberty [5-8].

The leptin and body fat theory explains the relationship between overweight children and early menarche. Modern science is suggesting that a combination of leptin and kisspeptin may activate GNRH and start the menstrual cycle. Leptin may promote kisspeptin production, which in turn activates the GPR54 hypothalamus receptor, which causes GnRH production. Figure 27.3 illustrates the proposed body fat, leptin, kisspeptin, GnRH model, with GnRH starting the menstrual cycle, GnRH, LH/FSH, Progesterone /Estrogens. Thus, the menstrual cycle is theoretically started [5-8].

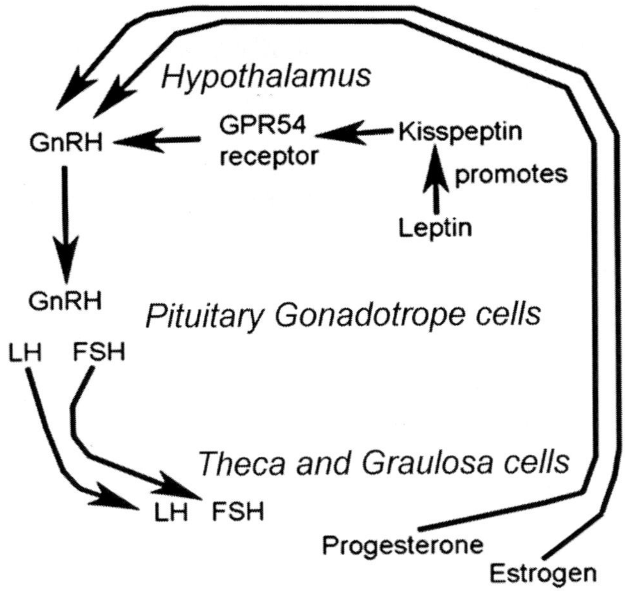

Figure 27.3. Leptin and kisspeptin starting the menstrual cycle.

References

[1] Ong KK, Potau N, Petry CJ, Jones R, Ness AR, Honour JW, de Zegher F, Ibáñez L, Dunger DB. Opposing influences of prenatal and postnatal weight gain on adrenarche in normal boys and girls. *J Clin Endocrinol Metab* 2004;89:2647-2651.

[2] Sopher AB, Thornton JC, Silfen ME, Manibo A, Oberfield SE, Wang J, Pierson RN Jr, Levine LS, Horlick M. Prepubertal girls with premature adrenarche have greater bone mineral content and density than controls. *J Clin Endocrinol Metab* 2001 86:5269-5272.

[3] Bordini B, Littlejohn E, Rosenfield RL. LH Dynamics in Overweight Girls with Premature Adrenarche and Slowly Progressive Sexual Precocity. *Int J Pediatr Endocrinol* 2010; http://www.ncbi.nlm.nih.gov/pmc/articles/PMC2945655/

[4] Saenger P, Dimartino-Nardi J. Premature adrenarche. *J Endocrinol Invest* 2001; 24:724-733.

[5] Wyshak G, Frisch RE. Evidence for a secular trend in age of menarche. *New Engl J Med* 1982;306:1033-1035.

[6] Błogowska A, Rzepka-Górska I, Krzyzanowska-Swiniarska B, Zółtowski S, Kosmowska B. Leptin, neuropeptide Y, beta-endorphin, gonadotropin, and estradiol levels in girls before menarche. *Gynecol Endocrinol* 2003;17:7-12.

[7] Blogowska A, Krzyzanowska-Swiniarska B, Zielińska D, Rzepka-Górska I. Body composition and concentrations of leptin, neuropeptide Y, beta-endorphin, growth hormone, insulin-like growth factor-I and insulin at menarche in girls with constitutional delay of puberty. *Gynecol Endocrinol* 2006;22:274-278.

[8] Comings DE, Gade R, Muhleman D, Peters WR, MacMurray JP. The LEP gene and age of menarche: maternal age as a potential cause of hidden stratification in association studies. *Mol Genet Metab* 2001;73:204-210.

Key Points

1. Adrenarche is important; it is the production of DHEA and DHEA-sulfate by the adrenal gland and the resulting production of low levels of estrogen.
2. Adrenarche involves early breast development, pubic hair and axillary hair growth, as well as muscle growth.
3. Menarche starts in girls at around age 10-11; it starts with breast budding, widening of the pelvis and growth of pubic hair.
4. At age 11-12 the ovaries mature, and the fallopian tube, vagina and breast areola become pigmented. At age 12-14, the breast fills, and axillary and pubic hair becomes coarse, curly and abundant; menses start.
5. At age 14-15 first ovulation occurs, making a woman fertile. Breast maturation completes and pubic hair become like that of an adult.
6. Tanner staging, Stages 1-5, is important. At Tanner Stage 5 puberty is over; the breast areola becomes part of the contours of the breast. The pubic hair at Stage 5 has formed and filled the feminine triangle, having spread to thighs; it is less coarse and curly.
7. Three mechanisms may initiate the menstrual cycle by promoting GnRH. There is the leptin-neuropeptide Y mechanism for activating GnRH, with body fat being the initiator, and the kisspeptin GPR54 receptor mechanism for activation of GnRH in the hypothalamus. Finally, a mechanism has been proposed that combines both procedures. Fat initiates leptin which promotes kisspeptin production. Kisspeptin then promotes or turns on GnRH by acting on the GPR54 receptor in the hypothalamus.

Chapter 28

Adrenarche and Puberty in Boys

Adrenarche

Adrenarche is a forewarning of ensuing menarche that occurs in boys. Adrenarche occurs at 7-9 years of age in boys or about 1 year later than it occurs in girls. It arises from adrenal gland production of dehydroepiandrosterone (DHEA) and DHEA-sulfate. Adrenarche is associated with a thickening of the zona reticularis, the innermost layers of the adrenal cortex. Some DHEA-sulfate can be converted to testosterone, a much more biologically potent androgen. The DHEA, DHEA-sulfate and testosterone lead to initial pubic hair growth and initial axillary hair growth (Figure 28.1). The DHEA and DHEA-sulfate effect the sexually dimorphic nucleus in the hypothalamus of the brain, promoting libido and aggressive behavior (Figure 28.1). Anabolic action of DHEA and DHEA-sulfate leads to muscle growth. Often parents become scared by adrenarche, thinking that something is wrong, and wondering why their child is going through puberty at such a young age [1-8].

Menarche

Menarche usually starts in boys approximately a year later than in girls, at ages 11 to 14 years. Menarche in boys is marked by maturation of the testes and the development of secondary sexual characteristics. Maturation of the testes includes the start of androgen production by the Leydig cells, the growth of seminiferous tubules and the start of spermatogenesis. All of these events are initiated by the production of luteinizing hormone (LH), and follicle stimulating hormone (FSH). During childhood FSH and LH concentrations in serum are low. Approximately one year before testicular enlargement occurs, pulses of LH and FSH increase in amplitude, suggesting the initiation of gonadotropin releasing hormone (GnRH). Table 28.1 and Figure 28.2 examine the stages of genital development and pubic hair development in boys [1-8].

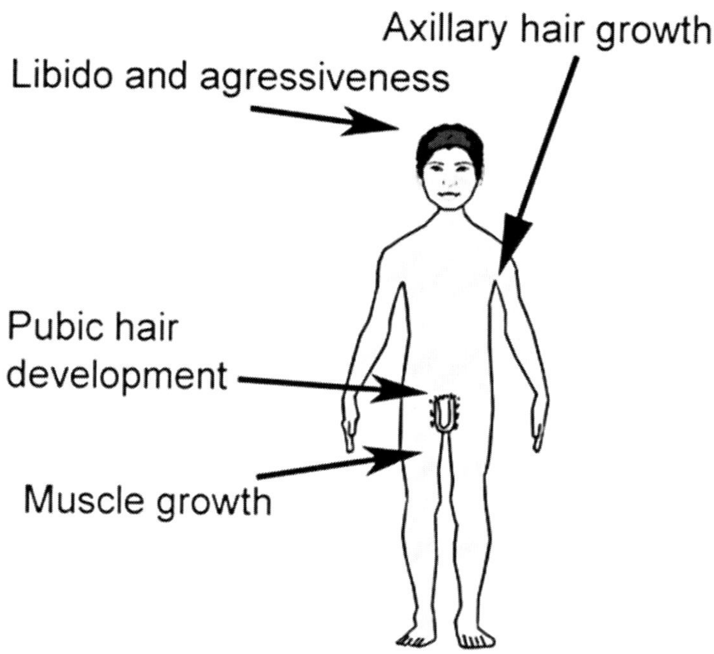

Figure 28.1. Adrenarche in boys.

Table 28.1. Markers of menarche

Genital development at menarche (Figure 27.2):	
Stage 1	Pre-puberty
Stage 2	Around age 11-12, testes and scrotum enlarge (see Figure 27.2)
Stage 3	Around age 12-13, penis has clearly grown, testes and scrotum continue to grow (see Figure 27.2)
Stage 4	Around mean age 13-14, penis, testes and scrotum continue to enlarge (see Figure 27.2)
Stage 5	Around mean age 14-15, genitalia reach adult size and shape
Pubic hair growth in menarche (Figure 27.2):	
Stage 1	Pre-puberty
Stage 2	Around age 13-14, light growth in pubic hairs is observed, mostly at the root of the penis (see Figure 27.2)
Stage 3	Around age 13½-14½, hair growth increases and becomes darker, mostly around the root of the penis (see Figure 27.2)
Stage 4	Around age 14-15, hair growth spreads wider, forming a bow-tie shape. There is no spread to the thighs (see Figure 27.2)
Stage 5	Around age 14½-16, adult hair growth is seen, forming a triangle (Figure 27.2)

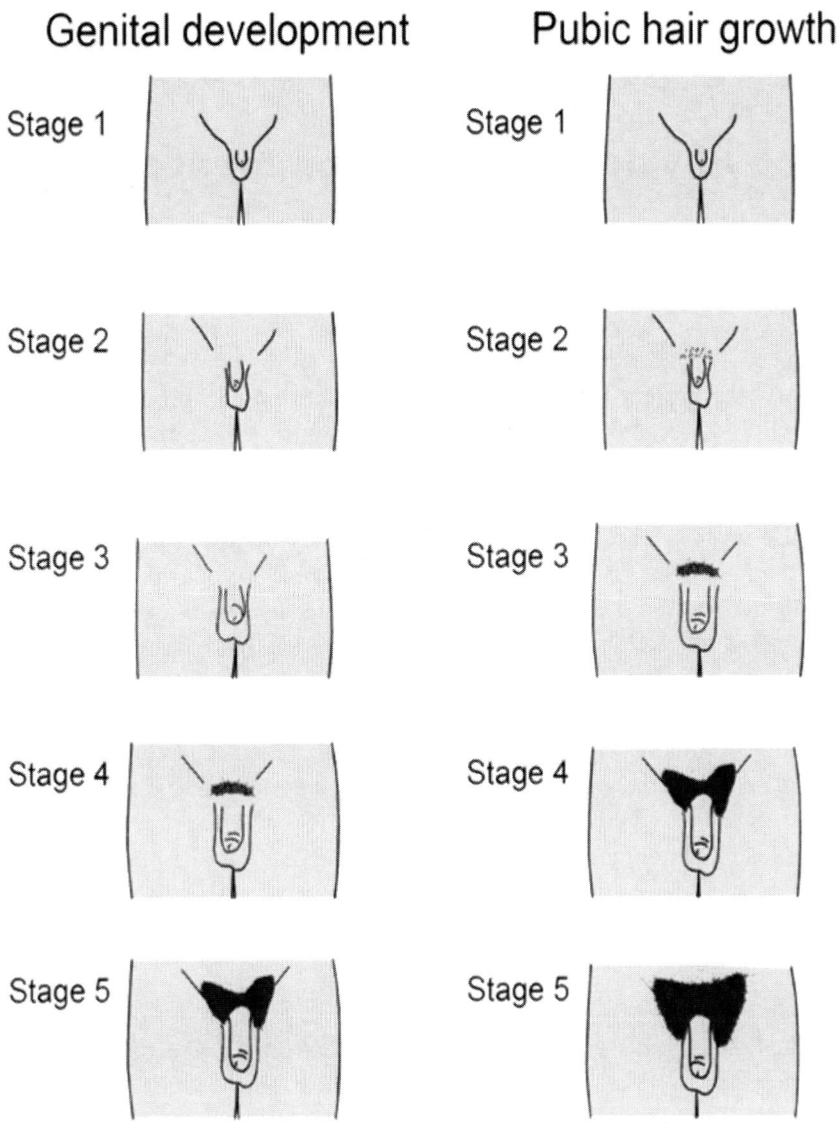

Figure 28.2. Staging of genital development in boys and pubic hair development in boys.

In terms of secondary sexual characteristics in boys, androgens cause clear somatic changes in boys. There is an increased laryngeal size, a deepening of the voice, a thickening of the skin and thickening of hair on the trunk, pubis, axillae and face. A combination of LH promotion of androgens and increase in growth hormone production by the pituitary causes the increase in growth, muscle mass and bone mass common to menarche, or to boys around 14-15 years of age. Androgen may also affect libido and the ability to erect the penis by modulating the sexually dimorphic nucleus and paraventricular nucleus in the hypothalamus, and the amygdala in the temporal lobe of the brain [1-8].

The timing of menstruation has been advancing with years. In 1835 a boy of average weight started puberty at age 16; in 1895 at age 14; in 1947 at age 13; in 1990 at age 12; and in 2010 at age 11. Menarche occurs up to two years earlier in overweight boys. It appears that throughout the ages children are being better fed and are increasingly becoming ready to enter menarche earlier.

The Physiology of the Commencement of Menarche

How does menarche get started? What turns on GnRH, which in turn promotes LH FSH production, which drives testosterone production? What starts the processes leading to the start of menarche? There are two theories being considered by numerous scientists today. In the KISS theory, the protein kisspeptin, a 53 amino acid protein produced by the KISS-1 gene, binds GPR54 receptor within the hypothalamus; this directly initiates GnRH production, starting menarche. Once GnRH starts, LH and FSH are produced by the pituitary, testosterone feedbacks controlling GnRH pulses [1-8].

There is also much science supporting the leptin theory. As the body builds up fat, leptin is produced. Leptin activates a neuropeptide Y, a neuroinhibitor of GnRH that keeps GnRH turned off until the leptin signal is received at menarche. It is well known that overweight children tend to mature earlier than lean children. This has led to the hypothesis that the degree of body fatness may trigger the neuroendocrine events that lead to the onset of puberty. The leptin and body fat theory explains the relationship between overweight children and early menarche. Modern science suggests that a combination of leptin and kisspeptin may activate GnRH and start the menstrual cycle. Leptin may promote kisspeptin production, which in turn activates the GPR54 hypothalamus receptor, which causes GnRH production. This theory is illustrated in Figure 27.3 in Chapter 27 [1-8].

References

[1] Ong KK, Potau N, Petry CJ, Jones R, Ness AR, Honour JW, de Zegher F, Ibáñez L, Dunger DB. Opposing influences of prenatal and postnatal weight gain on adrenarche in normal boys and girls. *J Clin Endocrinol Metab* 2004;89:2647-2651.

[2] Saenger P, Dimartino-Nardi J. Premature adrenarche. *J Endocrinol Invest* 2001; 24:724-733.

[3] Lazar L, Pertzelan A, Weintrob N, Phillip M, Kauli R. Sexual precocity in boys: accelerated versus slowly progressive puberty gonadotropin-suppressive therapy and final height. *J Clin Endocrinol Metab* 2001;86:4127-4132.

[4] *Puberty in boys.* http://www.nlm.nih.gov/medlineplus/ency/patientinstructions/000650.htm

[5] Oerter KE, Uriarte MM, Rose SR, Barnes KM, Cutler GB Jr. Gonadotropin secretory dynamics during puberty in normal girls and boys. *J Clin Endocrinol Metab* 1990; 71:1251-1258.

[6] Roy JR, Chakraborty S, Chakraborty TR. Estrogen-like endocrine disrupting chemicals affecting puberty in humans - a review. *Med Sci* Monit 2009;15:RA137-145.

[7] Yilmaz D, Ersoy B, Bilgin E, Gümüşer G, Onur E, Pinar ED. Bone mineral density in girls and boys at different pubertal stages: relation with gonadal steroids, bone formation markers, and growth parameters. *J Bone Miner Metab* 2005;23:476-482.

[8] Schoenau E, Neu CM, Mokov E, Wassmer G, Manz F. Influence of puberty on muscle area and cortical bone area of the forearm in boys and girls. *J Clin Endocrinol Metab* 2000;85:1095-1098.

Key Points

1. Adrenarche is important; it is the production of DHEA and DHEA-sulfate, two androgens by the adrenal gland.
2. Adrenarche involves early pubic hair and axillary hair development. In some cases the DHEA and DHEA-sulfate can affect the hypothalamus of the brain, promoting libido and aggressive behavior. Also, in some cases the anabolic action of DHEA and DHEA-sulfate can lead to muscle growth.
3. Menarche occurs approximately 1 year later in boys than in girls.
4. Menarche in boys is marked by maturation of the testes and the development of secondary sexual characteristics. Maturation of the testes includes the start of androgen production by the Leydig cells, growth of seminiferous tubules and the start of spermatogenesis. All of these events are initiated by the production of luteinizing hormone (LH), and follicle stimulating hormone (FSH).
5. A growth spurt occurs in boys at the mean average age of around 14-15. A combination of LH promotion of androgens and increase in growth hormone production by the pituitary causes the increase in growth, muscle mass and bone mass common to menarche.
6. Growth of the penis, testes and scrotum starts at around age 11 12 and continues on to age 14-15 (Stage 1 to Stage 5 of genital development).
7. Pubic hair growth starts at around age 13-14 and continues on to age 14½-16 (Stage 1 to Stage 5 of pubic hair growth).
8. Three mechanisms may initiate the menstrual cycle by promoting GnRH. There is the leptin-neuropeptide Y mechanism for activating GnRH, with body fat being the initiator, and the kisspeptin GPR54 receptor mechanism for activation GnRH in the hypothalamus. Finally, a mechanism has been proposed that combines both procedures. Fat initiates leptin, which promotes kisspeptin production. Kisspeptin then promotes or turns on GnRH by acting on the GPR54 receptor in the hypothalamus.

Menopause

Chapter 29

Perimenopause and Menopause

The Menopausal Process

As described in Chapter 3, the female body goes through an intricate process to initiate gonadotropin releasing hormone and to start the menstrual cycle. As described in Chapters 3-6, the female body also goes through an intricate process monthly to keep the menstrual cycle and ovulation running. Yet all these processes come to an absolute closure at menopause, or at approximately 45-58 years of age (average, 51.4 years). The ovary is the center or headquarters of the menstrual cycle, producing androgens, estrogens and progestogens, inhibin and most of all, producing the oocyte and corpus luteum. At menopause the ovary closes down, bringing the cycle to a complete halt.

The fertility of a woman varies very much with the age of starting puberty and extending to menopause (Figure 29.1). As a woman approaches menopause, her menstrual cycles may become increasing more anovulatory (Figure 29.1) and irregular in length or oligomenorrhea, and may lack or have an abbreviated luteal phase (Figure 29.1). Between age 40 and 55, or in the 10 years prior to menopause, fertility or the ability to achieve pregnancy drops significantly, peri-menooause (Figure 29.1). Fertility is highest when women are in their twenties and declines thereafter. This decline could be due to a reduction in fecundity that occurs with changes in sexual behavior, resulting in older women having less sexual intercourse [1-6].

Decline in regular menstrual cycles starts in women in their early forties and marks a climacteric or period of reproductive change that may last ten years before the onset of menopause (perimenopause). The climacteric is associated with a period of mood swings, irritability, loss of libido and hot flashes. The climacteric is related to the declining number of follicles in the ovaries and the associated reduction in estrogens and progestogens with the diminution of theca and granulosa cells and the increase of anovulatory cycles. The numbers of primordial follicles in each ovary decline significantly with age, leading to an overall decline in active follicles or to anovulatory menstrual cycles. Ovarian follicles are the tissues that make the ovary active; they make sex steroids and release the oocyte. Eventually, with the decline in ovarian follicles comes complete ovarian failure, known as menopause or cessation of reproductive life. These physical, functional and emotional changes of the climacteric and the eventual menopause are all driven by changes in the ovarian structure, loss of follicles, anovulation, loss of theca cells and loss of granulosa cells [1-6].

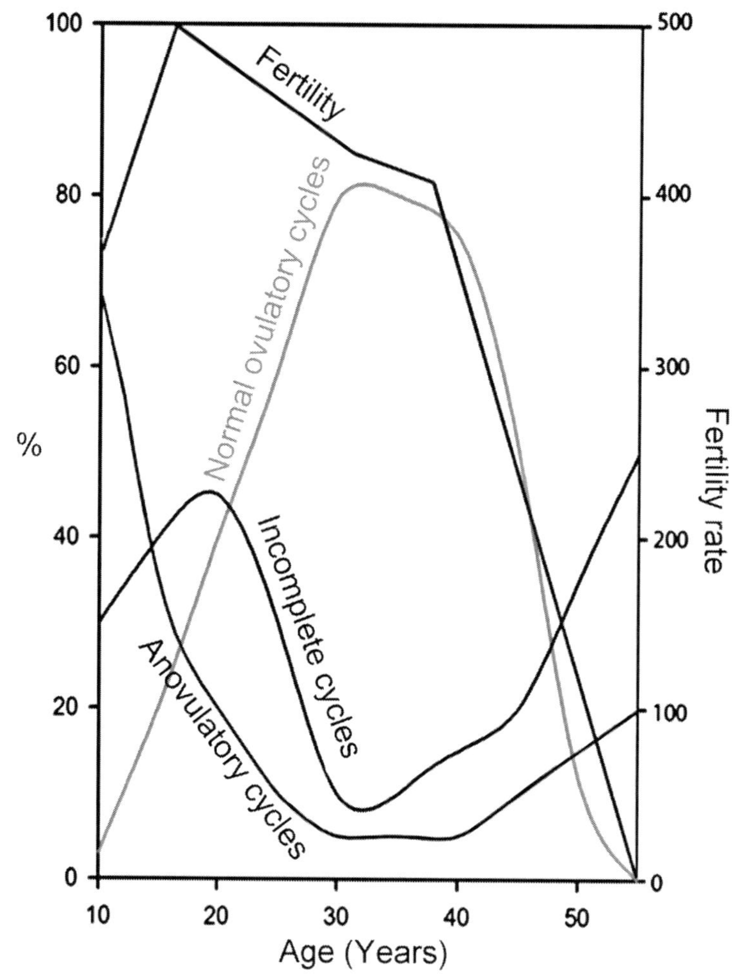

Figure 29.1. Fertility of women and age.

The ten years leading to menopause we call "perimenopause." During this perimenopause period, estrogen and progestogen output by granulosa and theca cells becomes diminished as the number of follicles diminishes. This is shown in Table 29.1. With the reduction in estrogen and progestogen feedback to the hypothalamus the gonadotropin releasing hormone (GnRH) pulses increase in number and increase in magnitude. With this increase in production of GnRH by the hypothalamus, LH, pituitary sulfated hCG), and FSH output from the gonadotrope cells of the pituitary increase accordingly (see Table 29.1). Interestingly, during perimenopause and menopause hCG levels rise out of the range undetectable by commercial serum pregnancy tests (sensitivity 1-3 IU/L), and into the detectable ranges. Most hospitals in the western world run hCG tests to check women for pregnancy prior to surgery and prior to many radiographic procedures. A perimenopausal or menopausal woman may yield a positive pregnancy test. A positive pregnancy test in an older woman may create a lot of needless confusion. Raised serum levels of hCG, FSH and LH are normal and natural in perimenopausal and menopausal subjects. Normally in the western world, perimenopause occurs between ages 37 and 47 and menopause between ages 45 and 58 (average, 51.4 years). We characterize perimenopause by irregular menstrual cycles (oligomenorrhea), and anovulatory menstrual cycles, and by menstrual cycles lacking a proper luteal phase [1-6].

Table 29.1. Reproductive endocrinology during the menstrual cycle, perimenopause and menopause

	E2 ng/L	**Progesterone µg/L**	**LH IU/L**	**FSH IU/L**	**Sulfated hCG IU/L**
Follicular phase of menstrual cycle	20 – 150	0.2 – 0.6	5.0 – 30	2.5 – 15	0.05 – 0.3
Luteal phase of menstrual cycle	30 – 350	5.0 – 30	3.0 – 40	1.5 – 9.1	0.03 – 0.4
Perimenopause	15 – 100	0.2 – 10	5.0 – 100	10 – 80	<1 – 12
Menopause	10 – 18	0 – 0.2	30 – 200	23 – 116	2.1 – 31.5

Menopause is marked by the complete failure of the ovaries to respond to LH or FSH and the end of menstrual cycles or amenorrhea. After menopause small amounts of estrogens and progestogens are made from dehydroepiandrosterone (DHEA) in the adrenal gland (see Table 29.1). As shown in Table 29.1, after menopause with the complete halting of theca and granulosa cell sex steroid hormone production hypothalamic GnRH becomes unregulated, leading to maximal hCG, LH and FSH production. The loss of ovarian sex hormones at menopause leads to hot flashes, night sweats and sleep disorders, loss of libido, mental depression and disorientation, mood swings and vaginal dryness [1-6].

Perimenopause and menopause occur in approximately 2% of women unduly early; some in their thirties and twenties and, in rare cases, as early as the teens.

References

[1] Dratva J, Gómez Real F, Schindler C, Ackermann-Liebrich U, Gerbase MW, Probst-Hensch NM, Svanes C, Omenaas ER, Neukirch F, Wjst M, Morabia A, Jarvis D, Leynaert B, Zemp E. Is age at menopause increasing across Europe? Results on age at menopause and determinants from two population-based studies. *Menopause* 2009;16:385-394.

[2] Rosano GM, Vitale C, Marazzi G, Volterrani M. Menopause and cardiovascular disease: the evidence. *Climacteric* 2007;10:19-24.

[3] Menopause. http://www.nlm.nih.gov/medlineplus/menopause.html

[4] Azizi H, Feng Liu Y, Du L, Hua Wang C, Bahrami-Taghanaki H, Ollah Esmaily H, Azizi H, Ou Xue X. Menopause-related symptoms: traditional Chinese medicine vs hormone therapy. *Altern Ther Health Med* 2011;17:48-53.

[5] *Aging changes in the female reproductive system* http://www.nlm.nih.gov/medlineplus/ency/article/004016.htm

[6] Nusrat N, Nishat Z, Gulfareen H, Aftab M, Asia N. Knowledge, attitude and experience of menopause. *J Ayub Med Coll* Abbottabad 2008;20:56-59.

Key Points

1. As women age beyond 35 (35-45) the menstrual cycle becomes anovulatory and irregular (oligomenorrhea) with incomplete cycles with short luteal phases. As the number of follicles in the ovaries declines, estrogen and progestogen levels decline. This is perimenopause.
2. The number of follicles in each ovary continues to decline leading to menopause, at which time the ovaries completely fail to produce sex steroids.
3. In perimenopause and in menopause GnRH pulses increase and pulse amplitude increases, leading to high pituitary production of hCG, LH and FSH.
4. Perimenopause is marked by changes in libido, mood swings, irritability and hot flashes with irregular menstrual periods (oligomenorrhea).
5. Menopause is marked by hot flashes, night sweats, a change in libido, mental depression or disorientation, and an absence of menstrual periods (amenorrhea).

Chapter 30

Managing Menopause

Starting Menopause

Menopause marks the end of a woman's natural reproductive life. The average age for menopause in the United States is 51.4 years, with 95% of women experiencing this event by age 55. The age of menopause is not influenced by the age of menarche, the number of ovulations or the number of pregnancies. Approximately 1% of women undergo menopause early, before age 40; this condition is referred to as premature ovarian failure. Contrary to popular belief, the ovaries at menopause are not quiescent. Under LH stimulation, theca cells will produce hormones, primarily androstenedione and testosterone. Testosterone appears to be a major product of the postmenopausal ovary. Estrone is the prominent form of estrogen produced. In the last two hundred years, the age of menopause, unlike the age of menarche, has not changed at all. However, the life expectancy of women has changed from 43 years on average, 200 years ago, to almost 80 years on average, showing that the age of menopause is not related to life expectancy.

As a woman approaches menopause, the frequency of ovulation decreases from 13-14 times per year to 11-12 times per year and then reduces continuously down to 3-4 times a year before coming to a complete halt at menopause. Recurrent hot flushes are common with the slow but sure disappearance of estradiol from the circulation. The hot flash is a hallmark symptom of menopause. Approximately 75% of women experience hot flashes. Other symptoms of menopause include sleep disorders (declining estradiol causes changes in a woman's sleep cycle), vaginal dryness and genital tract atrophy (with decreasing estradiol these estradiol-dependent tissues become atrophic), mood changes, depression and crying spells (related to estradiol interaction with central nervous system), skin and nail changes (estradiol influences skin thickness), osteoporosis (estrogen receptors are present on osteoblasts and have an essential role in bone formation), and cardiovascular lipid changes (total cholesterol increases and high density lipoproteins (HDL) increase at menopause.

Management of Menopause

The changes in menopause result from declining estradiol and 17ß estradiol production. These should possibly be administered in hormone replacement therapy. When 17ß estradiol is administered orally it is oxidized in the circulation to minimally active estrone. The administration of a mixture of estrogen derivatives or a synthetic estrogen agonist can result in endometrial hyperplasia and in increased risk of endometrial adenocarcinoma. Therefore, a progestogen must be prescribed in conjunction with estrogens, to prevent the estrogen side effects. Progestogens may include synthetic molecules such as medoxyprogesterone acetate or norethindrone.

There are two principals for hormone therapy. Estrogen replacement with accompanying progestogen results in excellent resolution of the symptoms of menopause (hot flashes, sleep disorders, vaginal dryness and genital tract atrophy, mood changes, depression and crying spells, skin and nail changes, osteoporosis, and cardiovascular lipid changes), with a monthly cyclic withdrawal of medication for menstrual bleeding. One of the difficulties of prescribing hormone replacement therapy is that many postmenopausal women today do not want to continue having the menstrual cycles that the steroid hormones would induce. As a result, many physicians avoid the problems of cyclic withdrawal bleeding by the daily administration of an estrogen and progestogen permitting no cyclic withdrawal or bleeding. Numerous preparations combining estrogen and a progestogen are available in both an oral and transdermal formulation.

Until recently, hormone replacement therapy was used by most women to treat menopausal symptoms and protect long-term health. Then a large clinical trial in 2002, the NIH WHI clinical trials (the National Institute of Health, Women's Health Initiative trials), unearthed hormone replacement therapy health risks. Hormone replacement therapy was thought to have the long-term benefits of preventing heart disease and osteoporosis. Attitudes changed abruptly in 2002 when this large clinical trial found that the hormone replacement therapy treatment posed major health risks for postmenopausal women. As the number of health hazards attributed to hormone replacement therapy grew, doctors have become less eager to prescribe this protocol.

What are the benefits of hormone replacement therapy? Women who choose standard hormone replacement therapy during menopause find that it can ease aspects of menopause such as the vaginal symptoms of menopause, hot flashes, sleep disorders, vaginal dryness and genital tract atrophy, mood changes, depression and crying spells, skin and nail changes; it can prevent the long-term occurrence of hip fractures and osteoporosis and prevent heart disease. It also decreases the risk of colorectal cancer.

What, however, are the risks of hormone therapy, as shown by the WHI study? In the largest clinical trial to date, the combination estrogen-progestin pill increases the risk of multiple conditions. According to the study, over one year, 10,000 women taking an estrogen plus progestogen combination hormone replacement therapy pill might experience a higher incidence of heart disease (7 in 10,000 cases, <0.1%), a higher incidence of breast cancer (8 in 10,000 cases, <0.1%), a higher incidence of cerebral vascular accidents (8 in 10,000 cases, <0.1%). The study found no increased risk of breast cancer or heart disease among women taking estrogen alone without progestogen. Over one year, however, 10,000 women taking estrogen alone might experience an increased incidence of cerebral vascular accidents (12 cases in 10,000 or 0.12%).

Despite the health risks, estrogen is still the gold standard for treating menopausal symptoms. The absolute risk to an individual woman taking estrogen only hormone replacement therapy is quite small. In summary, estrogen-progestogen combination hormone replacement therapy has significant but small risks (<0.1% per year) of heart disease, breast cancer and cerebral vascular accidents (Table 30.1). Estrogen only hormone replacement therapy has much less risk (Table 30.1); just a tiny risks for cerebral vascular accidents. There is also the small risk of endometrial cancer with an estrogen because of the estrogen problem with endometrial hyperplasia. In addition, hormone replacement therapy appears to reduce the risk of osteoporosis and cardiovascular disease. It is a woman's choice, careful advice is necessary as to whether to prescribe no hormone replacement therapy, estrogen only hormone replacement therapy or estrogen-progestogen hormone replacement therapy. You must consider whether the protective benefits of hormone replacement therapy may outweigh the risks, and discuss the risks carefully (Table 12.1).

Table 30.1. Risks and benefits of hormone replacement therapies

Issue	Estrogen-Progestogen therapy	Estrogen only therapy
Risks due to endometrial hypertrophy		Increased risk of endometrial adenocarcinoma
Risks shown by WHI study	Heart disease (<0.1% per year)	
	Breast cancer (<0.1% per year)	
	Cerebral vascular accident (<0.1% per year)	Cerebral vascular accident (<0.12% per year)
Menopause symptom benefits	Fixes hot flashes	
	Fixes sleep disorders	
	Fixes vaginal dryness and genital tract atrophy	
	Fixes mood changes, depression and crying spells	
Long-term benefits	Decreased risk of colorectal cancer	Decreased risk of colorectal cancer
	Prevents osteoporosis	Prevents osteoporosis
	Prevents heart disease	Prevents heart disease

Alternatives

With the revelation of these risks with hormone replacement therapy, women have been seeking out alternative medication for menopause. A combination of calcium and vitamin D is common for limiting osteoporosis onset. Soy and isoflavones may be helpful in the short-term (<2 years) treatment of hot flashes and night sweats. St John's Wort may be helpful in the short term (<2 years) for the treatment of mild depression. Black cohosh may be helpful in the short term (<6 months) for the treatment of hot flashes. One of the most commonly utilized off-label medication is progesterone. Numerous studies have indicated progesterone efficacy in the treatment of hot flashes. Lastly, patients should be advised of the potential relief achieved by lifestyle changes, such as eating a healthy low-fat diet, regular exercise, and avoidance of tobacco and alcohol intake. These practices may not only help to relieve some menopausal symptoms, but may help to prevent other health problems.

References

[1] Dratva J, Gómez Real F, Schindler C, Ackermann-Liebrich U, Gerbase MW, Probst-Hensch NM, Svanes C, Omenaas ER, Neukirch F, Wjst M, Morabia A, Jarvis D, Leynaert B, Zemp E. Is age at menopause increasing across Europe? Results on age at menopause and determinants from two population-based studies. *Menopause* 2009;16:385-394.

[2] Nusrat N, Nishat Z, Gulfareen H, Aftab M, Asia N. Knowledge, attitude and experience of menopause. *J Ayub Med Coll Abbottabad* 2008;20:56-59.

[3] Rosano GM, Vitale C, Marazzi G, Volterrani M. Menopause and cardiovascular disease: the evidence. *Climacteric* 2007;10:19-24.

[4] *Hormone therapy*. http://www.nlm.nih.gov/medlineplus/ency/article/007111.htm

[5] Troisi RJ, Speizer FE, Willett WC, Trichopoulos D, Rosner B. Menopause, postmenopausal estrogen preparations, and the risk of adult-onset asthma. A prospective cohort study. *Am J Respir Crit Care Med* 1995;152:1183-1188.

[6] Freedman MA. *Quality of life and menopause: the role of estrogen.* 2002;11:703-718.

Key Points

1. Menopause is commonly accompanied by hot flashes, sleep disorders, vaginal dryness and genital tract atrophy, mood changes, depression and crying spells, skin and nail changes. Without hormone replacement therapy menopause can lead to osteoporosis, and lipid changes that lead to heart disease.
2. The choices at menopause are: no therapy; estrogen only hormone replacement therapy; or estrogen-progestogen hormone replacement therapy. Physicians need to aid patients in making this difficult choice, weighing risks against benefits.
3. While estrogen-progestogen hormone replacement therapy optimally treats menopause and its symptoms, it reduces the patient's risk of colorectal cancer, and increases the risk for heart disease, breast cancer and cerebral vascular accident.
4. Estrogen only hormone replacement therapy optimally treats menopause. It reduces a patient's risk of colorectal cancer. It raises, however, a patient's risk for endometrial malignancy. Patients also have an increased risk of cerebral vascular accident.

Infections of the Reproductive Tract

Chapter 31

Pelvic Inflammatory Disease, Infections of the Reproductive Tract, and Endometriosis

Vulvovaginitis

Vulvovaginitis describes a wide range of conditions causing vaginal or vulvar symptoms, such as itching, burning and abnormal discharge. Vaginal and vulvar burning and discharges are a common reason for seeing a physician. Vulvovaginitis may create major concerns in terms of discomfort and pain, days lost from work, refraining from sexual activity and loss of self-esteem.

Vulvovaginitis is a broad diagnosis. The most common source, approximately half of all cases, is bacterial vaginosis. Other causes include vulvovaginal candidiasis, and vulvovaginal trichomoniasis. Vulvovaginal infections are easily mistaken for sexually transmitted disease lesions like herpes genitalis, papilloma virus infections and syphilis [1-2].

An evaluation of a patient with vulvovaginitis needs to include pertinent history, and pertinent symptoms, including discharges and changes in discharges. The location of symptoms and their duration needs to be carefully recorded. Sexual history can also be very useful. Samples obtained, such as discharges and swabs during vulvovaginal examination, should be examined by the laboratory. Laboratories can examine the samples by microscope and determine using specific tests on the associated organisms.

Treatments range from metronidazole (oral or topical) or clindamycin (oral or topical) for a bacterial vaginosis. Topical synthetic imidazoles or oral fluconazole can be used for treating candidiasis vaginovaginitis. Oral metronidazole or tinidazole can be used for treating trichomoniasis disease [1-2].

Pelvic Inflammatory Disease

Pelvic Inflammatory Disease (PID) can in some cases be considered a sexually transmitted disease. PID involves infection of the upper genital tract (endometrium, fallopian tubes and ovary) as a result of a broad spread of infectious organisms after initial infection of the cervix. The principal germs that cause PID are C. trachomatis and Neisseria gonorrheae. PID may also affect approximately 30% of women with poorly treated chlamydia or gonorrhea infections. The timing of PID in connection to the menstrual cycle can be important. In the luteal phase of the menstrual cycle, spread of infection can be limited due to the limitations of endocervical mucous [3-6].

Infertility is a complication of PID. It results from scarring of the fallopian tubes or adhesions. This causes infertility in approximately 15% of PID patients. This also increases the risk of having an ectopic pregnancy.

Symptoms of PID can be similar to those of ectopic pregnancy; acute appendicitis and diverticular abscesses. Patients with PID may also present with non-specific symptoms such as vaginal discharge or intermittent vaginal bleeding. A pus-ridden cervical discharge is commonly seen. Commonly, the adnexa are moderately to extremely tender, with a palpatable mass. Fever and chills are common. Because PID may not be associated with specific symptoms, empirical treatment is suggested. Normally, broad spectrum antibiotics are prescribed. Some extreme cases may need hospital care [3-6].

Endometriosis

Endometriosis is the presence of growing endometrial tissue at any extrauterine site. Just like endometrial tissue, from which endometriosis originates, endometriosis implants respond to the circulating estrogens and progestogens of the menstrual cycle. Laparoscopy can show an endometriosis lesion. However, because lesions can be very small and possibly result from other disorders, only proven tissue biopsies can be diagnostic for endometriosis. A lot of endometriosis cases can be asymptomatic. In these cases, endometriosis is only confirmed after surgery. Approximately 7-10% of women at any one time may have endometriosis. As shown, 6-43% of women undergoing tubal ligation actually have endometriosis; 21% to 48% of women undergoing laparoscopy for infertility may have endometriosis. It is a very common ailment. Endometriosis may have a genetic component. Women having endometriosis may find that their first-degree relatives are at high risk for endometriosis. Slides of women affected with endometriosis suggest that it may be an inherited disorder [7-10].

The misplaced tissue, as found in endometriosis, responds to estrogen and progesterone and the menstrual cycle in the same way as the endometrium does. Each month tissues build up, like the lining of the uterus, break down and are shed, as in menstrual periods. However, the endometriosis shedding has no exit through which to leave the body. This leads to inflammation and causes pain.

The methods by which endometriosis develops, or how endometrial tissue spreads to other areas of the body, is unclear. There are 4 clear hypotheses about how endometriosis occurs. All may be partially correct. The first hypothesis is "retrograde menstruation," or Samson's theory. Under this theory endometrial tissue backs up as it grows and fills the uterus. Excess tissue backs up into the fallopian tubes and backs up into the abdominal cavity, leading to endometriosis. Under the second hypothesis "coelomic metaplasia" or Meyer's theory, transformation may occur in chronically inflamed tissue, leading to endometrial tissue and endometriosis [7-10].

Under a third hypothesis, "vascular and lymphatic dissemination," or Halban's theory, endometrial cells may spread around the body like cancer cells and metastases, spreading through blood and through the lymphatic system, leading to endometriosis. In a fourth or final theory, "congenital factors," it is thought that congenital factors during fetal development may lead some people to develop endometrial tissue growth outside the uterus, or endometriosis. The biggest question that needs to be explained by these theories is: Why do some women develop endometriosis while others do not?

The gross appearance of endometriosis varies greatly among women. Commonly, lesions are small, about 1 mm clear white lesions, or dark red lesions. They can be cystic, or dark red or blue-domed lesions. Most commonly, lesions are found on the ovary or both ovaries, on the pelvic peritoneum over the uterus, on the cul-de-sacs, and in or on the fallopian tubes or the pelvic lymph nodes. Less commonly, lesions are found in or on the vagina or gastrointestinal tract. Rarely are lesions are found outside of the pelvic cavity.

Women with endometriosis present with a wide variety of symptoms. Endometriosis may also be asymptomatic. Symptoms include dysmenorrhea or painful menstruation, dyspareunia or painful sexual intercourse, and chronic pelvic pain or discomfort. Infertility may be common among women with endometriosis. Less common symptoms include gastro-intestinal problems, such as rectal bleeding. Pelvic examination may reveal uterosacral nodules.

The diagnosis of endometriosis can only be confirmed by laparascopy and biopsy. Magnetic resonance imaging may be useful in identifying the sight of endometriosis. The most effective treatment is surgical removal of the lesion. Because endometriosis tissue responds to estrogen and progesterone, and these are controlled by luteinizing hormone (LH) and follicle stimulating hormone (FSH), modulation of gonadotropins and sex steroids are a useful therapy. Combined estrogen-progesterone oral contraceptive can be useful, as can Denazol, a drug that suppresses pituitary LH and FSH production. Gonadotropin releasing hormone (GnRH) agonist can also be useful to down-regulate gonadotrope cells and stop production of LH and FSH [7-10].

References

[1] Carr PL, Felsenstein D, Friedman RH. Evaluation and Management of Vaginitis. *J Gen Intern Med* 1998; 13: 335–346.

[2] *Vulvovaginitis.* http://www.nlm.nih.gov/medlineplus/ency/article/000897.htm

[3] Soper DE. Pelvic inflammatory disease. *Obstet Gynecol* 2010;116:419-428

[4] Rees E. The treatment of pelvic inflammatory disease. *Am J Obstet Gynecol* 1980; 138:1042-1047.

[5] Jaiyeoba O, Lazenby G, Soper DE. Recommendations and rationale for the treatment of pelvic inflammatory disease. *Expert Rev Anti Infect Ther* 2011;9:61-70.

[6] Weström L, Joesoef R, Reynolds G, Hagdu A, Thompson SE. Pelvic inflammatory disease and fertility. A cohort study of 1,844 women with laparoscopically verified

disease and 657 control women with normal laparoscopic results. *Sex Transm* Dis 1992; 19:185-192.

[7] Viganò P, Parazzini F, Somigliana E, Vercellini P. Endometriosis: epidemiology and aetiological factors. *Best Pract Res Clin Obstet Gynaecol* 2004;18:177-200.

[8] Stilley JA, Birt JA, Sharpe-Timms KL. Cellular and molecular basis for endometriosis-associated infertility. *Cell Tissue Res* 2012;349:849-862.

[9] Giudice LC, Kao LC. Endometriosis. *Lancet* 2004;364:1789-1799.

[10] Yohannes P. Ureteral endometriosis. *J Urol.* 2003;170:20-25.

Key Points

1. Vulvovaginitis is a broad diagnosis. The most common source, approximately half of all cases, is bacterial vaginosis. Other causes include vulvovaginal candidiasis, and vulvovaginal trichomoniasis. Vulvovaginal infections are easily mistaken for sexually-transmitted disease lesions like herpes genitalis, papilloma virus infections and syphilis.
2. The principal germs that cause pelvic inflammatory diseases are C. trachomatis and N. gonorrhoeae. PID may also affect approximately 30% of women with poorly treated chlamydia or gonorrhea infections.
3. The misplaced tissue, as found in endometriosis, responds to estrogen and progesterone and the menstrual cycle in the same way as the endometrium does. Each month tissue builds up, like the lining of uterus, breaks down and is shed as in menstrual periods. However, the endometriosis shedding has no exit through which to leave the body. This leads to inflammation and causes pain.
4. Women with endometriosis present with a wide variety of symptoms. Endometriosis may also be asymptomatic. Symptoms include dysmenorrhea or painful menstruation, dyspareunia or painful sexual intercourse, and chronic pelvic pain or discomfort. Infertility may be common among women with endometriosis.

Chapter 32

Sexually Transmitted Diseases

Introduction

Numerous diseases are spread by sexual intercourse or anal or oral sex in humans. These range from bacterial infections, such as gonorrhea, to viral infection, or non-curable immunodeficient viral infections such as human immunodeficiency virus (HIV). Sexually transmitted diseases, or venereal diseases, are illnesses that have a significant chance of being transmitted between humans by means of sexual intercourse, oral sex, and anal sex. In the past, these diseases were referred to as venereal diseases. Today they are called sexually transmitted diseases or sexually transmitted infections. Some of these diseases can be transmitted via the use of drug needles after use by an infected person, as well as through childbirth or breastfeeding. Sexually transmitted diseases have been known about for thousands of years.

Table 32.1. Common sexually transmitted infectants

Bacterial
Neisseria gonorrhoeae (Gonorrhea)
Treponema pallidum (Syphilis)
Haemophilus ducreyi (Chancroid)
Chlamydia trachomatis (Chlamydia)
Klebsiella granulomatis (Granuloma)
Viral
Herpes simplex virus (Herpes simplex, Genital herpes)
Hepatitis B virus (Viral hepatitis B)
Human Immunodeficiency Virus (HIV)
Human Papilloma Virus (HPV)
Fungal
Tinea cruris (jock itch)
Candidiasis (yeast infection)
Parasitic
Sarcoptes scabiei (Scabies)
Pthirus pubis (Crab louse or crabs)
Trichomonas vaginalis (Trichomoniasis)

Public health officials introduced the terms sexually transmitted infection and sexually transmitted disease. These terms have been adopted widely. The term sexually transmitted disease refers only to infections with symptoms. The term sexually transmitted infection refers to a person who has been infected by a bacteria, virus or parasite, regardless of whether they have any symptoms. The infectious agents listed in Table 32.1 are classed as sexually transmitted infectants.

This list shown in Table 32.1 includes the most common sexually transmitted infectants or causes of sexually transmitted diseases. It should be noted that many common infectious diseases, including the common cold and influenza, can be transmitted during sexual contact, although they are not considered sexually transmitted diseases. Here we consider five of the most common sexually transmitted diseases. A sixth common sexually transmitted disease is human immunodeficiency virus (HIV); this is a book unto itself and is not dealt with here.

Gonorrhea

Gonorrhea is caused by Neisseria gonorrhoeae, a gram-negative coccal bacteria. Gonorrhea mostly affects younger men and women in the 18-24 age range. It is particularly evident in men and women of low socioeconomic standing, or among inner-city groups. The gonococcus bacteria grows best in warm and moist areas of the body, including the urethra that carries urine out of the body. In women, it may be found in the reproductive tract or the urinary tract. Health care workers in every state in the U.S.A. are required to tell their State Board of Health about anyone diagnosed with gonorrhea. This law is to make sure the patient gets proper health care and that their sexual partners are found and tested. Over 700,000 persons in the U.S.A. get gonorrhea every year [1-2].

Gonorrhea causes urethritis in men, leading to a urethral discharge. A high proportion of men with gonorrhea are also infected with chlamydia trachomatis. Other genital tract symptoms are uncommon in men, such as epididymal and prostatic infections.

Gonococcal infections in women are commonly asymptomatic. Gonorrhea may present as dysuria or painful urination. Gonorrhea can also cause pelvic inflammatory disease in women (see Chapter 31), leading to fallopian tube, endometrial and peritoneal infections. Salpingitis can lead to fallopian tube scar tissue and adhesions; these may lead to infertility or an ectopic pregnancy.

Gonorrhea can be quickly recognized by staining a sample of tissue or discharge and then looking at it under a microscope. This is called a gram stain; however, it is just an indicator and not proof. Cultures provide proof of gonorrhea. Cultures are taken from the cervix in women or urethra in men or women [1-2].

In treating sexually transmitted diseases such as gonorrhea, the objective is to firstly cure the patient and secondly to identify, test and treat others that have had sexual contact with the patient, to prevent further spread of the disease. A single shot of ceftriaxone or azithromycin is the recommended one-time antibiotic treatment [1-2].

Chlamydia

Chlamydia is caused by Chlamydia trachomatis. The bacteria invades the same cells a gonorrhea infections; the urethra in men, causing urethritis and discharges from the penis, and the urethra, endometrium and fallopian tubes in women, causing dysuria and pelvic inflammatory disease. Chlamydia infection may be asymptomatic in both men and women. As with gonorrhea, pelvic inflammatory disease may cause fallopian tube scar tissue and adhesions, leading to infertility and ectopic pregnancies. Like gonorrhea, chlamydia infections are a disease of the young in the 18-24 age range. It is particularly evident in men and women of low socioeconomic standing, or among inner-city groups. Chlamydia infection is the most common sexually transmitted disease in the United States. Sexually active individuals and individuals with multiple partners are at greatest risk [3-4].

Diagnosis of chlamydia infection involves sampling of cervical secretions in females and of the urethral discharge in males. If an individual is involved in anal sex, samples from the rectum may also be needed. The sample is sent for a fluorescent or monoclonal antibody test. The therapy for chlamydia infections is antibiotics, tetracyclines, and azithromycin, or erythromycin. In treating the disease, it is important to identify, test and treat others who have had sexual contact with the patient, to prevent further spread of the disease [3-4].

Genital Herpes

Genital herpes is a sexually transmitted disease that does not leave the patient, and cannot be cured; the patient has it for life. The responsible virus, herpes simplex virus, forms a latent infection in the lower end of the spinal cord or sacral dorsal root ganglia, from which the infection can be reactivated. The biggest complication of genital herpes is to the neonate who will acquire it from the genital tract of the mother during parturition. Research suggests that the herpes simplex virus in genital herpes, like human papilloma virus, can increase the risk of cervical malignancy [5-6].

There are two classes of herpes simplex virus (HSV), HSV-1 and HSV-2. HSV-1 virus is found in the spines of 80% of cadavers. An HSV-1 infection is commonly asymptomatic. It is transmitted primarily by respiratory tract infection and spreads through the body. HSV-1 activation commonly causes cold sores. In extreme cases, encephalitis and keratoconjuctivitis can develop from activation.

HSV-2 has the tendency to infect the reproductive tract and so is the cause of genital herpes. Occasionally, HSV-1 can infect the reproductive tract. A nationwide study shows that genital herpes affects 16.2% of the population of the U.S.A. in the age range 14 to 49 years. Genital HSV-2 infection is approximately two-fold more common in women than in men. HSV-1 and HSV-2 can be found in and released from the blisters or lesions on a man's penis or on a woman's vulva or vagina and then transmitted through sexual interactions [5-6].

Herpes infection can be asymptomatic. The first signs or symptoms are one or more blisters or lesions on the penis in men and vulva or vagina in women, or around the rectum. The lesions break, leaving tender areas that may take 2-4 weeks to heal. A second outbreak can appear weeks or months after the first, but it is less severe and shorter lasting. Although the infection stays in the body indefinitely, the number of outbreaks tends to decrease over years. Other symptoms in women are dysuria and vaginal or urethral discharges. Urethral discharges can occur in men. Fever, headache and malaise are often reported. Occasionally, a herpes infection can cause asceptic meningitis. Notwithstanding the severity of symptoms, genital herpes frequently causes psychological distress in people who know they are infected.

HSV infection can be diagnosed by visual inspection of the penis or vulva. Samples can be evaluated in the laboratory by DNA testing. HSV infections can be diagnosed between outbreaks by the use of a serum antibody test. The serum test detects antibodies to HSV-1 or HSV-2 infection. There is no treatment that can cure herpes, but antiviral medications can shorten and prevent outbreaks during the period of time the person takes the medication. Acylovir, a purine analog, is the drug of choice to treat symptoms of herpes infection. Treatment with Acylovir will stop viral DNA replication but will not prevent latent infections. Valtrex can diminish virus levels and limit herpes virus transmission [5-6].

Human Papilloma Virus

Genital warts deriving from human papilloma virus (HPV) are considered an inconvenient but relatively benign disease. They are seen in young people aged 16-25. It is now known that there is a range of HPV infections, or a range in the symptoms and effect of HPV infections. There are latent HPV infections, asymptomatic infections only detected by HPV DNA in tissue samples tested in epidemiological studies. There are subclinical HPV infections, such as genital warts, and evident or oddball genital warts known as condyloma aluminate, pink or pigmented papules. Warts on men are on the penis, and warts on women are mostly on the labia, and less commonly on the cervix and vagina. Most warts are simple irritations. The disease is commonly asymptomatic. However, HPV has been shown to be at the root of the majority of cases of carcinoma of the cervix and carcinoma of the vulva. Approximately 85% of women with cervical cancer have an HPV infection, as shown by HPV DNA testing. The prevalence of HPV infection, however, is very high compared to the small incidence of cervical cancer in the U.S.A. [7-8].

HPV cases are treated today with HPV vaccines or Cervarix or Gardasil. These block HPV growth and mitosis and limit genital wart formation and greatly lower the risks for cervical cancer and vulvar cancer. HPV is a virus present for life, and is not completely curable. HPV is detected today by DNA in situ hybridization analysis. In women, a Pap smear test is performed for cervical cancer. The Pap smear might also detect abnormal cells due to HPV infection. A similar cervical smear to that needed for the Pap smear is also used for testing for HPV. There is currently no FDA-approved test to detect HPV in men. That is because an effective, reliable way to collect a sample of male genital skin cells, which would allow detection of HPV, has yet to be developed.

Approximately 20 million subjects or 1 in 15 people in the U.S.A. have HPV. This incidence of HPV-associated malignancies is small. Female cervical cancer has an incidence of 12,000 cases a year in the U.S.A.; female vulvar cancer totals 3,700 cases and male penile cancer numbers 1,000 cases a year [7-8].

Syphilis

Syphilis is a system-wide disorder, yet it is strictly sexually transmitted through heterosexual intercourse and homosexual anal sex. It is believed that syphilis began in the New World. It is thought that Columbus and his crew caught the disease when visiting the New World and returned it to Europe, where it became widespread. Syphilis is caused by the bacteria Treponema pallidum, which enters the body through skin and breaks in the genitalia during sexual interactions [9-10].

Syphilis afflicts people through 4 advancement stages; a primary and secondary stage, a latent stage and a tertiary stage. In the primary, secondary and latent stages death can be prevented by antibiotic therapy. The primary stage of disease is the chancre. This develops close to the bacterial entry point, or the penis of men or labia of women, or rectum of homosexual men. Chancres are small non-painful papules that are very profound and persist for as long as two months.

Secondary syphilis is the result of the bacteria spreading around the body. It causes a rash, most commonly over the trunk and extremities of the body. Large papules develop in moist areas such as the vulva and anus. Fever, sore throat and headaches are common. Untreated disease resolves slowly over months leaving the patient symptom free. The third or latent stage of syphilis is asymptomatic and can only be identified by a blood test, the venereal disease research laboratory (VDRL) test. Latent disease can last for up to 40 years. What follows is the most advanced or deadly tertiary stage of syphilis [9-10].

Tertiary syphilis involves the skin, bones, cartilages, and possibly cardiovascular and nervous systems. Gummas or inflammatory granulomas form on the skin, soft tissues, bones, liver and testes. Gummas are very destructive lesions, leaving large ulcers in their place. Tertiary syphilis can affect the aorta leading to aortic valve insufficiency, left ventricular hypertrophy and congestive heart failure and possible death. Tertiary syphilis can cause aneurysms in the aorta, leading to death. Nervous system disease can lead to meningitis, hydrocephalus and dementia, numbness, and gradual blindness. About one-half of syphilis cases that progress to the tertiary stage lead to death from cardiovascular or nervous system complications.

Syphilis is diagnosed by examining material from a chancre using a dark-field microscope. Syphilis can also be diagnosed using the VDRL blood test. Syphilis is easily treated by intra-muscular injection of penicillin. A single injection of penicillin will cure a person who has had syphilis for less than a year. Additional doses are needed to treat someone who has had syphilis for longer than a year [9-10].

References

[1] Ohnishi M, Golparian D, Shimuta K, Saika T, Hoshina S, Iwasaku K, Nakayama S, Kitawaki J, Unemo M. Is *Neisseria gonorrhoeae* Initiating a Future Era of Untreatable Gonorrhea?: Detailed Characterization of the First Strain with High-Level Resistance to Ceftriaxone. *Antimicrob Agents Chemother* 2011; 55: 3538–3545.

[2] Kleist E, Moi H. Transmission of gonorrhoea through an inflatable doll. *Genitourin Med* 1993; 69: 322.

[3] Kissinger PJ, Reilly K, Taylor SN, Leichliter JS, Rosenthal S, Martin DH. Early repeat Chlamydia trachomatis and Neisseria gonorrhoeae infections among heterosexual men. *Sex Transm Dis* 2009;36:498-500.

[4] Paavonen J, Eggert-Kruse W. Chlamydia trachomatis: impact on human reproduction *Hum Reprod Update* 1999;5:433-447.

[5] Leone P. Reducing the risk of transmitting genital herpes: advances in understanding and therapy. *Curr Med Res Opin* 2005;21:1577-1582.

[6] Corey L, Adams HG, Brown ZA, Holmes KK. Genital herpes simplex virus infections: clinical manifestations, course, and complications. *Ann Intern Med* 1983;98:958-972.

[7] Burd EM. Human Papillomavirus and Cervical Cancer *Clin Microbiol Rev* 2003; 16: 1–17.

[8] Walboomers JM, Jacobs MV, Manos MM, Bosch FX, Kummer JA, Shah KV, Snijders PJ, Peto J, Meijer CJ, Muñoz N. Human papillomavirus is a necessary cause of invasive cervical cancer worldwide. *J Pathol* 1999;189:12-19.

[9] Mattei PL, Beachkofsky TM, Gilson RT, Wisco OJ. Syphilis: a reemerging infection. *Am Fam Physician* 2012;86:433-440.

[10] Lynn WA, Lightman S. Syphilis and HIV: a dangerous combination. *Lancet Infect Dis 2004*;4:456-466.

Key Points

1. Numerous diseases are spread by sexual intercourse or anal or oral sex in humans. These range from bacterial infections such as gonorrhea, to viral infection, and to non-curable immunodeficient viral infections such as HIV. Sexually transmitted diseases, or venereal diseases, are illnesses that have a significant chance of being transmitted between humans by means of sexual intercourse, oral sex, and anal sex. In the past, these diseases were referred to as venereal disease. Today they are called sexually transmitted diseases or sexually transmitted infections. Some of these diseases can be transmitted via the use of drug needles after use by an infected person, as well as through childbirth or breastfeeding. Sexually transmitted diseases have been known about for thousands of years.
2. Gonorrhea is caused by Neisseria gonorrhoeae, a gram-negative coccal bacteria. Gonorrhea mostly affects younger men and women in the 18-24 age range. It is particularly evident in men and women of low socioeconomic standing, or among inner-city groups. The gonococcus bacteria grows best in warm, moist areas of the body, including the urethra that carries urine out of the body. Over 700,000 persons in the U.S.A. get gonorrhea every year.
3. Chlamydia is caused by Chlamydia trachomatis. The bacteria invades the same cells as gonorrhea infections, causing urethritis in men and discharges from the penis, and the urethra, endometrium and fallopian tubes in women, causing dysuria and pelvic inflammatory disease. Chlamydia infection may be asymptomatic in both men and women. As with gonorrhea, pelvic inflammatory disease may cause fallopian tube scar tissue and adhesions leading to infertility and ectopic pregnancies. Like gonorrhea, chlamydia infections are a disease of the young in the 18-24 age range. It

is particularly evident in men and women of low socioeconomic standing, or among inner-city groups. Chlamydia infection is the most common sexually transmitted disease in the United States. Sexually active individuals and individuals with multiple partners are at highest risk.

4. Genital herpes is a sexually transmitted disease that does not leave the patient, and cannot be cured; the patient has it for life. The responsible virus, herpes simplex virus, forms a latent infection in the lower end of the spinal cord or sacra dorsal root ganglia, from which the infection can be reactivated. The biggest complication of genital herpes is to the neonate who will aquire it from the genital tract of the mother during parturition. Research suggests that herpes simplex virus in genital herpes, like human papilloma virus, can increase the risk of cervical malignancy.
5. Genital warts deriving from human papilloma virus (HPV) are considered an inconvenient but relatively benign disease. They are seen in young people aged 16-25. It is now known that there is a range of HPV infections, or a range in the symptoms and effect of HPV infections. There are latent HPV infections, asymptomatic infections only detected by HPV DNA in tissue samples tested in epidemiological studies. There are subclinical HPV infections, such as genital warts, and evident or oddball genital warts known as condyloma aluminate, pink or pigmented papules. Warts on men are on the penis, and warts on women are mostly on the labia, and less commonly on the cervix and vagina. Most warts are simply irritations. The disease is commonly otherwise asymptomatic. However, HPV has been shown to be at the root of the majority of cases of carcinoma of the cervix and carcinoma of the vulva. Approximately 85% of women with cervical cancer have an HPV infection, as shown by HPV DNA testing. The prevalence of HPV infection, however, is very high compared to the small incidence of cervical cancer in the U.S.A.
6. Syphilis is a system-wide disorder, yet is strictly sexually transmitted through heterosexual intercourse and homosexual anal sex. It is believed that syphilis began in the New World. It is thought that Columbus and his crew caught the disease when visiting the New World and returned it to Europe, where it became widespread. Syphilis is caused by the bacteria Treponema pallidum, which enters the body through skin breaks in the genitalia during sexual interactions.

Malignancies of the Reproductive Tract

Chapter 33

Hormones, Familial Factors and Breast Cancer

Breast Cancer

Breast cancer is the most common malignancy affecting women; approximately 1 in 8 women will get this cancer. Incidence ranges from 1 in 19,608 at age 25, down to 1 in 50 at age 50, down to 1 in 10 by age 80. Breast cancer incidence is very age-dependent. Most breast cancer cases occur in women (99% of cases). Breast cancer may be located in any part of the mammary gland. Cancers are classified according to whether cells are of lobular origin; lobular carcinomas (as in lobules of alveoli where milk is made); or ductal origin, ductal carcinoma (as in lactiferous ducts). Most breast cancers (about 85%) are of ductal origin [1-5].

Many breast cancers are sensitive to estrogen, meaning that estrogen causes the breast cancer to grow. These cancers are called estrogen receptor positive carcinomas. Some women have what's called HER2-positive carcinoma. HER2 refers to a gene that promotes growth causing cancer to grow faster, leading to more aggressive disease. Some people have genes that make them more prone to developing breast cancer. Such genes include BRCA1 and BRCA2. Women with BRCA1 and BRCA2 genes have up to an 80% chance of getting breast cancer during their lifetime. A person also has a higher risk for breast cancer when a close relative has had breast, uterine, ovarian, or colon cancer. Approximately one quarter of women with breast cancer have a family history of the disease. Other major risk factors for breast cancer include menarche before age 12, late menopause after age 55, significant alcohol use, being nulliparous or having no children, hormone replacement therapy, and obesity.

Early breast cancer is asymptomatic; regular mammograms are critical in identifying early stage disease. With advancing cancer, symptoms appear; a breast lump or mass, or lump in the armpit that is hard or has uneven edges may be a clear symptom. Other symptoms include changes in the size, shape, or feel of the breast or nipple, redness of the breast, dimpling or puckering of the breast, and fluid emitting from the nipple. Symptoms of advanced disease include bone pain, breast pain, skin ulcers and swelling of an arm.

Breast cancers metastasize first to the axillary lymph nodes, then to distant sites such as the bone, liver, lung, pleura and brain. Patients with histologically negative axillary lymph nodes have a much better survival rate than those with positive lymph nodes. The ultimate prognosis depends on the size of the tumor, the number of nodes and the presence or absence of lymphovascular invasion, so that the treatment depends on the cancer stage (see below). Surgical choices include radical mastectomy or lumpectomy. Radiation therapy is commonly used, as is chemotherapy. Tamoxifen, an anti-estrogen, is used for endocrine therapy to inhibit cancer cell growth [1-5].

Considering the cancer stage, in Stage 0 or ductal or lobular cancer *in situ*, a lumpectomy plus radiation is the standard treatment. In Stages I and II, a lumpectomy plus radiation or mastectomy with removal of the lymph nodes is standard treatment. Tamoxifen hormone therapy and chemotherapy may be recommended following surgery. In Stages III and IV standard treatment is a mastectomy followed by chemotherapy and tamoxifen therapy. In Stage III and Stage IV cancer therapy the use of mastectomy and targeted therapy together with chemotherapy is recommended. The targeted therapy is the drug trastuzumab (Herceptin). Trastuzumab is a monoclonal human antibody which limits HER-2 promotion of cancer tissue.

The 5-year survival rates refer to the number of patients who live at least 5 years after their cancer is found. According to the American Cancer Society (ACS), the 5-year survival rate is 100% for Stage 0 disease, 100% for Stage I disease, 92% for Stage IIA, 81% for Stage IIB, 67% for Stage IIIA 54% for Stage IIIB and 20% for Stage IV. Women at very high risk for breast cancer because of first-degree relative cancer and other risk factors can consider preventive (prophylactic) mastectomy. Frequent mammography or mammography and magnetic resonance imaging is the simplest option. Tamoxifen treatment is approved for breast cancer prevention in women aged 35 and older at high risk [1-5].

References

[1] Gonzalez-Angulo AM, Morales-Vasquez F, Hortobagyi GN. Overview of resistance to systemic therapy in patients with breast cancer. *Adv Exp Med Biol* 2007;608:1-22.

[2] Early Breast Cancer Trialists' Collaborative Group. Tamoxifen for early breast cancer. *Cochrane Database Syst Rev* 2001;(1):CD000486.

[3] King MC, Wieand S, Hale K, Lee M, Walsh T, Owens K, Tait J, Ford L, Dunn BK, Costantino J, Wickerham L, Wolmark N, Fisher B. Tamoxifen and breast cancer incidence among women with inherited mutations in BRCA1 and BRCA2: National Surgical Adjuvant Breast and Bowel Project (NSABP-P1) Breast Cancer Prevention Trial. *J Am Med Assoc.* 2001;286:2251-2256.

[4] Karabakhtsian RG, Johnson R, Sumkin J, Dabbs DJ. The clinical significance of lobular neoplasia on breast core biopsy. *Am J Surg Pathol* 2007;31:717-723.

[5] Chuba PJ, Hamre MR, Yap J, Severson RK, Lucas D, Shamsa F, Aref A. Bilateral risk for subsequent breast cancer after lobular carcinoma-in-situ: analysis of surveillance, epidemiology, and end results data. *J Clin Oncol* 2005;23:5534-5541.

Key Points

Approximately 1 in 8 women will have breast cancer. Incidence ranges from 1 in 19,608 at age 25 down to 1 in 50 at age 50, and down to 1 in 10 by age 80. Cancers are classified according to whether cells are of lobular origin (lobular carcinomas) or ductal origin (ductal carcinomas). Many breast cancers are sensitive to estrogen, meaning that estrogen causes the breast cancer to grow. These cancers are called estrogen receptor positive carcinomas. Some women have what's called HER2-positive carcinoma. HER2 refers to a gene that causes cancer to grow faster. Some people have genes making them more prone to developing breast cancer. Such genes include BRCA1 and BRCA2. Women with BRCA1 and BRCA2 genes have up to an 80% chance of getting breast cancer during their lifetime. Approximately one-quarter of women with breast cancer have a family history of the disease raising their risk for breast cancer. Other major risk factors for breast cancer include menarche before age 12, late menopause after age 55, significant alcohol use, being nulliparous or having no children, hormone replacement therapy, and obesity.

Chapter 34

Cervical, Ovarian and Endometrial Neoplasms

Introduction

Cervical, ovarian and endometrial malignancies are representative malignancies of most human cancers. As with all cancers, early detection, if possible, is important, and as with most cancers, incidence rises with age, with cancer being most common in women over 50 years of age. As with most malignancies, they express placental hyperglycosylated hCG β-subunit (see Chapter 1), which can both advance cancer growth and its invasion. Tumor markers are invaluable for early detection of malignancies. CA125 is a tumor marker specific to ovarian malignancies, particularly serous ovarian carcinoma. CA125 will detect some endometrial malignancies. Other endometrial malignancies may be detected by CA19-9 tumor marker. Squamous cell cervical (SCC) cell antigen is useful in marking cervical malignancies. Tumor markers can be used in patient screening, and in monitoring the progress and recurrence of malignancies.

Ovarian Neoplasms

Ovarian neoplasms affect approximately 2% of women. As with breast cancer (see Chapter 33), age is the most critical factor in determining the risk of ovarian cancer. Approximately 10% of palpatable adnexal masses turn out to be ovarian cancer, versus a benign neoplasm of the ovary, or ovarian cyst or polycystic ovary syndrome. The vast majority of ovarian cancer (85-90%) occurs in postmenopausal women, or after the ovary has completed its biological function [1-4].

There are multiple familial ovarian cancer factors. These include familial ovarian cancer hereditary factors (if another member of the family has had ovarian cancer), hereditary colorectal cancer syndrome, and Lynch cancer family syndrome. Many of the hereditary or genetic factors that make people susceptible to breast cancers may also make them susceptible to ovarian cancers (see Chapter 33). Most ovarian cancers occur in cases with

BRCA1 or BRCA2 gene mutations, just like breast cancers. Women with BRCA mutation have a 20-fold higher risk for ovarian cancer, and women with BRCA-2 factor have an 8-fold increased risk for ovarian cancer [1-4].

Most ovarian cancers are epithelial cell cancers; these are mostly serous carcinomas, and to a lesser extent mucinous and endometrioid carcinomas. These disseminate locally to the fallopian tube and uterus, to the other ovary and to the peritoneum. Metastases are commonly found in the cul-de-sac, bowel, peritoneum and diaphragm. Malignant ascites form from the diaphragm metastases and block the lymphatic drainage of the peritoneal cavity. Patients are generally asymptomatic until either the cancer advances to other organs or the ascites cause abdominal bloating, dyspepsia or urinary frequency. This lack of early symptoms leads to late cancer diagnosis with poor prognosis. Treatment of epithelial cancer involves cytoreductive surgery and aggressive chemotherapy. Only about 15% of woman first presenting with advanced disease, Stage III or Stage IV cancer, will survive (see Table 34.1).

Table 34.1. Staging ovarian cancer

Stage IA - involves one ovary, capsule intact, no tumor on ovarian surface
Stage IB - involves both ovaries, capsule intact, no tumor on ovarian surface
Stage IC - tumor limited to ovaries with any of the following: capsule ruptured, or tumor on ovarian surface
Stage IIA - extension or implants onto uterus or fallopian tube
Stage IIB - extension or implants onto other pelvic structures
Stage IIC - pelvic extension or implants with positive peritoneal washings
Stage IIIA - microscopic peritoneal metastases beyond pelvis
Stage IIIB - macroscopic peritoneal metastases beyond pelvis less than 2 cm in size
Stage IIIC - peritoneal metastases beyond pelvis > 2 cm or lymph node metastases
Stage IV - distant metastases to the liver or outside the peritoneal cavity

Other types of ovarian cancer include germ cell tumors (dysgerminoma, choriocarcinoma, yolk-sac carcinoma, and teratoma) and embryonal carcinoma. Germ cell malignancies are rare and are seen in young women or adolescent girls, and are generally curable if found and treated early. Use of combination chemotherapy after initial surgery can dramatically improve the prognosis for these tumors. Ovarian germ cell tumors can be difficult to diagnose early since they are often asymptomatic; the only symptoms may be a swelling or hard distended abdomen with or without pain. Tests which may be used to show this type of tumor are ultrasound or CT scan.

In the ovary, embryonal carcinomas are quite rare. Like germ cell malignancies, they mostly affect young adolescent women. The median age at diagnosis is just 15 years. Symptoms and signs are varied, and may include abnormal uterine bleeding. In 40% of cases there is extension of the tumor beyond the ovary. They are generally large tumors [1-4].

Cervical Neoplasms

Most cervical neoplasms are squamous cell malignancies. Unlike ovarian and endometrial cancers, which are more prevalent in industrialized countries, cervical malignancies are the biggest killer today in third world nations. Squamous cervical cancer is unique in that it can be prevented by regular Pap smear screening, along with concomitant screening for human papilloma virus. When one considers that most cervical cancer cases are associated with human papilloma virus (85% of women with cervical cancer have an HPV infection, as shown by HPV DNA testing), a sexually transmitted disease, cervical cancer itself might be considered a sexually transmitted disease [5-8].

Cervical cancer arises from a premalignant state, cervical intraepithelial neoplasia (CIN), which can be detected by a Pap smear; this transforms over 5-15 years to invasive cervical cancer. As such, an annual Pap smear should be able to prevent cervical cancer. The American Cancer Society estimates that in the United States 11,000 new cases of cervical cancer will be diagnosed each year. In addition, more than 50,000 cases of premalignant carcinoma *in situ* are diagnosed each year. It is estimated that 4,000 women will die from cervical cancer each year. Cervical cancers most commonly affect postmenopausal women.

Clinically, the first symptom of cervical cancer is abnormal vaginal bleeding. Vaginal discomfort, vaginal discharge, and dysuria may not be uncommon. The tumor disseminates upward to the endometrial cavity and downward to the vagina, and laterally to the peritoneum. Cervical cancer can invade the bladder and rectum directly. Common symptoms of cervical cancer are constipation, hematuria, fistula, and ureteral obstruction. Treatment is chemotherapy and surgery where needed [5-8].

Endometrial Neoplasms

Endometrial carcinoma is the most common pelvic malignancy in women. The U.S.A. has the highest incidence of endometrial carcinoma in the world. Developing countries like Japan have 5-fold lower incidences. Endometrial cancer is the most common type of uterine cancer. Although the exact cause of endometrial cancer is unknown, increased levels of estrogen can play a role. Estrogen helps stimulate the build-up of the lining of the uterus. Studies have shown that high levels of estrogen in animals result in excessive endometrial growth and cancer. Most cases of endometrial cancer occur between the ages of 60 and 70 years, but a few cases may occur before age 40 [9-12].

The following can increase risk for endometrial cancer: diabetes; estrogen replacement therapy without the use of progesterone; history of endometrial polyps; infertility; being nulliparous or never pregnant; obesity; starting menarche at an early age; and starting menopause after age 50. Symptoms of endometrial malignancy include: abnormal uterine bleeding, abnormal menstrual periods; bleeding during menstrual cycle; vaginal bleeding after menopause; vaginal bleeding after age 40; lower abdominal pain or cramping; vaginal discharge after menopause.

Treatment options involve surgery, radiation therapy, and chemotherapy. A trans-abdominal hysterectomy may be performed in women with the early stage disease. Removal of the fallopian tubes and ovaries (bilateral salpingo-oophorectomy) is also recommended.

Hysterectomy combined with radiation therapy is used to treat women with Stage 1 disease. Chemotherapy may be used in Stages 3 and 4 of the disease. The 5-year survival rate for endometrial cancer that has not spread is 95%. If the cancer has spread to distant organs, the 5-year survival rate drops to 23% [9-12].

Most endometrial cancers are carcinomas or adenocarcinomas, in that they originate from the single epithelial cells lining the endometrium or endometrial glands. There are subtypes of endometrial carcinoma, including endometrioid carcinoma, in which the cancer cells grow in patterns reminiscent of normal endometrium. There is the more aggressive papillary serous carcinoma and clear cell endometrial carcinomas. Type I cancers occur in patients with a history of estrogen exposure. These are often minimally invasive malignancies of the endometrioid type, and have a good prognosis. Type II cancers occur in older, postmenopausal women, and are not associated with increased exposure to estrogen. These cancers carry a poorer prognosis; they can be endometrioid cancer, uterine papillary serous carcinoma or uterine clear cell carcinoma.

References

[1] Cho KR, Shih IeM. Ovarian cancer. *Annu Rev Pathol* 2009;4:287-313.

[2] Pearce CL, Templeman C, Rossing MA, Lee A, Near AM, Webb PM, Nagle CM, Doherty JA, Cushing-Haugen KL, Wicklund KG, Chang-Claude J, Hein R, Lurie G, Wilkens LR, Carney ME, Goodman MT, Moysich K, Kjaer SK, Hogdall E, Jensen A, Goode EL, Fridley BL, Larson MC, Schildkraut JM, Palmieri RT, Cramer DW, Terry KL, Vitonis AF, Titus LJ, Ziogas A, Brewster W, Anton-Culver H, Gentry-Maharaj A, Ramus SJ, Anderson AR, Brueggmann D, Fasching PA, Gayther SA, Huntsman DG, Menon U, Ness RB, Pike MC, Risch H, Wu AH, Berchuck A. Association between endometriosis and risk of histological subtypes of ovarian cancer: a pooled analysis of case-control studies. *Lancet Oncol* 2012;13:385-394.

[3] Kurman RJ, Shih IeM. The origin and pathogenesis of epithelial ovarian cancer: a proposed unifying theory. *Am J Surg Pathol.* 2010;34:433-443.

[4] Genkinger JM, Hunter DJ, Spiegelman D, Anderson KE, Arslan A, Beeson WL, Buring JE, Fraser GE, Freudenheim JL, Goldbohm RA, Hankinson SE, Jacobs DR Jr, Koushik A, Lacey JV Jr, Larsson SC, Leitzmann M, McCullough ML, Miller AB, Rodriguez C, Rohan TE, Schouten LJ, Shore R, Smit E, Wolk A, Zhang SM, Smith-Warner SA. Dairy products and ovarian cancer: a pooled analysis of 12 cohort studies. *Cancer Epidemiol Biomarkers Prev* 2006;15:364-372.

[5] Walboomers JM, Jacobs MV, Manos MM, Bosch FX, Kummer JA, Shah KV, Snijders PJ, Peto J, Meijer CJ, Muñoz N. Human papillomavirus is a necessary cause of invasive cervical cancer worldwide. *J Pathol* 1999 Sep;189(1):12-9.

[6] Childers JM, Chu J, Voigt LF, Feigl P, Tamimi HK, Franklin EW, Alberts DS, Meyskens FL Jr. Chemoprevention of cervical cancer with folic acid: a phase III Southwest Oncology Group Intergroup study.*Cancer Epidemiol Biomarkers Prev* 1999; 4:155-159.

[7] Waggoner SE. Cervical cancer. *Lancet* 2003;36:2217-2225.

[8] Bosch FX, Lorincz A, Muñoz N, Meijer CJ, Shah KV. The causal relation between human papillomavirus and cervical cancer. *J Clin Pathol* 200;55:244-265.
[9] Amant F, Moerman P, Neven P, Timmerman D, Van Limbergen E, Vergote I. Endometrial cancer. *Lancet* 2005;366:491-505.
[10] Sorosky JI. Endometrial cancer. *Obstet Gynecol* 2008;111:436-447.
[11] Beiner ME, Finch A, Rosen B, Lubinski J, Moller P, Ghadirian P, Lynch HT, Friedman E, Sun P, Narod SA. The risk of endometrial cancer in women with BRCA1 and BRCA2 mutations. A prospective study. *Gynecol Oncol* 2007;104:7-10.
[12] Meyer LA, Broaddus RR, Lu KH. Endometrial cancer and Lynch syndrome: clinical and pathologic considerations. *Cancer Control* 2009;16:14-22.

Key Points

1. Ovarian cancer, like breast cancers, occurs in individuals with familial or genetic predispositions. BRCA1 and BRCA2 predispose a person to getting ovarian cancer. Most ovarian cancers are epithelial cell cancers; these are mostly serous carcinomas, and to a lesser extent mucinous and endometrioid carcinomas. These disseminate locally to the fallopian tube and uterus, to the other ovary and to the peritoneum. Metastases are commonly found in the cul-de-sac, bowel, peritoneum and diaphragm. Malignant ascites form from the diaphragm metastases and block the lymphatic drainage of the peritoneal cavity. Patients are generally asymptomatic until either the cancer advances to other organs or the ascites cause abdominal bloating, dyspepsia or urinary frequency. This lack of early symptoms leads to late cancer diagnosis with poor prognosis. Treatment of epithelial cancer involves cytoreductive surgery and aggressive chemotherapy. Only about 15% of woman first presenting with advanced disease, Stage III or Stage IV cancer, will survive (see Table 29.1).
2. Most cervical neoplasms are squamous cell malignancies. Most cervical cancer cases are associated with human papilloma virus (85% of women with cervical cancer have an HPV infection). Cervical cancer arises from a premalignant state, cervical intraepithelial neoplasia (CIN), which can be detected by a Pap smear; this transforms over 5-15 years to invasive cervical cancer. As such, an annual Pap smear should be able to prevent cervical cancer.
3. Endometrial carcinoma is the most common pelvic malignancy in women. Endometrial cancer is the most common type of uterine cancer. Although the exact cause of endometrial cancer is unknown, increased levels of estrogen can play a role. Estrogen helps stimulate the build-up of the lining of the uterus. Most cases of endometrial cancer occur between the ages of 60 and 70 years, but a few cases may occur before age 40.

Chapter 35

Hormones and Testicular and Prostate Malignancies

Testicular Cancer

Testicular cancer is the most common malignancy in young men aged 20-40. While approximately 8,400 cases of testicular malignancy are seen each year in the U.S.A., only 390 men (<5%), on average, die each year of this malignancy. Cryptorchidism, or undescended testes, places men at very high risk for testicular germ cell malignancy, with a 1 in 50 chance of developing testicular germ cell malignancy. Such men may be monitored regularly using ultrasound.

Testicular malignancies are, unlike most other cancers, comprised mostly of germ cells. Tumors are classified into testicular seminomas, and testicular non-seminomas. Non-seminomas include testicular choriocarcinoma, testicular yolk sac carcinoma, testicular embryonal carcinoma and testicular teratoma. These germ cell tumors arise from spermatogonial cells and exhibit embryonal-like differentiation. The non-seminoma malignancies take on a female choriocarcinoma-like trophoblastic nature, producing high levels of placental human chorionic gonadotropin (hCG), mostly producing hyperglycosylated hCG like female choriocarcinoma. Both alpha-fetoprotein and total hCG are excellent tumor markers for monitoring germ cell malignancy cases.

Most germ cell testicular malignancies are diagnosed at an early tumor stage when the malignancy is confined to the testis. A testicular mass can often be palpated by the physician. Symptoms may include one or more of the following: a lump in one testis; sharp pain or a dull ache in the scrotum; gynecomastia (breast enlargement) from hormonal effects of placental hCG. The nature of any palpated lump in the scrotum is evaluated by scrotal ultrasound. The extent of the disease is evaluated by CT scans, which are used to locate metastases. Blood tests are also used to identify and measure hCG and alpha-fetoprotein tumor markers.

While in a few cases removal of testicular cancer tumors from the testis may be satisfactory, most cases require orchidectomy. Men with spreading tumor masses are also treated with etoposide-cisplatin-based chemotherapy. Like choriocarcinoma or gestational trophoblastic neoplasm, germ cell testicular malignancy is very treatable with a high 5-year survival rate.

Prostate Cancer

Prostate cancer is the most common malignancy in men in the U.S.A. and is responsible for more deaths than any other cancer, except for lung cancer. The American Cancer Society (ACS) estimates that about 218,890 new cases of prostate cancer were diagnosed in the United States during 2007. About 1 man in 6 will be diagnosed with prostate cancer during his lifetime, but only 1 man in 34 will die of this malignancy. As men increase in age, their risk of developing prostate cancer increases exponentially. Although only 1 in 10,000 men under age 40 will be diagnosed, the rate shoots up to 1 in 39 for ages 40 to 59, and 1 in 14 for ages 60 to 69. More than 65% of all prostate cancers are diagnosed in men over the age of 65. African American men are 56% more likely to develop prostate cancer compared with Caucasian men and nearly 2.5 times as likely to die from the disease.

There is an excellent tumor marker for prostate cancer, but it is not perfect; it is prostate-specific antigen (PSA). PSA levels of less than 4 ng/mL are considered as negative or normal. PSA levels of 4 to 10 ng/ml represent a 20-30% risk of having prostate cancer, otherwise a high risk for having benign prostate hyperplasia (BPH). PSA of 10-20 ng/ml represents a high risk, 50-75% of having prostate cancer and a lesser risk for having BPH. PSA levels of over 20 ng/ml represent a very high risk, 90%, for having prostate cancer. The definitive test is prostate needle biopsy. The needle is placed in the anus, then across rectal tissue and into the prostate.

Prostate cancer may be asymptomatic in its early stages, which is why obtaining the PSA test is important. Prostate cancer that is more advanced may cause signs and symptoms such as trouble urinating, decreased force in the stream of urine, hematuria, blood in the semen, swelling in the legs and discomfort in the pelvic area. Ninety one percent of prostate cancer cases are diagnosed while the cancer is still confined to the primary site (early stage), and 5% of cases are diagnosed after the cancer has metastasized to distant sites (advanced stage). The 5-year survival rates are 100% for early stage and 33.3% for advanced stage disease. The most common pathology of prostate cancer is an adenocarcinoma of glandular epithelial origin (95% of cases). Approximately 4% of cases of prostate cancer have transitional cell morphology and are thought to arise from the urothelial lining of the prostatic urethra, prostatic intraplasia neoplasia.

Prostate cancer treatment options depend on several factors, such as the stage and grade of the malignancy. For men with an early stage prostate cancer, treatment may not be necessary right away. If tests show the cancer is progressing, radical prostatectomy may be recommended, combined with radiation therapy. Hormone therapy is also often used to block testosterone production and to shrink tumors, since testosterone can promote the growth of prostate adenocarcinoma tissue. Gonadotropin releasing hormone (GnRH) agonists may be used to block testosterone, testosterone antagonists (drugs such as Casodex or Nilandron) or an orchidectomy to stop testosterone.

References

[1] Huyghe E, Matsuda T, Thonneau P. Increasing incidence of testicular cancer worldwide: a review. *J Urol* 2003;170:5-11.

[2] Dieckmann KP, Pichlmeier U. The prevalence of familial testicular cancer: an analysis of two patient populations and a review of the literature. *Cancer* 1997;80:1954-1960.

[3] Einhorn LH. Treatment of testicular cancer: a new and improved model. *J Clin Oncol* 1990;8:1777-1781.

[4] Giles GG, Severi G, English DR, McCredie MR, Borland R, Boyle P, Hopper JL. Sexual factors and prostate cancer. *Brit J Urol Int* 2003;92:211-216.

[5] Catalona WJ, Richie JP, Ahmann FR, Hudson MA, Scardino PT, Flanigan RC, deKernion JB, Ratliff TL, Kavoussi LR, Dalkin BL. Comparison of digital rectal examination and serum prostate specific antigen in the early detection of prostate cancer: results of a multicenter clinical trial of 6,630 men. *J Urol* 1994;151:1283-1290.

[6] Schröder FH, van der Cruijsen-Koeter I, de Koning HJ, Vis AN, Hoedemaeker RF, Kranse R. Prostate cancer detection at low prostate specific antigen. *J Urol* 2000; 163:806-812.

Key Points

1. Testicular cancer is commonly a germ cell malignancy. Pathological types include testicular choriocarcinoma, testicular yolk sac carcinoma, testicular embryonal carcinoma and testicular teratoma. Testicular yolk sac carcinoma, testicular embryonal carcinoma and testicular teratoma can take on cytotrophoblast morphology and produce high concentrations of hyperglycosylated hCG.
2. Testicular germ cell malignancies commonly affect men aged 20-40.
3. Prostate cancer is the second most common malignancy (after skin cancer) to affect men. Prostate cancer primarily affects older men.
4. Prostate cancer is marked by prostate-specific antigen (PSA). PSA levels of less than 4 ng/mL are considered as negative or normal. PSA levels of 4 to 10 ng/ml represent a 20-30% risk of having prostate cancer, otherwise a high risk for having benign prostate hyperplasia (BPH). PSA of 10-20 ng/ml represents a high risk, 50-75% of having prostate cancer and a lesser risk for having BPH. PSA levels of over 20 ng/ml represent a very high risk, 90%, for having prostate cancer. The definitive test is prostate needle biopsy. The needle is placed in the anus, then across the rectal tissue and into the prostate. Most men over 50 today have a PSA test as part of their physical examination, annually.

Other

Chapter 36

Ethics, Morals and Much More

The whole field of human reproduction is plagued with random ethics, morals and much more. The church and politics do not accept human reproduction outside of marriage, teenage contraception, any aspects of assisted reproduction, pregnancy termination or a variety of other things.

The church and some states teach that conception comes about when the sperm meets an egg at fertilization. Is this true? Those first cells, 30-50 cells in the first week, form a zygote, morula or blastocyst. That is a tiny, encased, dying being - limited, in that they are encased by a solid zona pellucida case and cannot grow in size; and dying, in that it has no food source, no blood source and no nutritional source for life. Everyone is entitled to an opinion, but it is my expert belief that life does not start, or conception does not begin, until the blastocyst, about 30-50 cells, has hatched the zona pellucida and implanted itself into the uterus, or until it has a source of growth, or a source of life. Please consider that >40% of blastocysts, or possibly most blastocysts, fail due to biochemical pregnancy, spontaneous abortion or failure to associate with the endometrium and implant at this point (see Chapter 19). Life is clearly very questionable prior to implantation.

Some states, like the extremist Tea Party in the state of Texas, claim that killing a pregnancy, even preconception, as early as fertilization, is a murder, even though the fertilization zygote is a dying being. Somehow this seems to conflict with God's basic laws and the Bible. The only statement in the Bible regarding pregnancy and violent termination is Exodus Chapter 21, verse 22: "*If men strive, and hurt a woman with child, so that her fruit depart from her, and yet no mischief follow: he shall be surely fined, according as the woman's husband will lay upon him; and he shall pay as the judges determine*" (King James Bible). As stated in the Bible, killing somebody's unborn baby is a crime punishable by fine, and is not a murder.

I have had a fight with the state of Texas over these ridiculous extra-biblical laws. I am considered by many scientists as a world expert on the testing of placental hCG, or pregnancy testing. Back in 2004 Texas police needed the help of a pregnancy testing expert. I was contacted by Galveston, TX police asking if I could measure placental hCG in acidic abdominal remains from someone deceased. At first I saw no problem with this and agreed. Then I read the story on the internet of what was really happening in Galveston, TX.

A boy from the shady side of town had been having an affair with a young lady from the fancy properties in town. The upmarket parents were horrified by this rich-poor relationship and condemned the association. The upmarket parents went abroad for 3 weeks. The boy came to visit the girl, who was crying, claiming that she had just found out that she was pregnant and did not know how she could ever tell her parents. The boy came back the next night. He found the girl lying in bed, trying to position a noose that she had made over her head. After she requested, he helped her squeeze the noose over her nose. As she explained, she could not deal with life anymore, or with having to tell her parents that she was pregnant. The boy could not convince her to keep living and not kill herself and left the house. The girl hanged herself.

The parents returned home a couple of weeks later only to find the dead body of their daughter. They arranged with the local coroner for a quick and uneventful autopsy and for her body to be cremated. The abdominal acidic fluid was the only remains kept by the coroner. Nobody, including the coroner or the parents, ever found out that she was a couple of weeks pregnant. This story should have ended here, but for the innocent honesty that followed.

A couple of weeks later, the boy saw the new film "The Passion of Christ" starring Mel Gibson. The boy left the movie theater charmed by Christ and his religious feelings. With his religious feelings he said to himself that Christ would want him to tell the police and tell the parents what had really happened to the girl. He went to the Galveston police and related the whole honest story, hiding nothing. Under Texas law there is no assisted suicide provision. As the boy had related, he had aided the girl in pulling the noose over her nose, and in so doing, in getting it around her neck. The honest Jesus-loving boy was immediately arrested for murder. This is where the story started. If the police could demonstrate the presence of placental hCG in the remnant abdominal acidic fluids, they could prove that she was really pregnant as the boy had related. Under Texas law the boy could then be charged with two murders, the girl and her extremely early, barely implanted pregnancy. Two murders, a crime punishable in Texas by the death sentence.

Becoming familiar with the complete story of this boy and girl, from the internet, I contacted Galveston police, retracting my willingness to perform any testing. It was my opinion that the police should have just have given this Jesus-loving honest lad a spank on the bottom and said goodbye to him. How could I do placental hCG testing, and allow my testing to be used for sentencing him to death?

A few days later I received a subpoena from a New Mexico court ordering me to perform placental hCG testing on the abdominal fluid that I had been sent by Galveston police. My laboratory technicians, feeling similarly to me, all refused to do the testing. I had to do it myself. I used a sensitive test for hCG degradation products using antibody B204 to analyze the abdominal fluids, B204 tests for free ß-subunit, ß-core fragment and intermediate placental hCG degradation products. The test was marginally positive. I was not sure what to do. How could I produce test results that could cause an innocent young boy to be executed? I then went to see lawyers in Albuquerque, New Mexico. I wrote a report to Galveston police with help from the lawyers. It said that I had found that the fluids were marginally positive for placental hCG degradation products, but that I could not claim whether the positivity was due to pregnancy, or due to the acidity of the test fluids, or other degraded molecules in the test fluids. I sent the report.

From what I heard, the boy was charged with just one murder, and sent to prison for most of his life. I feel very relieved that he was not executed. I do believe, however, that Texas law can be very wrong, and that this boy is innocent of any major crime.

Can an obstetrician insist on terminating a doomed pregnancy? No! All the pregnancy issues and sexual issues raise questions - questions we do not know how to answer. Where do we stop?

Clearly, God's first commandment or principal commandment (Genesis 1:28) was "be fruitful and multiply." That surely means that we are to utilize the incredible intricate biology described in Chapters 3-25 of this book to the fullest degree possible. Enjoy life - why is anything else needed?

Author Contact Information

Dr. Laurence A. Cole, Ph.D.
USA hCG Reference Service Reference Service
P.O. Box 950, 34 Broadmoor Way Angel Fire NM 87710
E-mail: larry@hcglab.com

Index

B

C

D

G

H

I

J

K

L

M

N

O

P

R

S

T

U

V

W

X

Y

Z